USEFUL PROCEDURES

in

MEDICAL PRACTICE

ADVISORY BOARD

USEFUL PROCEDURES
in
MEDICAL PRACTICE

Compiled and Edited By:

PAUL W. ROBERTS, M.D. (Toronto),
M.D. (Quito), C.C.F.P.(C).

Associate Professor,
Department of Family and Community Medicine,
Faculty of Medicine,
University of Toronto;
Vice-Chairman,
Department of Family and Community Medicine,
Sunnybrook Medical Centre,
Toronto, Ontario, Canada

Lea & Febiger   *1986*   *Philadelphia*

Lea & Febiger
600 Washington Square
Philadelphia, PA 19106-4198
U.S.A.
(215) 922-1330

Library of Congress Cataloging in Publication Data
Main entry under title:

Useful procedures in medical practice.

  Includes bibliographies and index.
  1. Medicine, Clinical—Technique. I. Roberts, Paul W.
[DNLM: 1. Medicine. WB 100 U84]
RC48.U83   1985   616   85-4534
ISBN 0-8121-0985-6

PRINTED IN THE UNITED STATES OF AMERICA

Print Number: 5   4   3   2   1

Dedicated to
the most important person of all
—the patient.

Foreword

Increasing specialization has characterized medical practice since World War II. Each specialty seems to be going further in its own direction as if propelled by a centrifugal force. In the past 30 years, biomedical research has increased the informational base for medical practice several fold. New ideas and technology have improved old procedures and made new ones possible. This is one way health care progresses.

This progress has produced a problem. How can a patient get the best care when that care may relate to several specialties? It is tempting to have a recognized authority handle each aspect of medical care and to perform each procedure but past experience teaches us that there are many pitfalls associated with fragmented care.

How then can a patient receive the finest care? How can the medical profession make available to the patient the best that is known in its many specialties? Family Medicine and other specialties attempt to do this by embracing knowledge and procedures that relate to many other specialties.

The challenge of providing excellent care comes into sharp focus when a procedure is to be performed on a patient. Some procedures are performed frequently, others rarely. This makes little difference to the patient, who rightly expects the procedure to be done correctly. The physician is expected to use the latest methods and to perform the procedure deftly, safely, and effectively.

Many patients visiting a physician require a procedure as a part of the evaluation or treatment; but even the physician who reads regularly, selects articles wisely, and attends excellent continuing medical education courses cannot keep up with all the improvements and new information about every procedure. A handy reference book such as this compiled by Dr. Paul Roberts provides the key information needed for a quick review.

As I read the manuscript for this book, I was carried back to the 1950s to Jasper, Florida, where I did many procedures in my rural practice. My performance would have been better if I had had such a book. Were I returning to Jasper, I would have this book in my bookcase. This book will be equally useful to physicians in large cities, to those in frozen outposts in the Yukon, in sunny islands in the Caribbean, in hospital emergency rooms, and in military posts around the world.

Dr. Roberts has brought together descriptions of many procedures, written by experts, presented in a format that allows the busy physician to review quickly the essential information for each procedure. The authors have summarized the clinical uses for each procedure, reminded the operator of anatomic landmarks, clearly described the method, noted precautions, and outlined follow-up care. This type of information triggers the memory, updates one's information, and thereby helps the physician to carry out a procedure in an optimal manner.

Our task in medicine is to provide the best care known today and to do better tomorrow. One physician focuses on an approach to get a better history, another describes a new physical sign, and yet another tests a new drug.

Each health professional works within his or her area of expertise. Paul Roberts has perceived a need for physicians to have a ready source of reliable information about procedures. To persuade many experts to participate is no small feat; to persuade each one to follow a format that provides only essential information is remarkable. This book on procedures is indeed a fine contribution, and one which can improve medical care today and tomorrow.

Hiram B. Curry, M.D.
Professor and Chairman,
Department of Family Medicine;
Professor of Neurology,
Medical University of South Carolina,
Charleston, South Carolina

Preface

The nature of medical practice requires that most physicians perform a tremendous variety of procedures, some of which are done frequently, others infrequently. This manual is designed to provide detailed explanations of those procedures that may not be done frequently by some practitioners, or which may have come into use since completion of the practitioner's formal training. It is also intended as a resource for practitioners who may not have easy access to colleagues for answers or additional information.

Medical students and nurses will find this book helpful as they prepare to observe or assist in some of these procedures. In fact, it may enable them to find out all they ever wanted to know about common medical procedures but were afraid to ask.

It is intended, therefore, as a useful resource for medical professionals at several levels of training or experience to broaden the scope of procedures they feel comfortable in doing and to be sure that such activities are carried out competently and accurately, ultimately for the benefit of the patient.

This book covers a broad spectrum; however, it has been difficult at times to decide which procedures should be included and which should be omitted. Some subjects such as Dental Procedures may be inappropriate for urban physicians but extremely relevant for practitioners in remote areas where dental care may not be available. The readers will also note a spectrum of complexity. Some basic procedures will be helpful in the learning stage, while other more hazardous procedures should only be carried out in centers with adequate back-up resources. Each procedure has been carefully explained in detail by experts in the field so that it can be confidently carried out by following the steps as outlined, bearing in mind the indications and potential danger inherent in many procedures. Ultimately, of course, the physician bears the responsibility for any medical act performed.

In carrying out any procedure, the physician must always remember the nervousness and anxiety of the patient and do everything possible to make the patient as comfortable as possible. Each step should be explained and the patient reassured. Uncomfortable positions should be maintained only briefly and when unavoidable. Sufficient time must be allowed for local anesthesia to properly take effect, and if the patient says it hurts—believe him! Special care and gentleness must be shown to children. Such compassion and consideration will be amply rewarded by their cooperation and gratitude.

I wish to express special thanks to the Advisory Board of Family Physicians whose counsel and encouragement have been immeasurably helpful. Their contribution has helped to make this manual of Useful Procedures possible, and we all believe it will be of genuine assistance to many practitioners, both in urban and remote areas. If in some way this book contributes to better patient care and helps the physician in service to the community, I will feel rewarded for all my efforts.

Toronto, Ontario   Paul W. Roberts, M.D.

Acknowledgments

I would like to express special thanks to each contributor and author in this book. Without them it would have been impossible. Each has contributed in a significant and unique way, and I am deeply grateful for their help and encouragement.

Dr. Hiram B. Curry, Professor and Chairman, Department of Family Medicine, Medical University of South Carolina, has kindly honored me by writing the Foreword. I have thought of him as a rather special friend and colleague since we first met some years ago at a medical meeting in Spain. His words at that time were an inspiration to me, and this latest act of friendship is deeply appreciated.

The members of the Department of Family and Community Medicine, Sunnybrook Medical Centre, have kindly supported and encouraged me during the months of manuscript preparation. This too is appreciated, and I wish to formally thank them now.

The medical artists have given unstintingly of their time and talent. Their work has contributed enormously to the value and usefulness of this book. I thank each of them sincerely.

Lea & Febiger has been encouraging and helpful at every step, and I wish to acknowledge this as well, with special thanks to Mr. R. Kenneth Bussy, Executive Editor. This wonderful group of people has made the compilation and printing of this book possible, as well as making it an enjoyable experience.

The contribution and support of the resources of Sunnybrook Medical Centre and the University of Toronto Clinic have been invaluable, and I am deeply grateful to all who have had a part in this project. The assistance of Dr. Ruth Dunn in the final stages of the preparation of this book is also gratefully acknowledged.

To my wife Barbara go my gratitude and thanks for her patience, love and encouragement during the 3 years of preparation and work that have resulted in bringing this dream of mine to a final and happy completion.

Finally, but not least, I do not have sufficient words to thank Miss Jane Evans, who faithfully, carefully, and loyally worked over many months to transcribe and correct the many manuscripts related to the preparation of this book. She made it possible in a special way, doing all of the essential and tedious work of typing, month by month, so that this dream might become a reality. Thank you, Jane, most sincerely.

Paul W. Roberts, M.D.

Contributors

MARY E. ARCHIBALD, R.N.
Head Nurse, Intravenous and Blood Collection Team,
Sunnybrook Medical Centre, Toronto, Ontario, Canada

RONALD S. BAIGRIE, M.D., F.R.C.P.(C), F.A.C.C.
Associate Professor of Medicine, Faculty of Medicine,
University of Toronto; Consultant Cardiologist, Sunnybrook
Medical Centre, Toronto, Ontario, Canada

G.M. DAVIES, M.D., F.R.C.P., F.R.C.P.(C).
Associate Professor, Faculty of Medicine, University of
Toronto; Consultant Respirologist, Head, Division of
Respiratory Diseases, Sunnybrook Medical Centre, Toronto,
Ontario, Canada

JAMES D. DUBBIN, M.D., F.R.C.P.(C), F.A.C.C.
Assistant Professor, Division of Cardiology and Department of
Radiological Sciences, Faculty of Medicine, University of
Toronto; Consultant Cardiologist, Sunnybrook Medical Centre,
Toronto, Ontario, Canada

GRANT A. FARROW, M.D., F.R.C.S.(C), F.A.C.S.
*Assistant Professor, Department of Surgery, Faculty of
Medicine, University of Toronto; Urologist, Toronto General
Hospital, Toronto, Ontario, Canada*

CHARLES M. GODFREY, M.D., F.R.C.P.(C).
*Professor, Department of Rehabilitation Medicine, Faculty of
Medicine, University of Toronto; Physiatrist-in-Charge,
Wellesley Hospital, Department of Rehabilitation Medicine,
Princess Margaret Hospital; Consultant, Sunnybrook Medical
Centre, Toronto, Ontario, Canada*

W.H. HARRIS, M.D., F.R.C.S.(C), F.A.C.O.G.
*Assistant Professor, Department of Obstetrics and Gynecology,
Faculty of Medicine, University of Toronto; Consulting Staff,
Department of Gynecology, Sunnybrook Medical Centre;
Courtesy Staff, Department of Obstetrics, Wellesley Hospital,
Toronto, Ontario, Canada*

JAMES F. KELLAM, M.D., F.R.C.S.(C)
*Assistant Professor, Division of Orthopedics, Faculty of
Medicine, University of Toronto; Orthopedic Consultant,
Division of Orthopedics, Sunnybrook Medical Centre, Toronto,
Ontario, Canada*

PETER L. LANE, M.D.
*Assistant Professor, Department of Surgery, Faculty of
Medicine, University of Toronto; Head Emergency Physician,
Regional Trauma Unit, Sunnybrook Medical Centre, Toronto,
Ontario, Canada*

MARVIN G. LESTER, M.D., F.R.C.P.(C).
*Lecturer, Department of Medicine, Faculty of Medicine,
University of Toronto; Consultant Dermatologist, Sunnybrook
Medical Centre, Mount Sinai Hospital, Mississauga Hospital;
Workers' Compensation Board, Toronto, Ontario, Canada*

HUGH LITTLE, M.D., F.R.C.P.(C).
Associate Professor, Faculty of Medicine, University of Toronto; Head, Division of Rheumatology, Sunnybrook Medical Centre, Toronto, Ontario, Canada

JAMES H.P. MAIN, B.D.S., Ph.D., F.D.S.R.C.S.E., F.R.C. Path., F.R.C.D.(C).
Professor of Oral Pathology, Faculties of Medicine and Dentistry, University of Toronto; Head, Department of Dentistry, Sunnybrook Medical Centre, Toronto, Ontario, Canada

JAMES B.J. McKENDRY, M.D., F.R.C.P.(C).
Professor of Pediatrics, Faculty of Medicine, University of Toronto; Senior Physician, Hospital for Sick Children, Toronto, Ontario, Canada

COLIN F. MOSELEY, M.D., C.M., F.R.C.S.(C).
Assistant Professor, Faculty of Medicine, University of Toronto; Active Staff, Division of Orthopedics, Hospital for Sick Children, Toronto, Ontario, Canada

S.Z. NAQVI, M.D., F.R.C.P.(C).
Assistant Professor, Cardiology, Faculty of Medicine, University of Toronto; Director, Cardiovascular Laboratory, Consultant Cardiologist, Sunnybrook Medical Centre, Toronto, Ontario, Canada

JULIAN M. NEDZELSKI, M.D., F.R.C.S.(C).
Assistant Professor of Otolaryngology, Faculty of Medicine, University of Toronto; Consultant Otolaryngologist, Sunnybrook Medical Centre, Toronto, Ontario, Canada

RONALD E. NEEDS, MB. Bch., D.A., F.R.C.P.(C).
*Assistant Professor of Anesthesia, Faculty of Medicine,
University of Toronto; Consultant Anesthetist, Director, Nerve
Block and Pain Control Clinic, Sunnybrook Medical Centre,
Toronto, Ontario, Canada*

MICHAEL L. SCHWARTZ, M.D., M.Sc., F.R.C.S.(C).
*Assistant Professor, Department of Surgery, Faculty of
Medicine, University of Toronto; Staff Neurosurgeon,
Sunnybrook Medical Centre, Toronto, Ontario, Canada*

JOHN S. SENN, M.D., F.R.C.P.(C).
*Professor of Medicine, Faculty of Medicine, University of
Toronto; Head, Division of Clinical Hematology, Sunnybrook
Medical Centre, Toronto, Ontario, Canada*

T.F. SHAPERO, M.D., F.R.C.P.(C).
*Assistant Professor, Faculty of Medicine, University of
Toronto; Consultant in Gastroenterology, Sunnybrook Medical
Centre, Toronto, Ontario, Canada*

KENNETH P. SIREN, M.D., C.C.F.P. (EM).
*Assistant Professor, Department of Family and Community
Medicine, Faculty of Medicine, University of Toronto; Former
Head, Division of Emergency Services, Department of Family
and Community Medicine, Mount Sinai Hospital, Toronto,
Ontario, Canada*

JOHN SPEAKMAN, M.D., F.R.C.S.(C).
*Professor of Ophthalmology, Faculty of Medicine, University of
Toronto; Head, Department of Ophthalmology, Sunnybrook
Medical Centre, Toronto, Ontario, Canada*

GLEN A. TAYLOR, M.D., F.R.C.S.(C).
*Associate Professor of Surgery, Faculty of Medicine, University
of Toronto; Chief, Division of General Surgery, Consultant in
Thoracic and General Surgery, Sunnybrook Medical Centre,
Toronto, Ontario, Canada*

ENID H. WILSON, R.N., B.Sc.N., E.T.
*Nurse Clinician, Enterostomal Therapy, Department of
Nursing, Sunnybrook Medical Centre, Toronto, Ontario,
Canada*

Contents

Contents

1
Anesthesia

R.E. Needs

LOCAL ANESTHESIA AND REGIONAL NERVE BLOCK

The following techniques were selected because of their relative simplicity and usefulness to the physician with limited expertise in local anesthesia and nerve block. The list is not comprehensive but includes procedures covering a wide range of uses. These procedures, when applied with care and precision, should produce reliable results with minimal risk to the patient.

Major regional anesthesia, such as spinal and epidural block, and other blocks performed close to the neuraxis, are not considered as they require considerable expertise in the conduction of anesthesia and the management of potentially life-threatening complications. Before describing the various nerve blocks, general principles of preparation and performance of local anesthesia are considered along with precautions to avoid complications.

1

GENERAL PRINCIPLES

Although in the following techniques the total amount of anesthetic drug is well within the safe dosage limits, and serious reactions are rare, the facilities to manage all possible complications should be readily available. Many of the surgical procedures using these blocks require the facilities of the emergency department or the operating room. The room in which the procedure is performed should be well lighted and ventilated, and large enough to allow the physician easy access to all sides of the patient.

Equipment

Resuscitation Equipment

The following basic resuscitation equipment should be available to ensure the safe performance of a regional nerve block:

1. A table capable of tilting to the head-down position.
2. A means of providing a free airway and ventilation of the lungs with oxygen.
3. A simple kit containing airways and masks of various sizes and a self-inflating bag with a portable oxygen supply.
4. A suction apparatus (manual is preferred to electric because of possible power failure).
5. A selection of I.V. fluids and basic resuscitation drugs such as vasopressors, anticonvulsants, antihistamines, and I.V. steroids.

These items, together with additional materials such as laryngoscope, forceps, mouth gag, and tongue retractors are kept together in a box clearly labeled "Emergency Resuscitation Kit" and stored in a rapidly accessible central location. The box should be checked and restocked regularly.

Equipment

Syringes of 2, 5, 10, and 20 ml
Needles 20 to 27 gauge of 1.5 to 15 cm length

Disposable syringe and needle equipment are best for sterility and quality control; but where this is impossible or economically unfeasible, reusable equipment must be impeccably maintained for fit of syringes, patency and sharpness of needles, and for sterility. Failure to do this leads to frustration for the physician in the use of equipment and increased risk to the patient of added trauma during injection and possible infection.

Local Anesthesia Drugs. Although many local anesthetic agents are available, in practice all local anesthesia and nerve blocks can be performed effectively with only two or three agents:

1. For short periods of anesthesia and for patients with a history of malignant hyperthermia, 1% or 2% chloroprocaine is used.
2. For medium duration of action, 1% or 2% lidocaine with or without epinephrine is suitable.
3. For longer duration, postoperative analgesia, and therapeutic blocks, 0.25% to 0.5% bupivacaine with or without epinephrine is the drug of choice.

Miscellaneous Items. Materials for skin preparation include antiseptic and cleansing agents such as chlorhexidine and Cetrimide, and the appropriate sterile drapes. A sterile ruler and small rubber discs, acting as depth markers, are often helpful. For some nerve blocks, a peripheral nerve stimulator is useful to accurately locate the nerve and to avoid excessive nerve penetration with the risk of neurologic sequelae.

Selection and Preparation of the Patient

In addition to taking the routine medical history and performing a physical examination, the physician should ask the patient specifically about medication intake. The use of anticoagulants in therapeutic doses is an absolute contraindication to regional nerve block. When in doubt about the patient's medication intake, coagulation must be checked. Any drug allergies and previous experience with local anesthesia should be determined, as well as any family or personal history of conditions such as pseudocholinesterase deficiency, malignant hyperthermia, and neurologic disorders. Regional nerve block is contraindicated in patients suffering from certain neurologic conditions such as multiple sclerosis or peripheral neuropathies, although this may be more a medicolegal than a practical objection. Nerve block is also contraindicated if there is infection in the area.

Explain to the patient the nature of sensory and motor changes expected in the proposed nerve block. The patient must be cooperative and willing to undergo subsequent surgical procedures while awake or possibly with a minimum of additional sedation. Benefits gained by avoiding the risks and undesirable side effects of general anesthesia should be stressed.

In the case of minor surgical procedures, most patients will accept local anesthesia, but some are terrified by the thought of enduring an operation while awake. These fears can often be allayed by careful explanation of the procedure and the reassurance that the patient will experience no undue discomfort. A quiet, calm atmosphere during the operation and light sedation, which allows the patient to sleep, often overcome the problem.

Depending on the agent used and nerve block performed, the period for onset of anesthesia may range from 5 to 30 minutes. The patient should be asked about subjective sensations of warmth and numbness and observed for the presence of vasodilation and increased skin temperature that usually indicate the onset of block. Sensory loss is tested with an alcohol pledget and a safety pin (hypodermic needles are too sharp for this purpose and will give the patient unnecessary puncture marks). With some blocks of major nerves, motor paresis may become apparent with higher concentrations of anesthetic solution, further confirming the block.

The average time before surgery begins is 10 to 20 minutes. Incision or possible painful manipulation is not performed before both operator and patient are satisfied that anesthesia is adequate. The physician must remember that when the patient is awake during the procedure, a high standard of decorum and professional behavior is demanded.

If after 20 to 30 minutes the block anesthesia appears inadequate, an additional volume of anesthetic solution is injected at the original site, or by infiltration at the operative site if possible. In the event the anesthesia is insufficient, elect to switch to general anesthesia if the necessary expertise is available. Otherwise, if possible, postpone the procedure. Heavy sedation bordering on general anesthesia should be avoided because cardiorespiratory and airway management problems can lead to hazardous situations.

Although less rigorous conditions regarding food and drink consumption are often observed during local anesthetic procedures, advise the patient not to eat solid food for at least 4 hours prior to the procedure. Stress this when a nerve block is performed with large doses of local anesthetic; for example, multiple intercostal blocks or femoral/sciatic nerve block which increase the risk of adverse reactions.

Management of Complications and Side Effects

Complications resulting from the nerve blocks described are usually minor and transient. Hematomas occur occasionally and are avoided or minimized using careful technique and applying pressure over the injection site for a few minutes after the block. The most serious complications of regional block are seizure and cardiorespiratory collapse as a result of acute toxicity. This occurs most commonly from inadvertent intravascular injection or rapid absorption leading to high blood levels. These rare reactions must be managed quickly and efficiently.

Be aware of the potential for toxic reactions following high dose anesthetic injection or injection into vascular areas. Monitor the patient for prodromal signs such as dizziness, tinnitus, and agitation or minor twitching in the early post-injection period. Most minor reactions of this sort are self-limiting and resolve spontaneously.

In the event the reaction progresses, oxygen is administered and careful monitoring of heart rate, blood pressure, and respiratory activity maintained. If seizures occur, the airway must be secured and ventilated with oxygen. Incremental doses of diazepam or thiopental are given intravenously to control the seizure activity, and the airway is intubated if necessary with the aid of a short acting muscle relaxant such as succinylcholine and ventilation with oxygen is instituted. Cardiovascular collapse must be treated aggressively with I.V. fluids and vasopressors. Fortunately most reactions are short-lived. Because rapid I.V. access may be required, it is prudent to have a patent venous cannula or needle in place during most regional nerve blocks.

True allergic reactions of the anaphylactic type are rare. They occur more with ester-type anesthetics like procaine than with the amide group anesthetics like lidocaine. Intravenous steroid, antihistamines, and cardiorespiratory support must be administered if a reaction occurs.

Side effects such as motor paresis are expected with many blocks. No patient should be discharged from the hospital with motor paresis present, particularly in the lower limbs. Sensory impairment may persist for several hours after the surgery is completed; if the patient is to be discharged, he should be warned about the residual lack of sensation and have the affected area protected from accidental harm. Persistent parethesias following nerve block are rare but occasionally last for weeks or months before resolution. Rarely, depending on the nerve involved, permanent neurologic deficit with sensory impairment and motor paresis may result. This complication can be avoided by care and attention to technique, particularly the avoidance of injecting anesthetic directly into a nerve by withdrawing the needle slightly when parethesias are obtained and injecting the solution slowly and carefully.

Local Infiltration and Field Block

Clinical Uses

1. Suture of wounds and lacerations.
2. Excision of small cutaneous and subcutaneous lesions, e.g., papillomas, warts, nevi, sebaceous cysts, lipomas. Biopsies of subcutaneous lumps and nodules.
3. Incision of abscess. Aspiration of joints.

Equipment

2-ml and 10-ml syringes
27-gauge 1.5-cm needle, and a 22- or 25-gauge 8- to 10-cm needle
0.5 to 1% lidocaine with or without epinephrine or 0.25% bupivacaine with or without epinephrine
Materials for cleansing the skin and sterile draping for the area.

Method

Before the skin is injected, the area is cleansed with antiseptic and draped with sterile towels. At the site where a needle larger than 22 gauge is to be inserted, the skin is first desensitized by the injection of a small volume of an-

Anesthesia

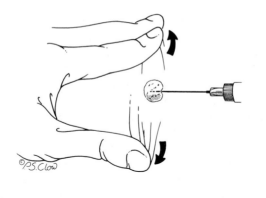

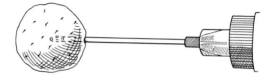

Fig. 1–1. Skin wheal. Note that the peau d'orange effect depends on the size of the wheal.

esthetic solution into the dermis, producing what is called the intradermal wheal. The wheal is raised by inserting a 25- or 27-gauge needle, bevel up, almost parallel to the skin being stretched by the thumb and forefinger of the other hand. The needle is gently inserted until all of the bevel is buried in the skin, and 0.1 to 0.25 ml of anesthetic solution is slowly injected.

The raised area produced usually has a characteristic pitted appearance similar to orange peel (peau d'orange) (Figure 1–1). The intradermal wheal not only serves to anesthetize the skin but also serves as a superficial landmark. The subcutaneous infiltration is performed by insertion through the skin wheal of a 4 cm or longer, 22- or 25-gauge needle attached to a 10-ml syringe containing the appropriate anesthetic solution. With the axis of the needle parallel to the skin, injection is made on advancing and withdrawing the needle through the subcutaneous area infiltrated (Fig. 1–2). Keeping the needle in motion minimizes the risk of inadvertent intravascular injection of a significant volume of solution (Fig. 1–2).

Field block is achieved by making subcutaneous and, if necessary, intramuscular injections around the area to be anesthetized. Thus, all the nerve supply is blocked a short distance from the required area. This is best done in a diamond-shaped pattern from two skin wheals at opposite sides of the area to be anesthetized. From the skin wheal, one side of the diamond is infiltrated to the appropriate distance (the length of needle is selected accordingly). (Fig. 1–3A). The needle is then withdrawn up to the subcutaneous point of the wheal but not removed. It is then redirected and additional infiltration carried out along the adjacent side of the diamond (Fig. 1–3B). The process is repeated through a skin wheal raised on the opposite side of the area to be anesthetized, thus completing the diamond (Fig. 1–3C). Infiltrating the proximal side of the dia-

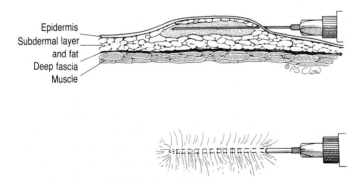

Epidermis
Subdermal layer
and fat
Deep fascia
Muscle

Fig. 1–2. Subcutaneous infiltration. Injection is made during advance and withdrawal of the needle.

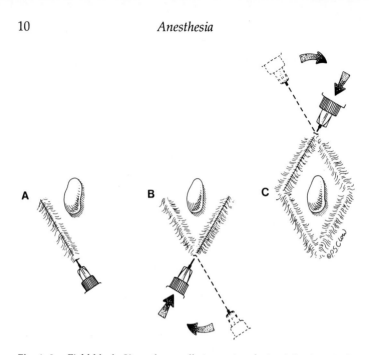

Fig. 1–3. Field block. Keep the needle in motion during injection. **A.** A wheal is raised, and the first side of the diamond is infiltrated. **B.** The needle tip is then withdrawn to just under the skin, the needle moved sideways, and the second side of the diamond infiltration is performed. **C.** The procedure is repeated on the other side of the lesion, completing the diamond-shaped field block.

mond first will make subsequent infiltration less uncomfortable (Fig. 1–3).

Precautions

Recommended maximum safe dosages (these apply to all nerve blocks):

1. 300 mg lidocaine without epinephrine and 500 mg with epinephrine 1:200,000 or 5 to 7 mg per kilo body weight, whichever is less.
2. Bupivacaine 150 mg without, 200 mg with, epineph-

rine 1:200,000 or 2 to 3 mg per kilo of body weight, whichever is less.

3. Aspirate frequently and keep the needle moving to avoid intravascular injection.

Follow-up Care

Remember that anesthesia may last 2 to 6 hours or more. Therefore, the patient should be warned to protect the area from accidental injury. Provide adequate analgesic medication for the patient before discharge because pain is likely to occur after the anesthesia wears off.

HEAD AND NECK

Occipital Nerve Block

Clinical Uses

1. Anesthesia of the posterior part of the scalp.
2. Relief of occipital neuralgia and other painful conditions affecting the posterior part of the scalp.

Equipment

5-ml syringe
25-gauge 4-cm needle
1% lidocaine with epinephrine or .25% bupivacaine with epinephrine

Anatomy

The greater occipital nerve is the medial (sensory) branch of the posterior division of C-2. The nerve becomes superficial by piercing the trapezius and deep fascia just below the superior nuchal line, about 3 cm lateral to the external occipital protuberance. The nerve runs upward to supply a wide area of the scalp; at the vertex, it ramifies with branches of the supraorbital nerve.

Landmarks

The greater occipital nerve is best blocked where it crosses the superior nuchal line, about midway between the mastoid and the external occipital protuberance. It is located at this point close to the occipital artery which is usually easily palpable (Fig. 1–4).

Method

The hair and scalp is thoroughly cleansed with antiseptic solution. The occipital artery is palpated at the level of the superior nuchal line. A 5-ml syringe with a 4-cm 25-gauge needle attached is inserted just medial to the palpating finger. If paresthesias are obtained, 2 ml of the solution are injected; otherwise, 5 ml are infiltrated around the artery. The lesser occipital nerve is blocked at the same time by injecting at the same level about 2.5 cm lateral to the greater occipital nerve.

Precaution

Aspirate carefully to avoid intravascular injection.

Supraorbital Nerve Block

Clinical Uses

1. Anesthesia of the forehead and anterior part of the scalp.
2. Treatment of certain painful conditions such as tic douloureux with first division trigger mechanisms and post-herpetic neuralgia of the first division of the trigeminal.
3. Diagnosis of painful disorders of the area.

Equipment

2-ml syringe
25-gauge 1.5-cm needle

Cutaneous Innervation

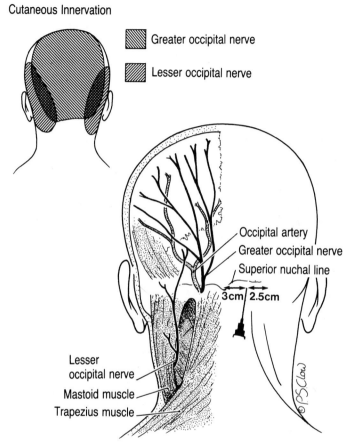

Greater occipital nerve

Lesser occipital nerve

Occipital artery
Greater occipital nerve
Superior nuchal line
3 cm / 2.5 cm

Lesser occipital nerve
Mastoid muscle
Trapezius muscle

Fig. 1–4. Cutaneous innervation. Occipital nerve block. Careful aspiration will avoid injection into the occipital artery.

1% lidocaine with epinephrine or 0.25% bupivacaine
  with epinephrine

Anatomy

The supraorbital nerve (together with the supratrochlear
nerve, the terminal branches of the frontal nerve, and a
branch of the ophthalmic division of the trigeminal nerve)
leaves the orbit through the supraorbital foramen or notch
of the superior orbital margin about 2.5 cm from the midline. It then passes upward to reach and supply the skin
of the forehead and the anterior two-thirds of the scalp.

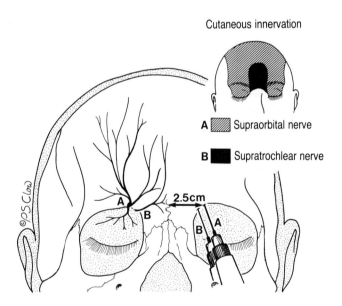

Fig. 1–5. Supraorbital nerve block. Subcutaneous infiltration along the
orbital margin will also produce adequate anesthesia. Cutaneous innervation.

Landmarks

The supraorbital notch or foramen can be palpated through the skin of the upper eyelid by retracting the eyebrow about 2.5 cm from the midline (Fig. 1–5).

Method

The skin of the eyebrow and upper lid is cleansed with suitable antiseptic (aqueous solution is used taking care to avoid entry of solution into the eye). The syringe with needle attached, held between forefinger and thumb like a dart, is gently thrust through the skin perpendicular to the orbital margin. Usually just before bone is contacted, paresthesias are produced and radiate into the frontal region. If these are not obtained, the advance is continued until gentle contact with the orbital rim is made. The needle is then redirected until it is felt to slip into the foramen. At this point, paresthesias are usually obtained, and .5 to 1 ml of the solution is injected after negative aspiration. The supratrochlear nerve may be blocked in the same manner and it lies about .5 to 1.75 cm medial to the supraorbital foramen. Gentle pressure on the site of the injection aids diffusion and helps prevent hematoma formation.

Precautions

1. Avoid getting antiseptic solution in the eye.
2. Aspirate to avoid intravascular injection.

Follow-up Care

Warn the patient that, if hematoma occurs, bruising or a black eye with a swollen lid are possible.

Infraorbital Nerve Block

Clinical Uses

1. Anesthesia of the lower eyelid, cheek, nasolabial fold, and upper lip.

2. Treatment of pain from neuralgic conditions involving the nerve (e.g., trigeminal neuralgia, post-herpetic neuralgia).

Equipment

2-ml syringe
25-gauge 5-cm needle
1% lidocaine with epinephrine or 0.25% bupivacaine with epinephrine

Anatomy

The infraorbital branch of the maxillary nerve, after traveling along the infraorbital canal, exits the maxilla via the infraorbital foramen, and divides into three branches:

1. The inferior palpebral branch supplying the lower eyelid.
2. External and internal nasal branches traveling medially to supply the skin on the side and tip of the nose, and the vestibule.
3. Superior labial branches descending to supply the skin of the anterior cheek and upper lip including the mucous membrane.

Landmarks

The infraorbital foramen faces medially. It is situated anteriorly and inferiorly about 1 to 1.5 cm below the inferior orbital margin on a line connecting the supraorbital notch, the infraorbital notch and the pupil (with the patient looking directly forward). The infraorbital foramen can be approached via the extraoral or intraoral approach. The intraoral approach is preferred because the risk of unsightly hematoma of the cheek is reduced (Fig. 1–6).

Method

The skin of the area is cleansed with the antiseptic solution. The index finger palpates the infraorbital foramen located by the above mentioned landmarks.

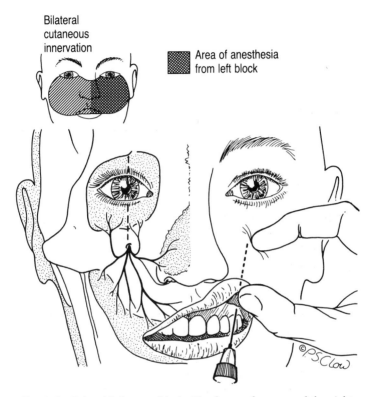

Bilateral cutaneous innervation

Area of anesthesia from left block

Fig. 1–6. Infraorbital nerve block. Hands may be reversed for right-handed operator. Bilateral cutaneous innervation. Area of anesthesia from the left block.

Keeping the finger in position, the physician retracts the upper lid by using his thumb; after suitable drying of the mucosa and topical analgesia with lidocaine jelly or ointment, the needle is inserted about 1 cm lateral to the midpoint of the nose ala, just above the premolar tooth. The needle is advanced in a superior, posterior, and slightly lateral direction guided by the externally palpating index finger. At a depth of about 1 to 1.5 cm, the bone of the inferior edge of the foramen is contacted, and paresthesias radiating into the upper lip are usually obtained. The needle is gently advanced until it is felt to slip into the foramen; here, paresthesias radiating in various directions may be elicited. The needle is advanced no more than .5 cm into the canal and 1 ml of anesthetic solution is injected slowly after negative aspiration. An additional 1 ml can be injected submucously on withdrawal of the needle. Pressure is maintained over the cheek for 2 to 3 minutes after withdrawal of the needle.

Precautions

Volumes larger than 1 ml injected into the infraorbital canal or rapid injection may cause anesthetic to track along the canal and into the orbit, which may produce block of orbital structures, particularly the ocular muscles, causing diplopia.

Follow-Up Care

Patient should be warned about the possible development of bruising in the cheek.

Mental Nerve Block

Clinical Uses

1. Mental nerve block is used to provide anesthesia of the lower lip. Accompanied by lingual nerve block, it is used for treatment or extraction of lower incisor, canine, or premolar teeth.
2. For procedures on the lip near the midline, bilateral block is required.

Anatomy

The mental nerve arises from the inferior alveolar nerve and exits from the mental foramen of the mandible on the level with the second premolar tooth. The nerve supplies the skin and mucous membrane of the lower lip and skin over the anterior one-third of the lower jaw. The nerve overlaps at the midline with branches from the other side.

Landmarks

The mental foramen is situated midway between the upper and lower borders of the mandible on a line drawn between the two lower premolar teeth.

Equipment

5-ml syringe
25-gauge 5-cm needle
1% lidocaine with epinephrine or .25% bupivacaine with epinephrine

Method (Fig. 1–7)

The lower lip is retracted and dried. Topical anesthetic agent is applied to the mucous membrane at the junction of the lip and the gum. The area of the mental foramen is palpated by the index finger, and the needle is inserted from the medial side until the point is felt to be close to the neurovascular bundle where it issues from the foramen. Paresthesias can be obtained but are not necessary. One to 2 ml of solution are injected after negative aspiration. If accurate localization of the foramen has not been obtained, infiltration with 2 to 3 ml of solution around the gum area is usually effective.

Precautions

Injection directly into the foramen must be avoided because of the risk of nerve injury and subsequent neuritis or prolonged numbness of the lip.

Superficial Cervical Plexus Block

Clinical Uses

To produce anesthesia of the skin in:
1. The occipitomastoid region of the head.

Bilateral
cutaneous
innervation

Area of anesthesia from
right block

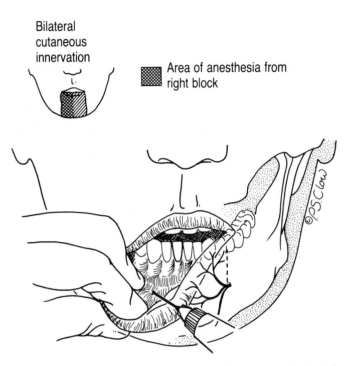

Fig. 1–7. Mental nerve block. Illustration shows approach for right-handed operator. Hands may be reversed for left-handed approach. Bilateral cutaneous innervation.

2. The posterior part of the ear and skin over the posterior part of the parotid region.
3. The anterior skin of the neck from the lower border of the mandible to the sternal notch.
4. The skin over the clavicle and pectoral region as far as the second rib,
5. The skin of the shoulder region over the deltoid and posteriorly as far as the spine of the scapula.

Anatomy

The superficial cervical plexus is formed from the superficial branches of the cervical plexus from the anterior primary rami of C-2-3 and 4. From their origin, the branches pass through the deep fascia about the midpoint of the sternocleidomastoid muscle to become subcutaneous. They curl around the posterior border of the muscle, proceeding upward, medially, and downward, to supply the area of skin previously described.

Landmarks

Injection is made at the midpoint of the posterior border of the sternomastoid, about one finger's breadth cephalad to the point where the external jugular vein crosses the muscle.

Equipment

10-ml syringe
25-gauge 1.5-cm needle
22-gauge 4- or 5-cm needle
0.5 to 1% lidocaine with epinephrine or 0.25% bupivacaine with epinephrine

Method (Fig. 1–8)

The skin is cleansed with suitable antiseptic and arranged with sterile drapes. A skin wheal is raised at the posterior border of the sternocleidomastoid muscle about midpoint as previously described. The 22-gauge 4- or 5-cm needle with syringe attached is then inserted through the wheal and advanced posteriorly behind the posterior border to the muscle until a slight click indicates its passage through the deep fascia (Fig. 1–8A). After negative aspiration, 3 ml of solution are injected subfascially. An additional 2 ml are injected as the needle is withdrawn to the subcutaneous layer. The needle is then redirected superiorly and inserted

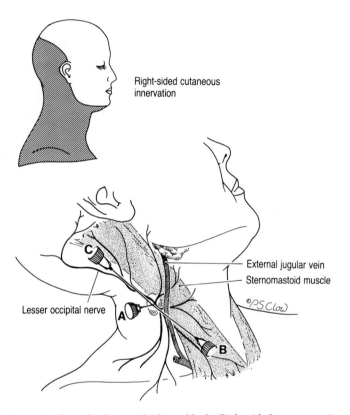

Right-sided cutaneous innervation

External jugular vein

Sternomastoid muscle

Lesser occipital nerve

Fig. 1–8. Superficial cervical plexus block. Right-sided cutaneous innervation. **A.** A skin wheal is raised, and the needle attached to the syringe is advanced until it passes through the deep fascia. **B.** The needle is then redirected superiorly and inserted through the fascia about 1 cm above the point at "**A.**" **C.** The needle is finally redirected inferiorly, through the fascia at the posterior border of the sternocleidomastoid muscle.

through the fascia at the posterior border of the muscle about 1 cm above the previous point (Fig. 1–8B). The needle is advanced 3 cm subfascially and 5 ml of solution are injected as the needle is withdrawn; aspirate frequently during the process to avoid intravascular injection. The needle is then redirected inferiorly and the process repeated injecting 5 ml of solution (Fig. 1–8C). Fifteen ml of anesthetic solution should be adequate for block of all branches of the superficial plexus.

Precautions

Frequent aspiration should be performed and the needle kept moving to avoid intravascular injection.

UPPER LIMB

Suprascapular Nerve Block

Clinical Uses

1. Anesthesia of the shoulder joint for manipulation or reduction of dislocations.
2. Diagnosis or treatment of painful shoulder conditions.

Anatomy

The suprascapular nerve arises from the supraclavicular portion of the brachial plexus and passes through the scapular notch to reach the supraspinous fossa where it supplies the supraspinatus muscle. After supplying sensory fibers to the shoulder joint and periscapular area, the nerve descends to supply the infraspinatus muscle.

Landmarks

The nerve is accessible from a point 1 cm above and lateral to a line bisecting the inferior angle of the scapula and the spine of the scapula.

Equipment

    10-ml syringe
    22- to 25-gauge 8-cm needle
    1% lidocaine with epinephrine
    0.25% bupivacaine with epinephrine

Method (Fig. 1–9)

The skin area is cleansed with appropriate antiseptic solution and draped. With the patient sitting with arms
folded across the chest, the angle of the scapula is bisected
and a line drawn upwards to cross a line drawn along the
spine of the scapula. The entry point for the needle is 1
cm above and lateral to the bisection point of these 2 lines.

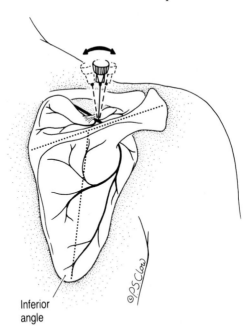

Inferior
angle

Fig. 1–9.   Suprascapular nerve block. The needle is gently walked along
the scapula until the notch is entered.

A skin wheal is raised at the previously determined entry point, and a 22- or 25-gauge 8-cm needle is inserted perpendicular to the skin then advanced in a direction anteriorly and slightly inferiorly and medially to contact the scapula in the supraspinous fossa close to the base of the coracoid process. The bone is contacted gently, usually lateral to the notch. The needle is then withdrawn and redirected slightly medially and gently reinserted. By repeating this process, the needle is gently walked along the scapula until paresthesias radiating to the tip of the shoulder are obtained, or the needle is felt to slip into the scapular notch. In this case, the needle should not be advanced more than 0.5 cm farther; after negative aspiration, 5 ml of solution are injected.

Precautions

1. Be gentle when contacting the bone as the periosteum of the area is very sensitive.
2. Do not advance the needle too far into the scapula notch. If the needle advances too far, it passes between the ribs with a consequent risk of pneumothorax.

Ulnar Nerve Block at the Wrist

Clinical Uses

1. To produce anesthesia in the ulnar distribution.
2. Used together with median and radial nerve blocks, this will produce anesthesia of the whole hand.

Anatomy

About 5 cm proximal to the wrist, in close proximity to the ulnar artery, the nerve divides into palmar and dorsal branches beneath the ulnocarpal tendon to reach the dorsal aspect of the wrist where it gives off branches to the ulnar side of the dorsum of the hand. The palmar branch continues along beneath the flexi carpi ulnaris tendon and divides at the level of the pisiform bone into a superficial branch that supplies cutaneous sensation to the ulnar side of the palm and little finger, and ulnar border of the ring finger. The deep branch supplies the intrinsic muscles of the hand.

Landmarks

The ulnar arterial pulse may be palpated at the level of the ulnar styloid at the radial side of the tendon of the flexor carpi ulnaris.

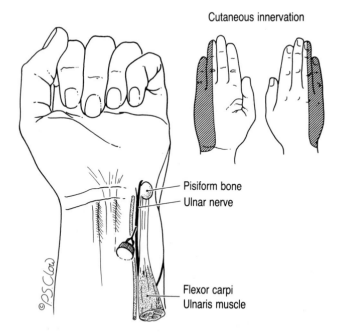

Cutaneous innervation

Pisiform bone
Ulnar nerve

Flexor carpi
Ulnaris muscle

Fig. 1–10.   Ulnar nerve block at wrist. Cutaneous innervation.

Equipment

5-ml syringe
25-gauge 4-cm needle
1% to 2% lidocaine without epinephrine or 0.25% to 0.5%
  bupivacaine without epinephrine (Fig. 1–10)

Method

The skin area is cleansed with suitable antiseptic. The needle is inserted on the radial side of the flexor carpi ulnaris tendon, between it and the ulnar artery, and directed beneath the tendon towards the pisiform bone. If paresthesias are elicited, the needle is arrested and 2 ml of the local anesthetic solution are injected after negative aspiration. If bone is contacted before paresthesias are obtained, 3 to 5 ml of solution are injected toward the surface on gradual withdrawal.

Precautions

1. Avoid intravascular injection through careful aspiration.
2. A solution containing epinephrine should be avoided in this area because of the frequent presence of small vessel arterial disease, particularly in the elderly patient.

Median Nerve Block at the Wrist

Clinical Uses

1. Anesthesia in the distribution of the nerve, together with ulnar and radial nerve block.
2. Wrist block anesthesia of the whole hand.

Anatomy

Just above the wrist, the median nerve lies superficially between the tendons of palmaris longus and the flexor carpi

Anesthesia

radialis. Passing into the palm, beneath the flexor retinaculum, the nerve supplies the small muscles of the thumb, the first and second lumbricals and cutaneous branches to the radial two-thirds of the palm, the index and middle fingers, and the radial side of the ring finger.

Landmarks

At the proximal flexor crease of the wrist between the flexor carpi radialis and palmaris longus tendons.

Equipment

5-ml syringe
25-gauge 3-cm needle
1% to 2% lidocaine without epinephrine or 0.25% or 0.5% bupivacaine without epinephrine

Method (Fig. 1–11)

The skin is cleansed with antiseptic. At the level of the proximal flexor crease, the needle is inserted between the tendons of the palmaris longus and the flexor carpi radialis or, in the absence of the palmaris longus, just on the ulnar side of the flexor carpi radialis tendon. The needle is kept perpendicular to the wrist and gently inserted toward the dorsal surface of the wrist. If paresthesias radiating into the fingers are obtained, the needle is arrested, and after aspiration, 2 ml of the local anesthetic solution are injected. Without paresthesias, 3 to 5 ml are injected toward the skin on gradual withdrawal.

Precaution

No epinephrine should be used.

Radial Nerve Block at the Wrist

Clinical Uses

For producing anesthesia in the distribution of the nerve, together with median and ulnar nerve block for anesthesia of the hand.

Cutaneous innervation

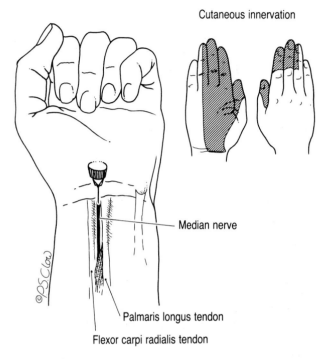

Median nerve

Palmaris longus tendon

Flexor carpi radialis tendon

Fig. 1–11. Median nerve block. Insertion is perpendicular to skin. Cutaneous innervation.

Anatomy

In the lower one-third of the forearm, the radial nerve passes under the tendon of the brachioradialis to run subcutaneously on the dorsal aspect of the wrist. It divides into several branches that supply sensation to the radial side of the dorsum of the hand, thumb, and proximal area of the index finger.

Equipment

5-ml syringe
25-gauge 4- to 5-cm needle

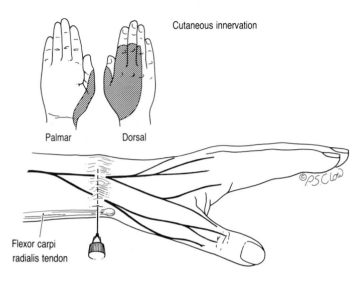

Cutaneous innervation

Palmar   Dorsal

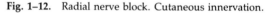

Flexor carpi
radialis tendon

Fig. 1–12. Radial nerve block. Cutaneous innervation.

0.5% to 1% lidocaine without epinephrine or 0.25% bupivacaine without epinephrine

Method (Fig. 1–12)

The skin is cleansed with the antiseptic. A subcutaneous
infiltration is performed from the flexor carpi radialis tendon that runs around the radial border of the wrist to the
dorsal aspect then up to the radial side of the ulnar styloid.
Approximately 5 ml anesthetic solution should be used.

Precautions

1. Aspirate carefully to avoid intravascular injection.
2. No epinephrine should be used.

Digital Nerve Block

Clinical Uses

Used for anesthesia of the fingers. Particularly useful for
procedures on the nail, nail bed, and pulp space.

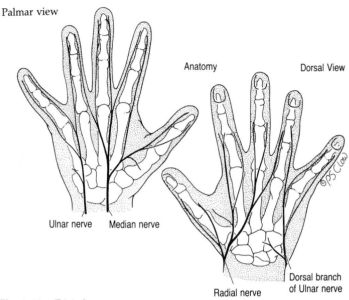

Palmar view

Anatomy

Dorsal View

Ulnar nerve   Median nerve

Radial nerve

Dorsal branch of Ulnar nerve

Fig. 1–13. Digital nerve anatomy.

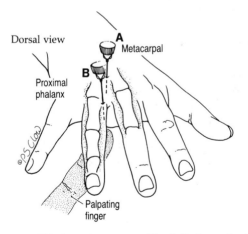

Dorsal view

A Metacarpal

B

Proximal phalanx

Palpating finger

Fig. 1–14. Digital block. *A.* At metacarpal head. *B.* At proximal phalanx.

Anatomy (Fig. 1–13)

The digital nerves arise from the median and ulnar nerves in the palm and supply adjacent sides of the fingers, the palmar surface, and terminal phalanx nail bed area. These run in the ventral-lateral aspect of the finger close beside the flexor tendons. Smaller dorsal digital branches derived from the radial and ulnar nerves run on the dorsal-lateral surface of the finger to supply the back of the fingers up to proximal phalangeal joint.

Equipment

5-ml syringe
3-cm 25- or 27-gauge needle and 1% lidocaine without epinephrine or 0.25% bupivacaine without epineph-rine

Method

Digital Block at the Metacarpal Head. The skin of the area is cleansed with antiseptic. The space between the metacarpal heads is palpated, and the needle is inserted from the dorsal surface and gently advanced until it is close beneath the palmar skin as felt by an examining finger placed on the palmar side of the hand (Fig. 1–14A). One ml of solution is injected at this point and an additional 1.5 to 2 ml injected on gradual withdrawal of the needle toward the dorsum of the hand. This is repeated between the metacarpal heads on the other side of the finger being blocked (Fig. 1–14).

Digital Nerve Block at the Proximal Phalanx. A 25- or 27-gauge needle is inserted on the dorsal aspect at the base of the finger and advanced towards the palmar surface close to the side of the proximal phalanx (Fig. 1–14B). When the operator's guarding finger feels the needle point close to the palmar skin, 1 ml of solution is injected. This is repeated on the other side of the same finger. The needle is withdrawn to a point just below the skin of the dorsal surface and an additional 0.5 ml injected to block the dorsal branch.

Precautions

Under no circumstances should epinephrine solutions be used for digital nerve block. Vasoconstrictors can produce intense arterial spasm in the end arterial circulation of the finger and lead to possible necrosis. Also, large volumes of solution or too rapid injection must be avoided due to the possible ischemic effects of pressure on the vessels.

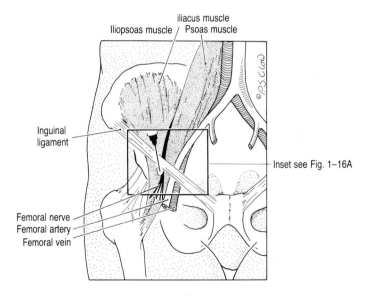

Fig. 1–15. Femoral nerve block.

LOWER LIMB BLOCKS

Femoral Nerve Block

Clinical Uses

1. Used in combination with lateral femoral cutaneous nerve block it provides anesthesia for the anterior thigh.
2. Used with sciatic nerve block it provides anesthesia for the lower leg and foot.
3. Also useful in the diagnosis and treatment of painful conditions of the anterolateral thigh and knee.

Anatomy (Fig. 1–15)

The femoral nerve, a branch of the lumbar plexus, enters the thigh by passing deep to the inguinal ligament that lies anterior to the iliopsoas muscle and just lateral to the femoral artery. At this point, the nerve may have already divided into several branches that supply the anterior thigh muscles, the knee joint, and skin of the anterior thigh. The terminal branch, the saphenous nerve, runs down the medial calf and supplies the skin down to the medial malleolus.

Landmarks

A line drawn between the anterior superior iliac spine and the pubic tubercle marks the inguinal ligament. Just below this line, the femoral artery is palpated and the femoral nerve located approximately 1 cm lateral to the artery.

Equipment

  10- or 20-ml syringe
  5-cm 22- or 25-gauge needle
  1% lidocaine with epinephrine or 0.25 bupivacaine with epinephrine

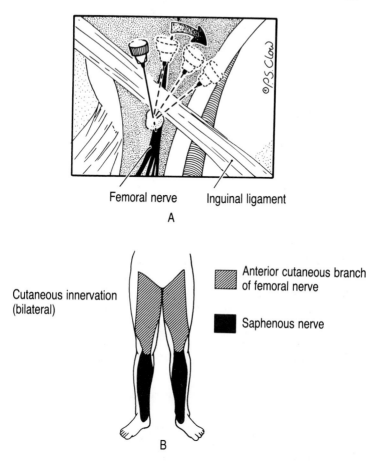

Femoral nerve   Inguinal ligament

A

Cutaneous innervation
(bilateral)

Anterior cutaneous branch
of femoral nerve

Saphenous nerve

B

Fig. 1–16. **A.** Femoral block on right side. Note the fanwise injection around the nerve. **B.** Bilateral cutaneous innervation.

Method (Fig. 1–16)

The skin of the groin area is cleansed with antiseptic. The femoral artery is palpated just below the inguinal ligament, and a skin wheal is raised 1 cm lateral to it. Using a 5-cm 22- or 25-gauge needle with syringe attached, the needle is inserted perpendicular to the skin and slowly advanced until paresthesias radiating into the thigh or knee are obtained; then, after negative aspiration, 8 to 10 ml of solution are injected.

If paresthesias are not obtained, the syringe is detached and the needle carefully reinserted until pulsations transmitted from the artery are observed. After careful aspiration, 10 ml of solution are injected and an additional 10 ml injected in a fanwise fashion below the deep fascia, directed laterally along the line parallel to the inguinal ligament.

Precautions

Careful aspiration will usually avoid intravascular injection. If the femoral artery is inadvertently punctured, the needle must immediately be withdrawn, and arterial compression must be maintained by the operator for 5 to 10 minutes in order to prevent hematoma formation.

Lateral Femoral Cutaneous Nerve Block

Clinical Uses

1. Used together with femoral nerve block to provide anesthesia of the anterior thigh.
2. Also useful for anesthesia in donor areas of skin grafting.
3. Used in diagnosis and management of meralgia paresthetica.

Anatomy (Fig. 1–17)

This nerve arises from the lumbar plexus and runs downward and forward on the side of the iliac muscle to pass

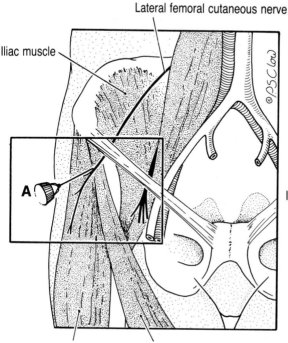

Lateral femoral cutaneous nerve

Iliac muscle

A

Inset see Figure 1–18

Tensor fascia lata muscle   Sartorius muscle

Fig. 1–17.   Lateral femoral cutaneous nerve block.

beneath the inguinal ligament at a point approximately 1
to 2 cm medial to the anterior superior iliac spine. It descends to supply skin over the lateral thigh down to the
knee.

Landmarks

Found at a point approximately 2 cm below and medial
to the anterior superior iliac spine in a groove between the
origins of the sartorius and tensor fascia lata muscles.

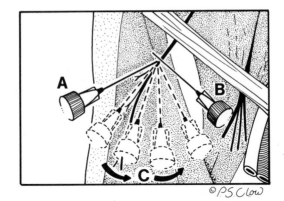

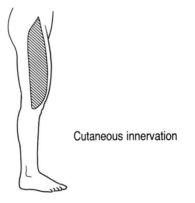

Cutaneous innervation

Fig. 1–18. Lateral femoral cutaneous nerve block. Right-sided block. Note the fanwise injection around the nerve. Cutaneous innervation. **A.** At a point approximately 2 cm below and medial to the anterior superior iliac spine, the needle is advanced with a slightly superior angulation. **B.** Further infiltration is made 0.5 cm laterally and superiorly. **C.** If necessary, a series of further injections of local anesthetic may be made in a fanwise fashion to complete the arc.

Equipment

   10- or 20-ml syringe
   5-cm 22- or 25-gauge needle
   1% lidocaine with epinephrine or 0.25 bupivacaine with
      epinephrine

Method (Fig. 1–18)

The skin of the area is cleansed with antiseptic. The needle, with syringe attached, is inserted at the point described above and advanced with a slightly superior angulation (Fig. 1–18A). If paresthesias are obtained, the advance is arrested and, after negative aspiration, 5 ml of solution are injected. If bone is contacted before paresthesias are elicited, the needle is withdrawn to the skin and redirected 0.5 cm farther laterally and superiorly (Fig. 1–18B). If difficulty is obtained in gaining paresthesias, 10 to 15 ml of solution deposited beneath the fascia lata, in a fanwise fashion, medially and laterally around the original point of entry, will usually provide adequate block (Fig. 1–18C). Penetration of the fascia is usually easily recognized by a slight click as the needle is advanced.

Precautions

If this block is combined with femoral or sciatic nerve blocks, there is a risk of overdosage. For such combined blocks, maximum safe dosages should be calculated and strictly adhered to in order to avoid toxic reaction.

Sciatic Nerve Block

Clinical Uses

1. Anesthesia in the distribution of the nerve.
2. In combination with femoral nerve block for anesthesia of the lower leg and foot in surgical procedures not requiring tourniquet.

3. Relief of pain from fracture of the tibia.
4. Vascular procedures on the lower leg.
5. Differential diagnosis of sciatica.

Anatomy

The sciatic nerve arises from the sacral plexus and leaves the pelvis with the posterior cutaneous nerve of the thigh through the greater sciatic notch. These nerves provide sensory supply to the posterior thigh and lateral leg. Below the knee, the sciatic branch is posterior. The tibial, sural, and peroneal nerves provide complete innervation below the ankle.

Landmarks (Fig. 1–19)

Several approaches to the sciatic nerve block have been described and used successfully for many years. The anterior approach is described here because it requires no special positioning of the patient. The sciatic nerve block, with the femoral and lateral femoral cutaneous nerve blocks, if necessary, can be performed with the patient in supine position.

A line is drawn from the anterior superior iliac spine to the pubic tubercle. A second line is drawn perpendicular to the first from the junction of the medial and middle one-third. This line is extended down and across the thigh. A third line is drawn parallel to the first from the greater trochanter medially across the thigh. Where it bisects the second line lies a suitable entry point for the needle.

Equipment

20-ml syringe
15-cm 22-gauge needle
1% lidocaine with epinephrine or 0.25 bupivacaine with epinephrine. A peripheral nerve stimulator, if available, is useful in helping to locate the nerve accurately.

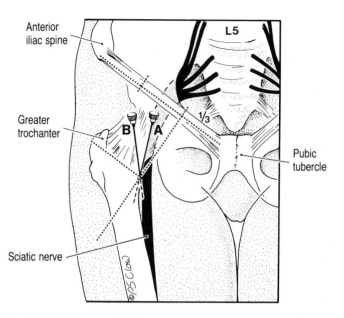

Fig. 1–19. Sciatic nerve block.

Method (Fig. 1–19)

The upper thigh is cleansed with antiseptic. A skin wheal is raised at the previously determined entry point. The 15-cm 22-gauge needle is then inserted through the wheal and advanced slightly laterally until gentle contact with the anterior surface of the femur is detected (Fig. 1–19A). A note of the depth is made. This can be performed by using a small rubber disc as a depth marker attached to the needle. The needle is withdrawn through the subcutaneous tissue and reinserted slightly medially so it slides past the femur and is then advanced a farther 5 cm beyond the previous point of bone contact (Fig. 1–19B).

By 1 to 2 cm readjustment of the angle and depth of the needle, the fascial plane containing the sciatic nerve can be denoted by a reduction in resistance to advance of the

needle and to injection of a trial volume of anesthetic solution (Fig. 1–19B). If paresthesias radiate into the foot,
positive confirmation of accurate position is obtained. In
the absence of paresthesias, a nerve stimulator is helpful.
Using minimal stimulating current at 2 cycles per second,
close approximation to the nerve is indicated by rhythmic
plantar flexion of the foot. When satisfactory localization
is obtained, 20 to 25 ml of anesthetic solution are injected.
At this level, the posterior cutaneous nerve of the thigh
may not be blocked (Fig. 1–20).

Precautions

1. Even when accompanied by femoral block, there can
   be insufficient anesthesia of the thigh for the patient
   to tolerate a tourniquet for any significant length of

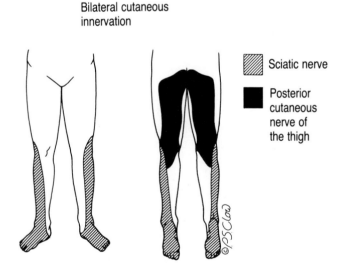

Fig. 1–20. Sciatic nerve block. Bilateral cutaneous innervation. Note that
the posterior cutaneous nerve is not always blocked with anterior approach to sciatic nerve block.

time. In addition, the dosages of drug required are high, and the risk of toxic reaction is considerable.
2. Adequate precautions must be followed as described in patient preparation.
3. Twenty to 30 minutes may elapse before anesthesia is fully established.

FOOT (ANKLE) BLOCK

Block of the posterior tibial, sural, superficial and deep peroneal, and saphenous nerves will give complete anesthesia of the foot. When only partial anesthesia of the foot suffices, block of the appropriate nerves is adequate.

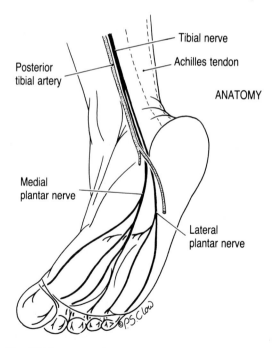

Fig. 1–21. Tibial nerve anatomy.

Tibial Nerve Block

Anatomy (Fig. 1–21)

At the ankle, the tibial nerve lies posterolateral to the posterior tibial artery between the medial malleolus and the Achilles tendon. It divides beneath the flexor retinaculum into the medial and lateral nerves that supply the skin of the sole and plantar aspect of the toes.

Landmarks

The medial malleolus, the Achilles tendon and the posterior tibial artery.

Equipment

5-ml syringe
5-cm 25-gauge needle
1% lidocaine or 0.25% bupivacaine without epinephrine

Method (Fig. 1–22)

With the patient supine, a padded roll is placed underneath the calf to elevate the foot; the foot and ankle are externally rotated. The ankle and foot are cleansed with antiseptic. At the midpoint between the posterior margin of the medial malleolus and the Achilles tendon, the posterior tibial pulse is palpated and serves as a guide to the insertion point. In the absence of a palpable arterial pulse, the point midway between the tendon and medial malleolus is selected. The needle is inserted here, is guided by the palpating finger over the posterior tibial artery, and is advanced anteriorly toward the posterior border of the tibia. Paresthesias may be obtained close to the posterior tibial artery. At this point, the needle is fixed and 2 to 3 ml of the anesthetic solution are injected after negative aspiration. If paresthesias have not been obtained, the tibia is contacted and then the needle withdrawn 1 cm and 3 ml of anesthetic injected and a further 2 ml injected on slow

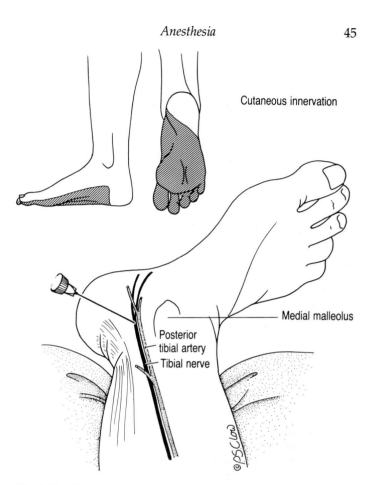

Cutaneous innervation

Medial malleolus

Posterior
tibial artery
Tibial nerve

Fig. 1–22. Cutaneous innervation. Tibial nerve block.

withdrawal to the skin. The area is gently massaged, and pressure is maintained for 2 to 3 minutes in order to spread the solution and reduce possible hematoma formation if a vessel is inadvertently punctured.

Sural Nerve Block

Anatomy (Fig. 1–23)

At the ankle, the sural nerve lies subcutaneously with the short saphenous vein behind and below the lateral malleolus. It supplies the lateral border of the heel and foot as far forward as the fifth metatarsal head.

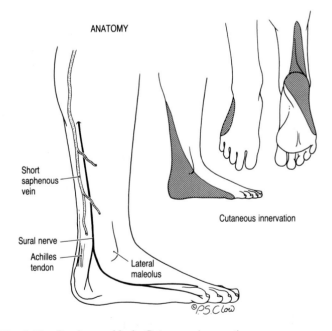

Fig. 1–23. Sural nerve block. Cutaneous innervation.

Landmarks

The nerve can often be palpated subcutaneously at the point midway between the lateral malleolus and the calcaneum just below the insertion of the Achilles tendon.

Equipment

Same as tibial nerve block.

Method (Fig. 1–24)

The foot is prepared the same way as in the tibial block, but is rotated internally and inverted. A 25-gauge 5-cm needle, with a 5-ml syringe attached, is inserted at the site overlying the nerve, and if paresthesias are obtained, 2 to 3 ml of solution are injected after negative aspiration (Fig. 1–24A). A good block can also be obtained without paresthesias by infiltrating subcutaneously in a fanwise fashion, between the Achilles tendon and the lateral malleolus

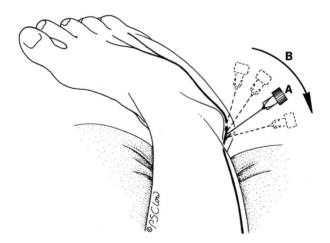

Fig. 1–24. Sural nerve block. Having located the sural nerve, block is performed at point **A. B.** An alternative method of blocking is by infiltrating subcutaneously in a fanwise fashion.

(Fig. 1–24B). Five ml of local anesthetic solution should be sufficient.

Superficial Peroneal Nerve Block

Anatomy (Fig. 1–25)

The superficial peroneal nerve runs subcutaneously in the anterolateral aspect of the lower one-third of the leg, passing in front of the lateral malleolus, to supply the skin of the dorsum of the foot and toes excluding the adjacent surfaces of the big toe and second toe.

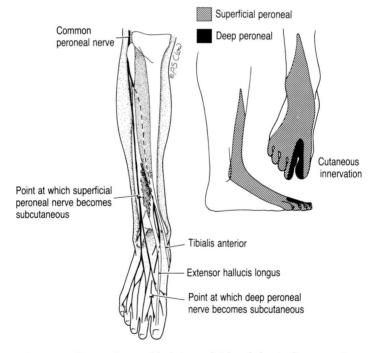

Fig. 1–25. Peroneal nerve block (superficial and deep). Cutaneous innervation.

Landmarks

The extensor hallucis longus tendon and the lateral malleolus.

Equipment

Same as tibial nerve block.

Method (Fig. 1–26)

The ankle and foot are prepared just as in the tibial nerve block, but with the foot pointing straight upward. A subcutaneous infiltration of 5 ml of anesthetic solution between

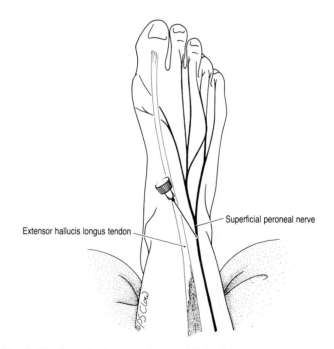

Fig. 1–26. Superficial peroneal nerve block. Subcutaneous infiltration between extensor hallucis longus and lateral malleolus is usually effective.

the extensor hallucis longus tendon and the superior aspect
of the lateral malleolus will provide adequate block.

Deep Peroneal Nerve Block

Anatomy (Fig. 1–25)

At the ankle, the nerve lies between the anterior tibial
and the extensor hallucis longus tendons, on the lateral
side of the anterior tibial artery. It descends to the dorsum
of the foot under the extensor retinaculum and pierces the
deep fascia to become subcutaneous between the first and
second metatarsals. It supplies the short extensors of the
toes and the skin over the contiguous surfaces of the first
and second toes.

Landmarks

The tibialis anterior and the extensor hallucis longus tendons at the level of the ankle joint.

Equipment

Same as the tibial nerve block except that a 3-cm needle
usually suffices.

Method (Fig. 1–27)

The foot is prepared and positioned just as in the superficial peroneal nerve block.

A 25-gauge needle is inserted between the tibialis anterior tendon and the tendon of the extensor hallucis longus
at the level of the line between the malleoli. If the anterior
tibial artery can be palpated, the needle is inserted just
lateral to it. The needle is advanced toward the tibia and
after negative aspiration, 5 ml of solution are injected.

Saphenous Nerve Block

Anatomy

The saphenous nerve at the ankle runs subcutaneously,
accompanying the long saphenous vein just anterior to the

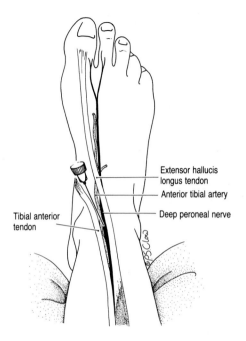

Fig. 1–27. Deep peroneal nerve block.

medial malleolus. It supplies skin over the medial malleolus and foot below it, occasionally as far as the first metatarsophalangeal joint.

Landmarks

The medial malleolus and the saphenous vein.

Equipment

Same as for tibial nerve block.

Method (Fig. 1–28)

The ankle and foot are prepared and positioned just as in the peroneal nerve block. Using a 25-gauge needle, 3 to

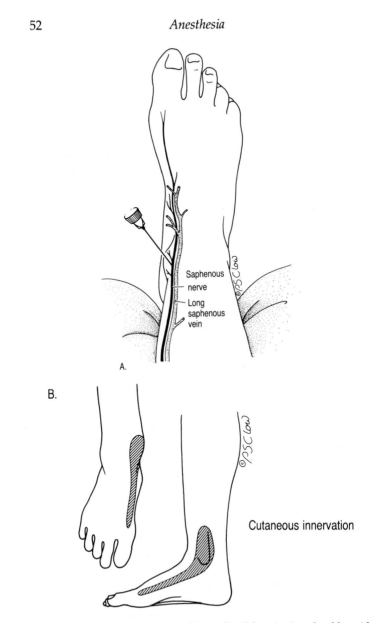

Saphenous
nerve

Long
saphenous
vein

A.

B.

Cutaneous innervation

Fig. 1–28. **A.** Saphenous nerve block. Careful aspiration should avoid injection into the saphenous vein. **B.** Cutaneous innervation.

5 ml of local anesthetic solution are infiltrated around the saphenous vein just anterior to the medial malleolus.

Precautions

Because varying degrees of arterial disease frequently occur in the region, it is better to avoid epinephrine-containing solutions for these blocks. For similar reasons, excessive volumes and rapid injections must be avoided. Twenty ml should suffice for an ankle block.

Digital Block of the Toes

The anatomy and technique of digital nerve block in the toes is similar to that described for fingers. Refer to that section. The same precautions should be observed. Avoid excessive volume; epinephrine-containing solutions should *never* be used for fingers or toes.

THORAX

Intercostal Nerve Block

Clinical Uses

1. Relief from pain of fractured ribs
2. Post-operative pain relief for thoracic and abdominal wounds, permitting early physiotherapy and removal of secretions.
3. Anesthesia of the abdominal wall.
4. Diagnosis and treatment of intercostal neuralgia.

Anatomy (Fig. 1–29)

The intercostal nerves arise from the anterior primary rami of the thoracic spinal nerves. Leaving the intervertebral foramen and traveling through the paravertebral space close to the endothoracic fascia, the nerve at the angle of the rib enters the neurovascular groove on the inferomedial aspect of the rib lying between the internal and

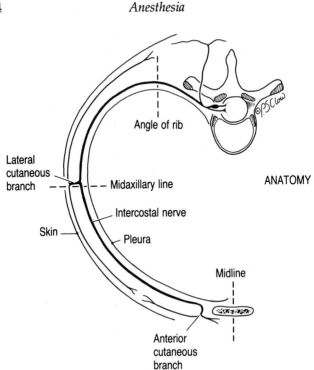

Fig. 1–29.   Intercostal nerve branches.

external intercostal muscles. In the midaxillary line, the nerve gives off a lateral cutaneous branch; near the midline it gives off an anterior cutaneous branch.

The upper six nerves are distributed to the intercostal muscles and skin of the anterolateral chest wall. The lower six nerves continue around the abdomen to supply the muscles and skin of the anterior abdominal wall.

Equipment

  5- to 10-ml syringe
  3- to 5-cm 25-gauge needle

1% lidocaine with epinephrine or 0.25% bupivacaine with epinephrine

Method (Fig. 1–30)

The patient is placed in the lateral or prone position with the arm drawn up over the head to bring the scapula forward away from the rib angles. The skin of the chest wall is cleansed with antiseptic. The lower edge of the rib is palpated at or close to the angle. The skin is retracted up-

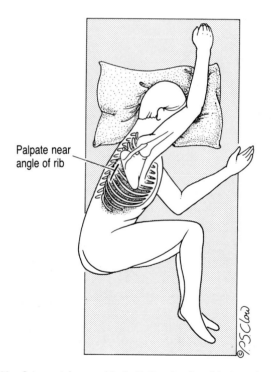

Palpate near angle of rib

Fig. 1–30. Intercostal nerve block. Patient is placed in lateral or prone position with arm elevated to bring the scapula forward and away from the rib angles.

ward, and a 25-gauge needle with syringe attached is inserted toward the rib, in a slightly upward direction, until bone is gently contacted. As the retracted skin is slowly allowed to relax, the needle is walked down the ribs until it slips off the inferior edge. Keeping a definite cephalad incline to the needle, advance it between 3 and 5 mm under the rib. After negative aspiration, inject 5 ml of solution. The number of nerves blocked depends on either the requirements of the procedure or the extent of the painful area. Unless three consecutive nerves are injected, objective evidence of cutaneous anesthesia is difficult to obtain because of the overlapping nerve supply in the thoracic and abdominal wall (Fig. 1–31).

Precautions

1. Deep needle penetration between the ribs risks penetration of the pleura or lung with the possible production of pneumothorax. Similarly, a puncture of an intercostal vein or artery is also possible.
2. Careful aspiration will reveal the presence of air or blood; thus intrapleural or intravascular injection can be avoided.
3. If many nerves are injected, large doses are required and the risk of toxic reaction is inherent. Adhere to maximum safe dosages.

ABDOMEN

Ilioinguinal and Iliohypogastric Nerve Block or Iliac Crest Block

Clinical Uses

1. Anesthesia in the distribution of these nerves.
2. Diagnosis and treatment of neuralgias and entrapment neuropathies of these nerves.

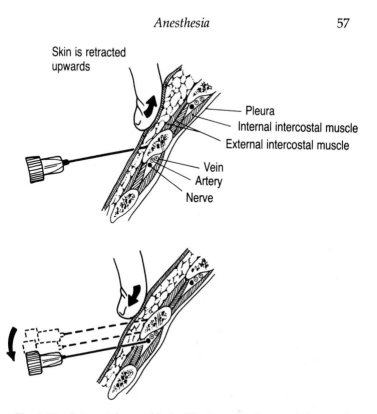

Skin is retracted upwards

Pleura
Internal intercostal muscle
External intercostal muscle
Vein
Artery
Nerve

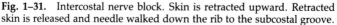

Fig. 1–31. Intercostal nerve block. Skin is retracted upward. Retracted skin is released and needle walked down the rib to the subcostal groove.

3. Inguinal hernia repair accompanied by local infiltration field block of the inguinal region.

Anatomy (Fig. 1–32)

The iliohypogastric nerve arises from the lumbar plexus and its anterior cutaneous branch runs downward and medially between the transversus abdominis and the internal oblique muscles. It enters the lower part of the anterior abdominal wall, 2 to 3 cm medial to the anterior superior

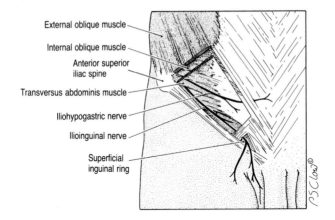

External oblique muscle

Internal oblique muscle

Anterior superior
iliac spine

Transversus abdominis muscle

Iliohypogastric nerve

Ilioinguinal nerve

Superficial
inguinal ring

Fig. 1–32.   Iliac crest anatomy.

iliac spine, to supply the skin just above the inguinal ligament.

The ilioinguinal nerve also arises from the lumbar plexus and runs parallel to, but slightly below, the iliohypogastric nerve. It emerges through the external inguinal ring and supplies the adjacent skin of the scrotum or labium majorum.

Landmark

The anterior superior iliac spine.

Equipment

10- or 20-ml syringe
8-cm short bevel needle
0.75% lidocaine with epinephrine or 0.25% bupivacaine
    with epinephrine

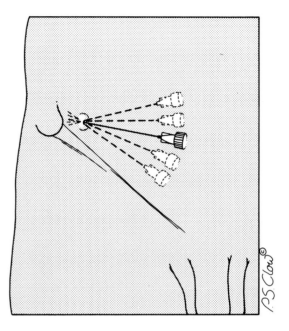

Fig. 1–33. Iliac crest block. Note the fanwise injection.

Method (Fig. 1–33)

The patient lies in the supine position, and the operator stands on the side opposite the one to be blocked. The skin of the inguinal area is cleansed with antiseptic. A point is marked 2 to 3 cm medial to the anterior superior iliac spine, and a skin wheal is raised. A short beveled 8-cm needle, 22- or 25-gauge (a spinal needle is useful for this purpose), is inserted through the skin wheal and directed laterally through the external and internal oblique muscles to contact the inner surface of the iliac crest external to the transversus abdominis. Ten ml of solution are injected and a further 10 ml injected as the needle is moved in a fanwise fashion back through the muscle layers. If inguinal hernia repair is to be performed, further subcutaneous infiltration is performed superiorly, inferiorly, and medially. Further subcutaneous/intramuscular infiltration is made from a skin wheal just above the pubic tubercle. The diamond-shaped field block blocks all nerves entering the area (Fig. 1–34). Infiltration of the internal inguinal ring and neck of the hernial sac is best left until the area has been exposed. This avoids possible damage to the contents of the hernial sac. A total volume of 50 to 60 ml of solution is required.

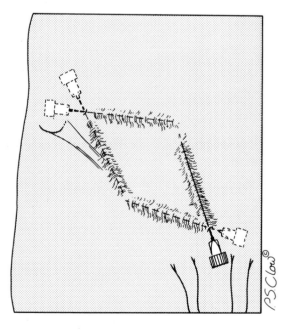

Fig. 1–34. Inguinal field block.

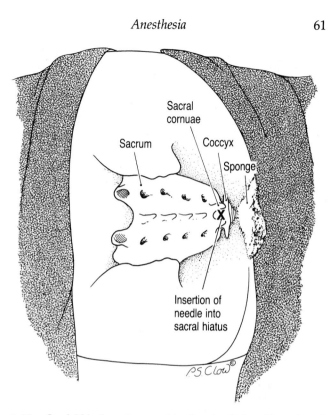

Fig. 1–35. Caudal block anatomy and landmarks. Point of insertion of needle into sacral hiatus.

Precautions

Avoid deep injection in a medial direction as peritoneal puncture and intra-abdominal injection can occur.

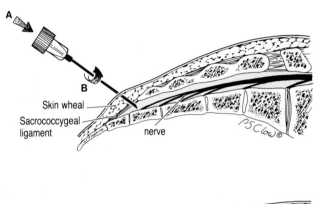

Skin wheal

Sacrococcygeal
ligament

nerve

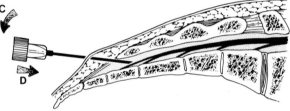

Fig. 1–36. Caudal block: After piercing sacrococcygeal ligament, the bevel of needle is turned ventrally. **A.** The needle is introduced with the bevel posterior. **B.** The needle is then rotated so the bevel is ventral or anterior. **C.** The hub of the needle is depressed toward the anal cleft. **D.** The needle, with bevel ventral, is advanced into the sacral canal.

PERINEUM

Low Caudal Block (Sacral Epidural Block)

Clinical Uses

1. Anesthesia of the perineal area and anorectal region, low vagina and vulva.
2. Useful for surgery of the anal region, hemorrhoids, fissures, fistula, vulvar cysts, and perineal repair.

Anatomy

Caudal block is produced by inserting a needle through the sacral hiatus into the sacral extradural space. The laminae and spinous processes of the upper four sacral vertebra are fused to form the posterior wall of the sacral canal. As a rule, however, the spinous process of the fifth sacral vertebra is absent, leaving behind two vestigial laminae which form the sacral cornuae; between these an arched opening, the sacral hiatus, is covered by the elastic sacrococcygeal ligament. The sacral canal communicates with the rest of the epidural space that extends up to the foramen magnum (Fig. 1–35).

Landmarks

Sacral hiatus, sacral cornuae, and the coccyx

Equipment

1% or 1.5% lidocaine with epinephrine or 0.25% bupivacaine with epinephrine
20-ml syringe
4-cm 20- or 22-gauge needle

Method (Fig. 1–36)

The patient is placed prone with hips raised on a pillow or in the lateral Sims' position. The buttocks are held apart with adhesive tape, and the sacral hiatus is located and marked with an indelible pen. A sponge is placed in the anal cleft to protect the anus and genitalia from the antiseptic solution and the sacrococcygeal area is carefully cleaned. A skin wheal is raised over the marked area of the sacral hiatus with a 25- or 27-gauge needle, which is then inserted through the sacrococcygeal ligament and, after aspiration, 2 to 3 ml of solution are injected to anesthetize the lower area of the sacral canal (subcutaneous infiltration only obscures the landmarks). A 20-gauge 4-cm needle is inserted through the skin wheal in the previously determined direction to pierce the sacrococcygeal ligament and contact the ventral wall of the sacral canal. The bevel of the needle is then turned ventrally and the hub of the needle depressed towards the anal cleft, and the needle is advanced, cephalad, 2 to 3 cm into the sacral canal. After aspiration to ensure a blood vessel has not been entered, a test dose of 3 ml of solution is injected (dural puncture is most unlikely to occur with a short needle). In the absence of evidence of intravascular injection (transient rise in pulse and blood pressure) or subarachnoid injection (rapid onset of anesthesia in the legs) 10 to 15 ml of solution are *slowly* injected. There should be little or no resistance to injection. A finger over the sacrum will identify any injection dorsal to the sacral canal, while resistance to injection may indicate subperiosteal puncture. In either case the needle must be repositioned. When the needle is withdrawn, the site should be sealed with a small waterproof dressing. Anesthesia of the saddle area will usually develop within 15 to 30 minutes.

Precautions

This block should not be performed if local infection is present. Sacral abnormalities make this procedure difficult or impossible in approximately 15 per cent of patients.

Avoid larger doses than suggested because this increases the risk of side effects from more extensive epidural anesthesia and from possible toxic reactions. In the elderly, the dose must be reduced.

REFERENCES

Texts

Bonica, J.: Management of Pain. Lea & Febiger, Philadelphia, 1953.
Cousins, M.J., Bridenbaugh, P.O.: Neural Blockage in Clinical Anesthesia and Management of Pain. Lippincott, Philadelphia, 1980.

Eriksson, E.: Illustrated Handbook in Local Anaesthesia. 2nd Ed. W.B. Saunders Co., Philadelphia, 1980.

Moore, D.C.: Regional Block: A Handbook for Use in Clinical Practice of Medicine and Surgery. 4th Ed. C.C. Thomas, Springfield, Illinois, 1981.

Anesthetic Drugs and Manufacturers

Bupivacaine: Wintrop Laboratories
Chloroprocaine: Pennwalt Corporation
Lidocaine: Astra Pharmaceutical Products, Inc.

Equipment Manufacturers

Needles and Syringes

Becton-Dickinson, Ltd.
Monoject/Sherwood Medical

Nerve Stimulators

Burrough Wellcome Co.
Bard Biochemical
Dupaco, Ltd.

$\overline{\underline{2}}$
Cardiology

The Resting Electrocardiogram
James D. Dubbin

UNDERSTANDING THE ELECTROCARDIOGRAM

The electrocardiogram (ECG) is a graphic recording of electrical forces that are rhythmically generated in each cardiac cycle. It is a graph of cardiac electrical voltage or potential (which may be positive or negative) plotted against time.

Pacemaker cells in the heart discharge electrical impulses, which are transmitted along an intricate conducting system to the heart muscle. These impulses cause cellular depolarization, initiating a chain of events which result in mechanical contraction of myocardial muscle. The depolarization and subsequent repolarization of the cardiac tissue produce weak electric currents that diffuse throughout the body, which acts as a conductor. Application of electrodes to various positions, usually on the body (but occasionally within the body, for example the esophagus), and the connection of the electrodes to an electrocardiographic apparatus (a galvanometer) allow for the production of the ECG.

The standard 12-lead ECG is an essential component of the evaluation of the cardiovascular system. Although there are many different types of electrocardiographic equipment available, by becoming familiar with the specific device available and by performing ECGs with attention to only a few technical matters, excellent studies may be obtained in the vast majority of situations.

OBTAINING THE ELECTROCARDIOGRAM

In order to obtain an electrocardiogram, the patient should lie quietly on a comfortable bed. Any muscular motions or twitchings by the patient can result in a poor record.

Proper skin contact is obtained by using electrical paste in contact with skin. In certain situations, it may not be possible to use traditional electrodes, and for those situations, needle electrodes are available.

The standard 12-lead ECG uses both unipolar and bipolar leads. The bipolar leads are lead I, II, III and the augmented limb leads aV_R, aV_L, and aV_F. These leads are generated by measuring a difference in electrical potential between two selected sites. Lead I represents the difference in potential between an electrode connected to the left arm and one connected to the right arm. Lead II is the difference in potential between the left leg and the right arm, and lead III is the difference in potential between the left leg and the left arm. The augmented limb leads are unipolar leads that use electrodes on the left and right arms as well as on the left leg.

Precordial leads that are routinely obtained are V_1 to V_6.

The selector dial on the electrocardiographic instrument is turned to the V lead position. Older electrocardiographic instruments require that a single lead be moved sequentially from lead position V_1 through to V_6. More modern instruments are equipped with six different precordial electrodes and wires, making it possible to take simultaneous precordial leads from V_1 to V_6.

The standard precordial lead positions are defined in terms of surface anatomy (Figs. 2–1 and 2–2). Lead V_1 is taken at the fourth intercostal space at the right sternal border. V_2 is the fourth intercostal space at the left sternal border. Lead V_3 is obtained by placing the electrode mid-

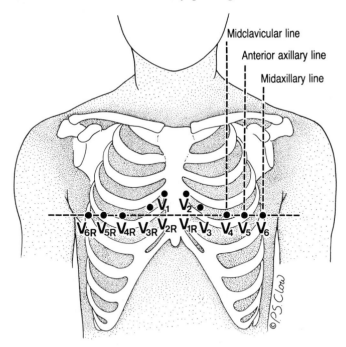

Fig. 2–1. Standard precordial lead positions.

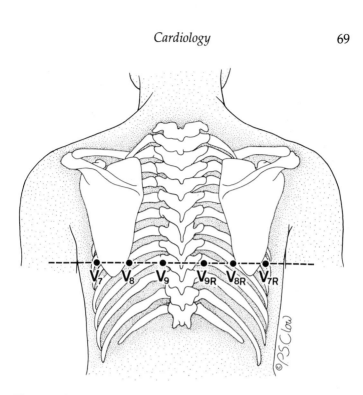

Fig. 2–2. Standard precordial lead positions.

way between leads V_2 and V_4. Lead V_4 is taken at the fifth intercostal space in the left midclavicular line. Lead V_5 is taken at the anterior axillary line and V_6 at the midaxillary line. Both V_5 and V_6 are taken in the same horizontal plane as lead V_4. Additional precordial leads are not part of the standard electrocardiogram. However, standard positions for leads V_7 to V_9 as well as for right unipolar precordial leads V_{1R} to V_{9R} have been defined. Lead V_7 is taken in the posterior axillary line, V_8 at the posterior scapular line, and lead V_9 at the left border of the spine. Leads V_7 to V_9 are taken in the same horizontal plane as lead V_4.

The right unipolar precordial leads (V_{2R} to V_{9R}) are obtained by using positions on the right chest wall that correspond to those defined above for the left chest wall.

STANDARDIZING THE ELECTROCARDIOGRAM

At the time that each electrocardiogram is obtained, it should be standardized. Modern electrocardiographic instruments are permanently standardized at the factory and will deviate 1 cm for 1 mV. Further calibration or standardization is needed only to indicate if the ECG has been recorded at normal, one-half, or two times standard sensitivity and, more importantly, to check the shape of the calibration mark for evidence of over or under damping.

It should be stressed that an ECG requires standardization only once at the initiation of the study. On occasion, it may be necessary to change sensitivities in some leads, namely to one-half sensitivity if very large QRS excursions are encountered or to twice normal sensitivity when it is necessary to bring out very small wave amplitudes. The latter situation often occurs when very small P waves appear when normal standardization is used. Whenever standardization is changed to one-half or two times normal sensitivity, the calibration marker should be repeated.

In the more modern ECG recorders, where three leads are recorded simultaneously (usually the standard limb leads I, II and III, then the augmented limb leads, aV_R, aV_L and aV_F; then the right precordial leads V_1 to V_3 and finally the left precordial leads V_4 to V_6) the sensitivity calibration is taken at the end of the 12-lead ECG. The first half of the sensitivity calibration refers to the limb leads and the second half to the precordial leads.

Most electrocardiographic instruments offer three different paper speeds. The routine speed at which 12-lead ECGs are obtained is 25 mm per second. Paper speeds of one-half and double that rate are available.

Exercise Stress Testing
James D. Dubbin

The following is an overview of the methodology of standard exercise stress testing. It is not to be considered comprehensive.

Exercise stress testing has become an integral part of the evaluation and management of many forms of cardiac disease. It provides the physician with an objective assessment of the patient's response to exercise, by measuring several parameters.

A survey of clinical exercise facilities has shown exercise testing to be a safe procedure with approximately one death and five nonfatal complications per 10,000 tests. Nevertheless, the risk of undergoing exercise testing to coronary artery disease patients cannot be disregarded, and the importance of adhering to the various safety precautions and procedures outlined below must be emphasized.

The indications for exercise testing are listed in Table 2–1. These indications have evolved over the last decade, and controversy still remains about some of them. However, a more accurate understanding of the proper use of exercise stress testing has emerged from some of these

Table 2–1.   Indications for Exercise Stress Testing

To Aid in Clinical Evaluation of:
A. Patients with chest, arm, or neck pain syndromes.
B. Patients with known exertional angina pectoris.
C. Patients receiving medical therapy for coronary artery disease.
D. Patients after surgical therapy of coronary artery disease.
E. Patients after myocardial infarction.
F. Patients with known or suspected arrhythmias.
G. Individuals in high risk professions (e.g., airline pilots).
H. Previously sedentary patients who are embarking on a fitness program.

controversies. In particular, a crucial concept has been recognized: the exercise stress test is valuable as an aid in the diagnosis of chest pain only when applied to the appropriate patient population. Later, this concept will be reviewed briefly.

Prior to the initiation of the exercise test, the physician must secure certain patient information that will optimize the usefulness of the study and ensure that the procedure is performed with the lowest possible risk. Clinical review of the patient's status, with both history and cardiac physical examination, will alert the physician to any possible contraindications, relative or absolute, to conducting the study (Table 2–2). For example, recent prolonged chest pain highly indicative of myocardial ischemia or physical findings suggestive of critical left ventricular outflow obstruction require further clarification prior to exercise testing. The clinical assessment allows the physician who is responsible for the exercise study an opportunity to review the indications for the test. These aspects must be stressed because the patient's primary physician, who requests the

Table 2–2.   Contraindications to Exercise Stress Testing

Absolute
A. Inability of patient to cooperate.
B. Acute myocardial infarction.
C. Unstable angina, refractory to medical therapy.
D. Acute myocarditis, pericarditis, or endocarditis.
E. Rapid arrhythmia.
F. 3° AV heart block.
G. Severe left ventricular outflow obstruction.
H. Heart failure (untreated).
I. Any acute or serious noncardiac disorder (e.g., pulmonary embolus, infection, severe anemia, thyroid disease).

Relative
A. Known important left main coronary artery disease.
B. 2° Mobitz type II AV block.
C. Severe arterial or pulmonary hypertension.

study, is usually not the one who performs it. Some exercise laboratories have found it advantageous to have the referring physician either complete a request exercise-testing form or provide a referral letter indicating the patient's status, with a description of a recent 12-lead ECG, a list of the patient's medications, and an explanation of the reason for the test. These documents facilitate the pretest assessment of the patient by the physician responsible for the procedure.

INSTRUCTING THE PATIENT

The patient requires specific instructions regarding any medications he or she may be using. These instructions may vary depending on the reason the exercise test is being performed. For example, the patient being referred for exercise stress testing to aid in the diagnosis of ischemic heart disease will probably be taking medications (such as beta-blockers) that might delay or mask the signs or symptoms of ischemia. Discontinue these medications at an appropriate time prior to the test. However, the patient with known ischemic heart disease, who is being studied to assess the effect of medications on his or her cardiac symptomatology, should be instructed to continue his or her usual antianginal medication regimen.

Patients undergoing exercise testing should receive simple, clear instructions, before they arrive in the laboratory. Not only should they be aware of the reason that the test is being conducted, but they should also have been given an overview of what to expect. The patients, in general, should be asked to fast for 2 or 3 hours immediately prior to the scheduled test. They should wear comfortable walking shoes and exercise clothing (women are advised to wear slacks). Immediately prior to the test, the physician conducting the study must emphasize to the patient the importance of promptly reporting any symptoms that develop during the exercise portion of the study. Of course, specific symptoms such as light-headedness or chest discomfort, which may be considered reasons for terminating the study (Table 2–3), must be emphasized. Finally, the patient must be made aware that although there are risks to the procedure, these are very small and can be further minimized by complete patient cooperation during the test. Some laboratories require that the patient sign a standard consent form prior to the test.

USING THE TREADMILL

In North America, most exercise stress testing uses a motor-driven treadmill with operator-adjustable speed and elevation. By selecting the treadmill speed and grade, and altering these over specified time intervals, the physician

Table 2–3. Indications for Termination of Exercise Stress Testing

A. Patient's request to stop.
B. Fall in heart rate or systolic blood pressure with continuing exercise accompanied by any of the following:
   1. Chest, neck, or arm discomfort suggestive of angina pectoris but more severe than usual for particular patient.
   2. Complaints of dizziness, or light-headedness, or severe fatigue.
   3. Pallor or cyanosis.
   4. Severe dyspnea.
   5. Development of either ventricular or supraventricular arrhythmias (i.e., ventricular ectopy consisting of ventricular bigeminy or couplets or more complex forms, or atrial fibrillation or flutter with rapid, greater than 150 per minute ventricular response).
   6. Disabling claudication.
   7. Marked ST-segment depression (3.0 mm beneath resting baseline) or ST-segment elevation (2.0 mm above resting baseline).
   8. Technical problems with patient monitoring (e.g., loss of continuous ECG oscilloscope read out).
   9. Achievement of pretest set target heart rate.

can exercise patients according to one of several standard protocols.

The initial work load should be light enough to serve as a warm-up period. Many patients have initial difficulty walking comfortably on a treadmill; the low-level warm-up period can provide a needed opportunity for adaptation to smooth walking (Figs. 2–3 and 2–4).

It is important that subsequent increments in the work load are not excessive; each increment should be such that the patient tolerates it, at least initially. Most widely used exercise protocols allow three minutes at each work load stage, thus allowing the patients to achieve a steady state before being challenged with a greater work load.

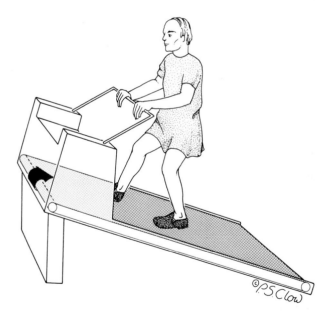

Fig. 2–3. Correct posture on treadmill.

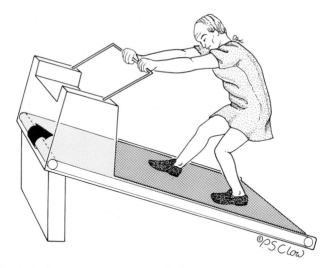

Fig. 2–4. Incorrect posture on treadmill.

MONITORING THE PATIENT

Electrocardiographic and blood pressure monitoring of the patient begins prior to the exercise portion of the study. A 12-lead ECG and blood pressure measurement should be recorded in both supine and standing positions. These are inspected for resting abnormalities that must be considered when interpreting the response of the ECG and the blood pressure to exercise. Moreover, these ECGs should be compared to any previous tracings that are available.

Unusual increases in standing heart rate or blood pressure may provide a clue to the existence of a vasoregulatory abnormality.

Some laboratories perform ECGs after short periods (30 seconds) of hyperventilation. These ECGs are inspected for ventricular repolarization changes (ST-segment or T-wave abnormalities) that may mimic ischemia and thus confound the electrocardiographic interpretation of the test.

Satisfactory monitoring and analysis of electrocardiographic responses during exercise may be obtained with a single bipolar precordial lead with one electrode at the V_5 position and the other at the lower tip of the right scapula or alternatively near the manubrium sternum. A third electrode is used as a ground.

In recent years, though, most laboratories have used multi-lead (12-lead electrocardiographic) monitoring not only before and after, but also during the exercise portion of the test. This has required relocation of the electrodes for bipolar limb leads to the subclavicular fossa and the iliac crests. The use of additional leads (beyond the single V_5) has been repeatedly demonstrated to increase the value of the test in detecting electrocardiographic abnormalities that may occur with exercise.

Skin should be cleansed and resistance reduced either by using a dental burr or by rotating a cotton swab moistened with electrode jelly to remove the outer layer of the epidermis. Stainless steel electrodes with the disc 1 mm below the plastic rim, 1 cm in diameter, and filled with electrode paste, should be attached firmly to the skin with double-sided adhesive discs and stabilized with adhesive tape. Disposable cloth mesh vests over the chest electrodes provide further stabilization. Lightweight wire cables with grounded shielding should be used and suspended near the patient to avoid interference with walking.

During the exercise test, selected leads should be displayed continuously on an oscilloscope and blood pressure measurements made every 60–120 seconds. A complete multi-lead ECG should be obtained in the last 30 seconds of each work load stage. These are retained for review and inclusion in the permanent stress test record. The capability for recording in hard-copy form any arrhythmia detected on the rhythm strip oscilloscope is ideal.

Blood pressure measurements and ECGs after exercise should be recorded during the recovery period. Optimally, after exercise recording should continue intermittently (every 1 to 2 minutes) until the supine ECG and blood pressure results return to their pretest baselines. Vigilant observation during the postexercise test is obligatory since not only ischemic changes, but also hypotension and high-grade blocks or arrhythmias may manifest during this period.

TERMINATING THE EXERCISE TEST

Termination of the exercise portion of the test is a most important aspect of the study. Premature termination, not necessitated by signs or symptoms, will result in an inadequate study (Table 2–3). In the patient who exercises without developing any sign or symptom requiring termination, the test is ideally continued until a certain pretest determined heart rate is achieved. Tables are available which can be used to calculate the patient's maximum heart rate relative to sex and age.

It was shown that heart rate limited testing, where the target heart rate is established at 85–90% of the patient's age-predicted maximum heart rate, is adequate to detect signs or symptoms of even previously occult ischemic heart disease in the majority of individuals. Terminating the exercise test on the basis of heart rate requirements often, however, rests on the judgment and experience of the physician performing the test. Some individuals can easily reach the 85–90% maximum predicted heart rate, whereas others, even though asymptomatic and not on medications, cannot.

TAKING PRECAUTIONS

All exercise laboratories must be equipped with readily accessible safety equipment and cardiac medications. Moreover, all laboratory personnel, in addition to the physician responsible for the test, must be thoroughly familiar with basic cardiopulmonary resuscitation procedures. The cardiac medications and defibrillation equipment must be meticulously maintained. Most manufacturers of defibrillation equipment provide maintenance specifications. If the laboratory is a facility or service of a general hospital, the mechanisms for alerting the cardiac arrest team must be clearly indicated and known by all personnel. These aspects of the exercise testing laboratory function must be stressed.

TYPES OF TEST ABNORMALITIES

Rigid electrocardiographic criteria should be used for classifying a tracing as indicating myocardial ischemia. These criteria include the following three patterns of exercise-induced electrocardiographic abnormalities: first, 1 mm or more of J-junction depression combined with downward sloping or horizontal ST-segment depression; second, slowly upward sloping ST-segment depression remaining 2 mm below the isoelectric line, 80 milliseconds after the J-point; and third, ST-segment elevation above the isoelectric line greater than or equal to 1 mm for at least 80 milliseconds duration in the absence of prior myocardial infarction.

The development of any of these abnormalities would suggest the presence of myocardial ischemia. These criteria cannot be extended to include the entire patient population; this represents one of the limitations of using the electrocardiographic component of an exercise stress test to establish a diagnosis of myocardial ischemia. In patients on certain medications, most notably digitalis preparations, it has been repeatedly demonstrated that ST-segment abnormalities may develop with exercise when there is no other functional or structural evidence of coronary artery disease. In these cases, the test gives a false-positive electrocardiograph result. In patients with ST-segment abnormalities on the resting ECG (e.g., patients with ventricular conduction defects, left and right bundle branch block, previous myocardial infarction, valvular, cardiomyopathic or hypertensive heart disease), electrocardiographic evidence for myocardial ischemia is either difficult or impossible to determine during an exercise stress test.

However, there are other response parameters to be considered in the analysis of the exercise test. The most important of these are listed in Table 2–4.

TWO HYPOTHETICAL CASE STUDIES

It is worthwhile contrasting two hypothetical cases to demonstrate this multi-variable approach to exercise test interpretation. In each of these hypothetical cases, the patient is a 50-year-old male with a three month history of

Table 2–4.   Response Parameters Other Than ST-Segment Changes to be Assessed with Exercise Stress Testing

A. Heart rate (i.e., chronotropic incompetence, failure for heart rate to increase in a smooth, gradual fashion with continuing exercise).
B. Blood pressure.
C. Marked increase in R-wave amplitude or QRS duration.
D. Patient complaint, especially description of any chest, neck, or arm discomfort.
E. Patient appearance.
F. Post exercise evidence of exercise-induced heart failure (gallop rhythm, mitral regurgitation murmur or pulmonary crepitations).

chest discomfort "moderately suggestive of angina pectoris." In both cases, the histories were otherwise unremarkable and the physical examinations were normal. The pre-exercise ECGs were both normal. Neither patient was on medication.

The first of the patients exercised for 11 minutes using the Bruce protocol (a standard protocol). The test was terminated by fatigue. There were no other symptoms. The patient achieved a heart rate of 170 (i.e., 95% of his age-predicted maximum heart rate). His blood pressure rose gradually from 120/80 to 200/70 at peak exercise. There were no arrhythmias. During the tenth minute of exercise, 1 mm ST-segment horizontal depression was observed in lead V_6 only. The immediately after exercise, supine ECG showed sinus tachycardia at 140 per minute with no ST-segment abnormalities. Cardiac auscultation revealed no new sounds or murmurs. Five minutes after exercise, the heart rate was 100/minute, blood pressure 140/80, and the ECG pattern was normal.

The second of these patients exercised for 3.5 minutes using the Bruce protocol. The test was terminated because of a combination of the following signs and symptoms. The patient complained of central anterior chest pain at 2.5 minutes of exercise, and this gradually increased in intensity with continuing exercise. He reported vague light-headedness at 3.5 minutes of exercise. His initial blood pressure was 120/80, and at one minute of exercise, it was 160/90, unchanged at two minutes and at three minutes. At 3.5 minutes, his blood pressure had fallen to 130/95. The patient appeared pale and unwell. The maximum heart rate achieved was 130 (i.e., 75% of his age-predicted maximum). There were no exercise-induced arrhythmias. At two minutes, 1 mm horizontal ST-segment depression was present in leads V_2–V_6. At one minute after exercise, the chest pain was diminishing, and the light-headedness had vanished. Cardiac auscultation revealed an apical systolic murmur and a clearly audible gallop rhythm. His heart rate was 120 beats/minute and his blood pressure 150/90. The ECG showed sinus rhythm with 3 mm ST-segment downward sloping depression in leads V_2–V_6. These ECG abnormalities persisted until five minutes after exercise and then began to abate gradually. At 12 minutes after exercise, the ECG and the cardiac auscultatory findings had returned to normal. The patient felt well.

It is strikingly clear that the exercise test has provided different information about these patients. However, if the exercise test had been reported only as either negative or positive with respect to ECG abnormalities, both tests should be considered positive based on the development of at least 1 mm ST-segment depression during exercise. Such reports would be misleading.

There is little doubt that the second patient has exercise-induced myocardial ischemia and probably extensive and severe coronary artery disease. The postexercise physical examination abnormalities, though transient, were clearly suggestive of exercise-induced left ventricular dysfunction (the gallop rhythm) and papillary muscle dysfunction (the systolic apical murmur). In the first patient, the good exercise tolerance, the lack of chest pain, the appropriate increase in blood pressure and heart rate, and the development of only transient 1 mm ST-segment depression in only one lead, after a full ten minutes of exercise, suggests that if coronary artery disease is present in this individual, it is unlikely to be extensive or severe. These two cases demonstrate the need to consider several variables from the exercise stress test, in order to put the results in perspective and hence guide patient management.

DEFINING TERMS

Certain groups of patients can benefit more than others from exercise stress testing. In order to facilitate this discussion, knowledge of three terms "sensitivity," "specific-ity," and "predictive accuracy" are required. "Sensitivity" refers to the percentage of all patients *with* disease who manifest an abnormal test. Sensitivity is determined by calculating the number of true-positive tests divided by the total number of true-positive tests plus false negative tests. "Specificity" refers to the patient *without* disease who manifest a negative test. Specificity is determined by calculating the number of true-negative tests divided by the number of true-negative tests plus false-positive tests. "Predictive accuracy" refers to the percent of positive tests that are truly positive and is determined by calculating the number of true-positive tests divided by the number of true-positive tests plus false-positive tests.

Within the last 6 years, the importance of the relationship between predictive accuracy of exercise stress testing in the diagnosis of coronary artery disease and the prevalence of coronary artery disease in the population being studied has been well recognized. The predictive accuracy of the ex-ercise stress test is highly dependent on the prevalence of the disease in the population tested; this is the concept formulated in Bayes' theorem of probability. Where the disease is uncommon, the test will not be accurate; how-ever, the test can become accurate if the disease prevalence is high.

UNDERSTANDING RESULTS

As a practical matter then, the frequency of false-positive and false-negative studies is related to the "population" from which an individual is selected. Thus, a "positive" electrocardiographic response in an exercise stress test on a young woman with atypical chest pain is more likely to be a false-positive result than a true-positive. Alternatively, a "negative" electrocardiographic response of an exercise stress test of a middle-aged male with a history suggestive of angina pectoris is more likely to be a false-negative than a true-negative result. Obviously, a patient's primary physician must be aware of these practical implications of Bayes' theorem when ordering an exercise test as well as when incorporating the results into a patient's management scheme.

This discussion is intended to acquaint the family physician with the general methods, as well as uses and limitations of exercise stress testing. Any of several excellent monographs will provide the physician with further details of this increasingly used technique.

Representative Electrocardiograms
James D. Dubbin

A comprehensive description of normal and abnormal electrocardiograms is beyond the scope of this book. It may be helpful, however, to study these representative cardiograms to note certain abnormalities in the tracings in the specific examples which follow. Although the examples are valid and taken from real patients, remember that tracings with obvious and clear findings have been chosen to help the physician make a probable interpretation of an ECG tracing when expert advice is not immediately available. Thus, electrocardiograms taken in actual practice might not be as clear-cut as those presented here.

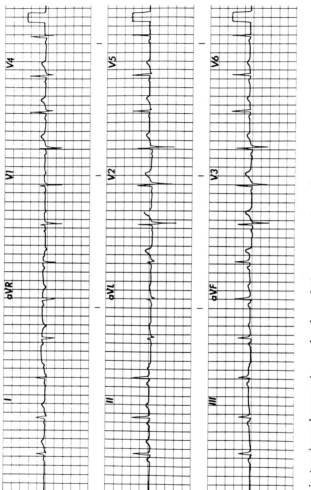

1. This tracing shows sinus rhythm. It is a normal study.

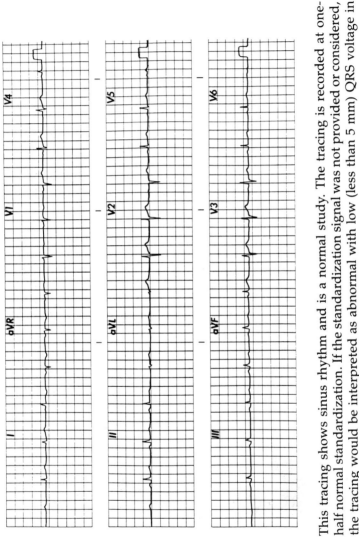

2. This tracing shows sinus rhythm and is a normal study. The tracing is recorded at one-half normal standardization. If the standardization signal was not provided or considered, the tracing would be interpreted as abnormal with low (less than 5 mm) QRS voltage in the limb leads.

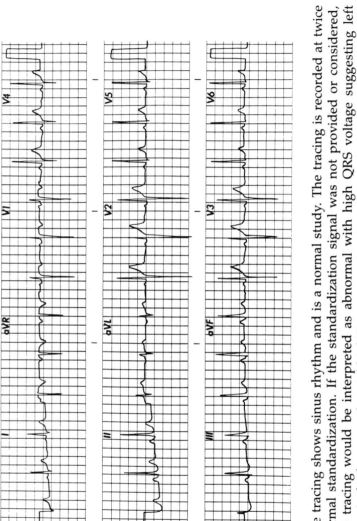

3. The tracing shows sinus rhythm and is a normal study. The tracing is recorded at twice normal standardization. If the standardization signal was not provided or considered, the tracing would be interpreted as abnormal with high QRS voltage suggesting left ventricular hypertrophy and high P-wave amplitude suggesting right atrial enlargement.

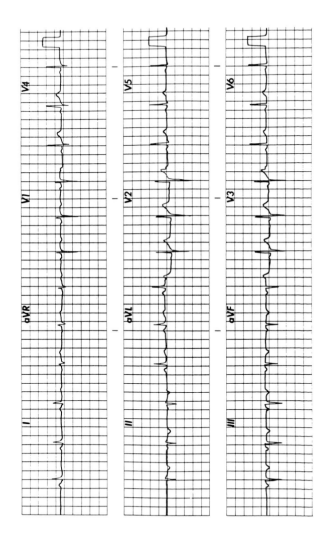

4. This tracing shows sinus rhythm. There is left axis deviation of both the P waves and QRS complexes in the frontal plane. In the precordial leads, the QRS complexes and P waves are normal.

   The discordant P wave axis suggests lead placement problems. Indeed the limb leads are incorrectly placed; the left arm lead is on the left leg, the right arm lead is on the left arm, and the left leg on the right arm. When the leads are placed correctly, the tracing is normal (see No. 1).

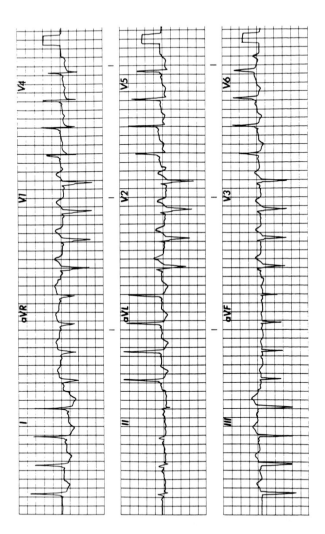

5. This tracing shows sinus rhythm with pre-excitation (in this case Wolff-Parkinson-White syndrome).

The PR interval is short (less than 0.08 seconds). The initial deflection of each QRS is slurred with a typical delta wave. The R waves in lead I and aV_L are tall, and the S waves in III and V_1 are deep. The ST segments and T waves are inverted in leads I, aV_L, V_4, V_5 and V_6. Both these abnormalities in QRS voltage and in repolarization (ST segment and T waves) can be secondary to the pre-excitation of the ventricular myocardium and do not necessarily imply left ventricular hypertrophy or myocardial ischemia.

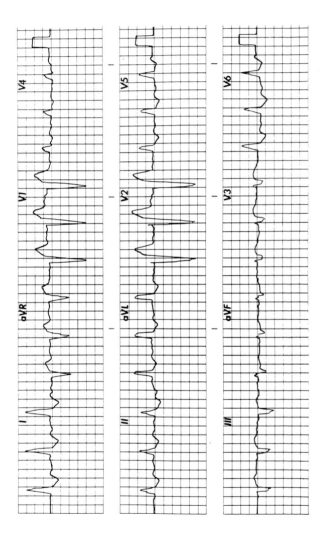

6. This tracing shows complete left bundle branch block (LBBB).

   The essential electrocardiographic features include a prolonged QRS interval (0.12 seconds or more). QRS complex is upright in lead I and downward in lead III. Large T waves are diverted opposite to the major QRS deflections as in leads I and V_1. The R waves in V_1 and V_2 when present are small.

   Atypical variations in LBBB pattern may occur, but the precordial leads either V_1 or V_6 clarify the picture.

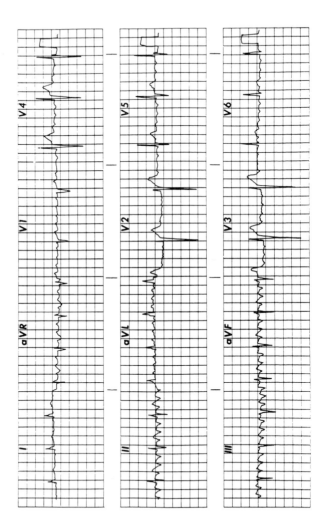

7. This tracing shows atrial flutter (flutter waves at 300/minute) with a variable and high degree AV block. The ventricular rate averages approximately 60 beats per minute.

The f, or flutter waves, in leads II, III, and aVf show a typical "inverted saw-tooth" pattern. The QRS axis in the frontal plane is abnormally leftward (more negative than −30°). The flutter waves are at times superimposed on the ST segment and T waves, thereby deforming their usual pattern and making comment on them not possible.

The degree of AV block of the flutter waves in this tracing is somewhat unusual, and reflects co-existent AV node disease (this patient was not on any medications).

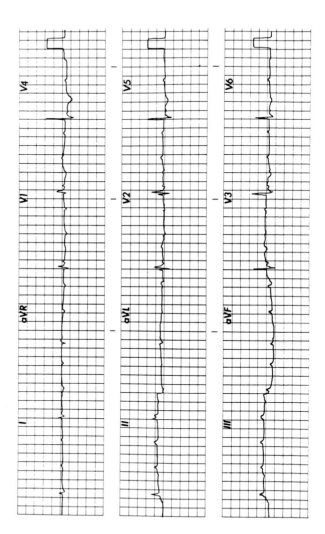

8. This tracing shows complete heart block (3° AV block). The atrial rate is at 100 beats per minute and the regular ventricular escape rhythm at 35 beats per minute.

In all leads, P waves unrelated to QRS complexes can be seen. The QRS complexes are in the pattern of a RBBB as seen in V_1 and V_2 where a typical RSR complex exists.

The QRS voltage in the limb leads (in this normally-standardized tracing) are of low voltage (less than 5 mm). This abnormality can occur with pericardial effusion, chronic lung disease, diffuse myocardial disease or as in this case with marked obesity.

Cardiology

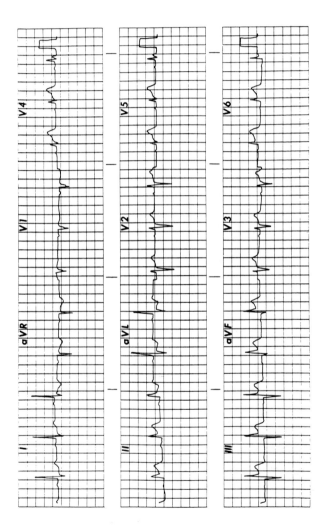

9. This tracing shows evidence for an inferolateral wall myocardial infarction that is acute. In the limb leads II, III, and aV$_F$, ST-segment elevation exists in association with significant Q waves. In lead I and aV$_L$, ST-segment depression may indicate either myocardial ischemia or reflect (electrical recipient) the inferior wall ST segment.

In the precordial leads, there is ST-segment elevation in leads V$_5$ and V$_6$, suggesting that the area of infarction may include some of the lateral wall.

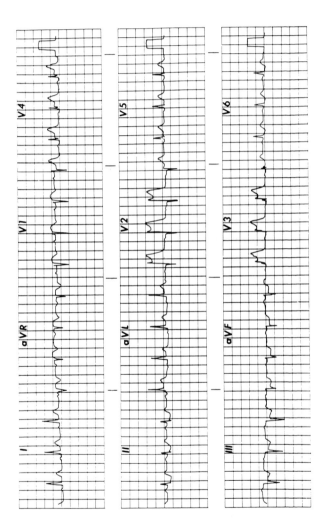

10. This tracing shows evidence of an anteroseptal lateral wall myocardial infarction which is acute.

   In the precordial leads, V_1 to V_4, ST-segment elevation is seen. In V_2 a significant Q wave exists. In lead V_6, there is ST-segment depression. Similarly in the limb leads, ST-segment depression is seen in leads II, III, and aV_F.

   The ST-segment depression in the inferolateral leads may be either a reflection (the electrical reciprocal) of the ST-segment elevation in V_1 to V_4 or may indicate ischemia inferolaterally. A single ECG cannot distinguish these two possibilities.

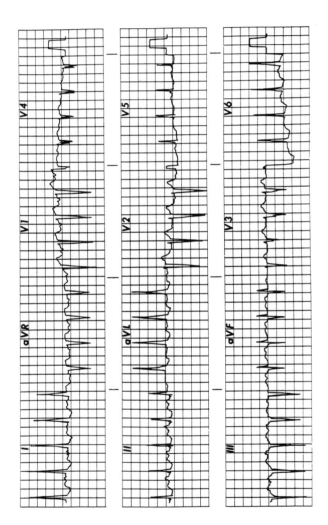

11. This tracing demonstrates evidence for left ventricular hypertrophy (LVH) and left atrial enlargement (LAE).

LVH. The R wave in lead I is abnormally high; the S wave in lead III is abnormally deep, and their sum exceeds 25 mm. In the unipolar limb leads, aV_L shows a tall R wave (greater than 11 mm). In both lead I and aV_L, the ST-segments are depressed (in a downward sloping fashion). In the precordial lead V_1, the S wave is deep and in V_6 the R wave tall. Their sum exceeds 35 mm. In V_6, the ST-segment is depressed. There is clockwise rotation in the horizontal plane (the R to S ratio does not become greater than unity until V_5; in a normal study, this occurs in V_4). These aspects are consistent for LVH.

LAE. In lead V_1 the terminal aspect of the P wave is deep (greater than 1 mm) and wide (greater than 1 mm). The area of the terminal P wave is negative and greater than 1 mm × 1 mm. These aspects are typical for LAE.

Note: The ECG was obtained at normal standardization.

Temporary Transvenous Cardiac Pacing
S.Z. Naqvi

Clinical Uses

1. High grade AV block (3rd degree or 2nd degree).
2. Sino atrial nodal disease, e.g., sick sinus syndrome.
3. Uncontrolled tachyarrhythmias, e.g., ventricular tachycardia associated with long QT intervals.

Equipment

Fluoroscope

External demand pacemaker pulse generator and extension wire cable

100-cm #6 French bipolar pacing electrode catheter

#6 introducer and sheath, 40-cm long 0.32 stainless steel guide wire

Equipment required for femoral venous catheterization is the same as listed in the chapter on Vascular Access

Seldinger needle (or equivalent)

Oscilloscope for continuous monitoring of cardiac rhythm

Routes Used

Any venous route can be used, e.g., antecubital vein, internal jugular vein, or femoral vein.

Method

The femoral vein approach is described here. The area is shaved, prepped, and covered with a laparotomy sheet, and the femoral vein is catheterized as described in the section on vascular access (page 576) using a Seldinger needle.

The distal 5 cm of the electrode catheter is gently, manually curved. The catheter is then inserted through the sheath in the femoral vein and advanced under fluoroscopic control via the inferior vena cava to the right atrium and ultimately to the apex of the right ventricle (Fig. 2–5). If the electrode does not pass directly across the tricuspid valve, the catheter is withdrawn into the inferior vena cava. The distal end is then advanced gently into one of the hepatic veins, to form a small loop at the distal end of the catheter. The loop is advanced upward into the right atrium

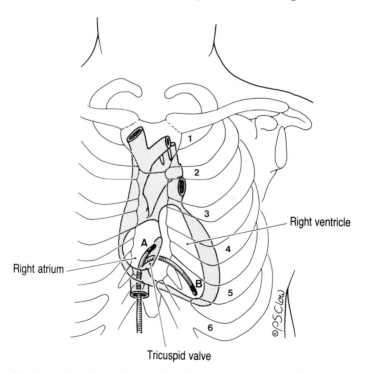

Fig. 2–5. **A.** Catheter tip in right atrium, directed at tricuspid valve. **B.** Catheter tip at apex of right ventricle.

Cardiology

with the catheter tip directed towards the tricuspid valve. Gentle maneuvering allows the catheter tip to cross the valve. Final positioning places the catheter tip near the apex of the right ventricle, anteriorly placed when viewed in the lateral plane (Fig. 2–6). The electrode terminals are then attached to a pacemaker pulse generator that is initially turned off.

The sensing and pacing components of the system are

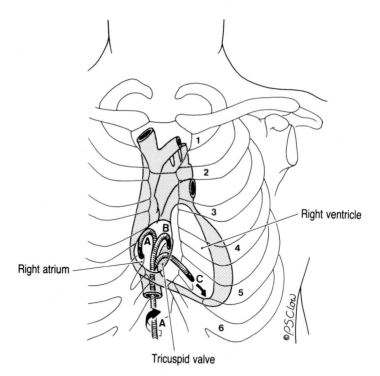

Fig. 2–6. **A.** Catheter in right atrium forming loop. **B.** Loop rotated such that tip is facing tricuspid valve. **C.** Final positioning toward apex of right ventricle.

checked with the pacemaker in the demand mode, and the unit is turned on at a rate greater than the underlying heart rate. The initial pacemaker output is set at 3.0 mAmp. Once consistent capture is obtained, the output should be turned down gradually to 2.0, 1.5, 1.0, and 0.5 mAmp. When pacing is lost, the threshold for pacing has been reached. The threshold should also be tested at the lowest output that will consistently pace the patient during deep inspiration and coughing.

The sensing circuit can be tested by pacing the patient at a rate somewhat less than the patient's intrinsic heart rate. Gradually decreasing the degree of sensitivity allows the pacemaker to become a fixed-rate unit and abolishes sensing. The millivolts shown on the dial at which the pacemaker becomes a fixed rate unit is equivalent to the ventricular output. Pacing threshold and ventricular output are recorded for future reference.

A reasonable threshold for ventricular pacing is usually 3 mAmp and never more than 10 mAmp. If the threshold is greater than this, repositioning is suggested. Finally, the optimal pacing rate and energy necessary should be preset. It is wise to use approximately 2 to 5 mAmp more than the resting pacing threshold. The pacemaker is then changed to the demand mode. The electrode is held at the proximal end while the introducer in the vein is gradually removed. Make sure that the tip is not displaced when the introducer is withdrawn. The pacemaker wire is secured to the skin with No. 4 silk sutures. The electrode is bandaged to the thigh to prevent it from being pulled accidentally, thereby causing loss of contact with the ventricular floor. Do not use tape for securing the electrode to the skin; it ruins the electrode, thus preventing re-use. The pacemaker threshold and position of the tip should be checked prior to leaving the fluoroscopy room.

Precaution

Strict sterile technique should be observed during the entire procedure.

Pericardiocentesis
Ronald S. Baigrie

Needle aspiration of the pericardial space is usually performed for either diagnostic (removal of pericardial fluid for laboratory analysis) or therapeutic (relief of tamponade) reasons. This is a major procedure with serious potential complications and therefore should not be performed in a cavalier fashion by the untrained. Several approaches are possible, including left or right parasternal or subxiphoid, or the cardiac apex. I prefer the left subxiphoid approach, which is probably the safest.

During the procedure, it is wise to observe blood pressure in case of a vasovagal episode that would require intravenous atropine. A cardiac defibrillator should be available. An intravenous line should be in place to allow administration of any necessary therapy. It is wise to perform this procedure in an environment equipped to monitor the patient closely and respond to any untoward events. A cardiac care unit or intensive care unit is preferred to a general ward if feasible.

Equipment

ECG machine with oscilloscope
5- or 10-ml syringe, and one 25-gauge needle or one 22-gauge needle for anesthetic
2% lidocaine
Sharp pointed scalpel
Pericardiocentesis needle (French No. 18 or No. 20)
One 5- to 10-ml syringe for aspiration

One 50-ml syringe for aspiration
Sample bottles or tubes for specimens
Sterile normal saline
Cardiac defibrillator should be available

Method

This procedure must be done under sterile conditions. The patient is attached to the limb leads of an ECG machine which lies ready to record the cardiac rhythm. When possible, the patient *should also* be attached to an oscilloscope for continuous ECG monitoring. The patient should be in bed with the thorax upright 30° to 60° if possible.

The xiphisternal area is widely prepped with iodine and alcohol and draped with a sterile spinal sheet. A No. 25 hypodermic needle is used to infiltrate the left xiphisternal area with local anesthetic (2% lidocaine). A No. 22 needle is then used to infiltrate the deeper subcutaneous tissue with anesthetic. Once local anesthesia is effective, a 1 to 2 mm scalpel incision is made in the skin only large enough to allow easy passage of the pericardiocentesis needle. The pericardiocentesis needle is inserted at the site in the left xiphicostal angle about 1 to 2 cm below the costal margin and directed upward toward the lower inner aspect of the costal margin (rib cage) (Fig. 2–7).

The precordial lead wire of a single channel ECG (V_1) machine (or the V_1 lead of a multiple channel ECG machine) is then attached by sterile alligator clip to the needle. Continuous monitoring of this V lead by monitor or ECG strip chart recorder is begun. This V lead is now recording the ECG activity as seen by the exploring pericardiocentesis needle. If significant ST-segment elevation is seen on this lead at anytime, the needle should be partially withdrawn until the ST elevation disappears.

This ST elevation implies that the needle is recording an epicardial signal and is in contact with the ventricle. This

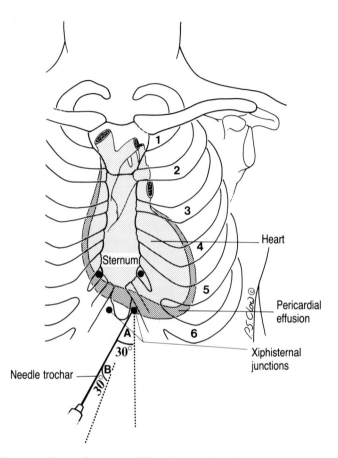

Fig. 2–7. Pericardiocentesis: left xiphisternal angle approach.

must be avoided to prevent cardiac laceration and trauma. The needle is angled such that it is directed toward the left shoulder at about a 30° angle from the skin and 30° angle from the midline (Figs. 2–7 **A**, 2–7 **B**). The needle stylet is left in place while the needle is advanced 5 to 10 mm at a time, guided by the electrocardiograph V lead control. After each short advance, the stylet is removed and the needle held rigidly in place by the left hand and aspirated using a 5- to 10-ml syringe held by the right hand. If no fluid is obtained, the syringe is removed, stylet replaced, and the needle advanced a farther 5 to 10 mm.

When the parietal pericardium is punctured, there may be a "giving" sensation. This puncturing of the pericardium may not be obvious. Once fluid is obtained, a 25- to 50-ml syringe is attached to the needle and aspiration performed. It is important to stabilize the aspiration needle at all times, usually, with the left hand.

Fluid samples are taken for biochemical, bacteriological, and other required studies. It is possible to attach a short length of tubing to the needle vial Luer-lok and aspirate at a stop-cock at the other end but I prefer to aspirate directly from the needle with syringe. Continuous ECG observation is mandatory.

When the pericardiocentesis is completed, the needle is removed, and the skin puncture site is dressed. The patient is assessed with regard to symptoms, vital signs, and cardiac rhythm. The clinical circumstances will dictate the duration of observation.

In the event that grossly bloody fluid is aspirated, it is important to minimize the possibility that a cardiac chamber has been entered. If the blood is bright red and spurts out with each heart beat, the needle should be removed and the patient observed for tamponade. If the flow does not spurt, the use of a microhematocrit device quickly ensures that it is much less than systemic blood and therefore a bloody pericardial effusion. Also bloody pericardial fluid usually does not clot and appears less viscous than blood. Echocardiography can be used for clarification. Saline flush through the needle may produce a cloud of echos in the pericardial space or a cardiac chamber. The patient will taste an injection of chemicals such as saccharin or dehydro-cholic acid (which have been used to measure circulation time) if a cardiac chamber is entered. If a fluoroscope is readily available, an injection of radiopaque contrast may help determine the needle location. As an alternative, some authorities suggest that the stylet of the pericardiocentesis needle be removed and a 10- to 20-ml syringe be attached; the subsequent insertion of the needle is done with gentle suction on the syringe. When the pericardial space is entered, the syringe fills with fluid and aspiration continues.

3
Dentistry

J.H.P. Main

EXAMINATION OF THE MOUTH

Good illumination is essential for oral examination. The light source may be either a special dental light fixture or a head mirror and naked bulb. The lips, cheeks, and tongue are readily displaced, extended, or reflected by the fingers or by means of a mouth mirror which is necessary to see behind and between the teeth and to reflect light into hidden areas. A polished stainless steel tongue depressor will also reflect light, displace soft tissues, and can be used as a mirror to some extent. Every part of the mouth may be illuminated, visualized, and palpated either under direct vision or by means of a mouth mirror.

LOCAL ANESTHESIA FOR THE MOUTH

In many circumstances, emergency procedures in the mouth necessitate local anesthesia. Hypodermic needles of

113

3.5 to 4 cm in length and gauge 26 or 27 should always be used intraorally so that in the unlikely event of needle breakage, which usually occurs at the hub, enough is left protruding from the mucosa to allow easy recovery of the broken part. Lidocaine is the anesthetic of choice because it has the lowest incidence of side effects. A 2% solution with 1:100,000 epinephrine is the preparation of choice, unless there are contraindications to the use of a vasoconstrictor in a particular patient. Application of a 5% topical lidocaine ointment to the mucosa prior to injection will lessen the discomfort. This requires 1 minute to take effect.

Intraoral Infiltration Anesthesia

Equipment

Syringe with gauge 26 or 27, 3.5- to 4.0-cm long hypodermic needle
2% solution of lidocaine with 1:100,000 epinephrine
Mouth mirror
Topical lidocaine in spray or ointment form
Source of suction to remove accumulations of saliva

Clinical Uses and Method

1. Anesthesia of maxillary teeth in adults and children.
2. Anesthesia of mandibular teeth in children only:
   The point of penetration is directly over the apex of the relevant tooth on the labial side of the alveolar ridge. Having already applied the topical anesthetic now puncture the mucous membrane with the needle lying at an angle of approximately 45° to the surface and penetrate to a depth of 3 to 4 mm. Slowly deposit the solution, initially aspirating to avoid intravascular injection (Fig. 3–1). Slow injection is important to allow diffusion of the solution and to minimize pain. A rate of 1 ml per 20 seconds should not be exceeded.

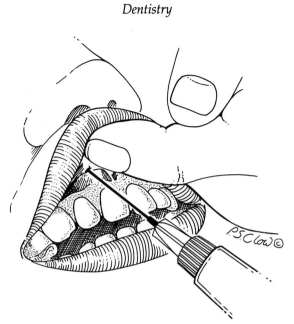

Fig. 3–1. Infiltration local anesthesia for a maxillary incisor.

One to 1.5 ml of 2% lidocaine is needed for a single tooth. 0.25 ml of the solution should then be injected similarly on the palatal or lingual aspect of the tooth, to anesthetize the gingiva on that side.

3. Anesthesia for incision and drainage or other minor soft tissue surgery:

Using the same technique, the anesthetic solution should be deposited around the incision site and 1 cm away from it. Two or three injection sites using a total volume of 1 ml is adequate.

Inferior Dental Nerve Block

To achieve anesthesia of mandibular teeth in adults, nerve block is required in most cases, although infiltration will suffice in some.

Using a syringe containing 2 ml of the anesthetic solution, grasp the middle of the vertical ramus of the mandible between the thumb and forefinger; the former is inside the mouth, and the latter is on the skin at the posterior border of the ramus. Aim the point of the needle at the midpoint of these two fingers, and puncture the mucosa just anterior to the pterygomandibular raphe at the level of the occlusal plane. The body of the syringe should lie over the first mandibular molar on the opposite side. Advance the needle 1 to 2 cm until it contacts the medial aspect of the mandible at the lingula (Fig. 3–2). Aspirate to avoid injecting into the pterygoid venous plexus, and slowly deposit 2 ml of the solution. This injection produces anesthesia of all the mandibular teeth on that side and also anesthetizes the lingual nerve, thus producing anesthesia of the ipsilateral half of the anterior two-thirds of the tongue.

Precaution

Rare cases of allergy to lidocaine exist. Question the patient regarding this prior to administering the drug. An alternative drug is 3% mepivacaine with 1:100,000 epinephrine.

TOOTHACHE

Physicians will often encounter a patient who complains about a toothache. There are four common causes for this symptom, and the precise cause must be determined in order to give appropriate and effective treatment.

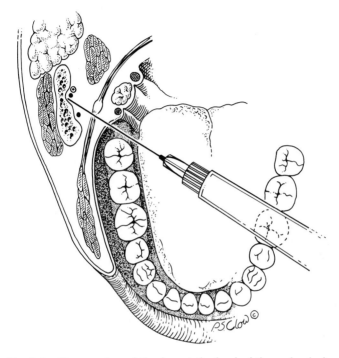

Fig. 3–2. Cross section of the face at the level of the occlusal plane showing the correct position of the hypodermic needle for an inferior dental nerve block.

Pulpitis

This is the most common cause of toothache and usually results from an inflammation of the tooth pulp caused by bacterial irritants from dental caries. Pulpitis can also result from the splitting of a tooth, sometimes without displacement being evident. The symptoms are poorly localized pain that is exacerbated or precipitated by hot or cold fluids; the latter symptom is unique. On examination, a carious tooth is usually found in the quadrant of the mouth where the pain is felt. The tooth is not tender to gentle percussion, although direct pressure into the carious cavity may cause pain.

Placement of Sedative Dressing in a Carious Tooth

Clinical Uses

This is only effective for toothache caused by pulpitis.

Equipment

Cotton wool
Dental tweezers
Eugenol (oil of cloves)
Blunt probe
Mouth mirror
Suction equipment

Method

First, dry the cavity with cotton wool held by tweezers. Then, take a fresh pledget of cotton wool, about 4 mm in diameter; holding it with tweezers, dip it into the oil of cloves and place it directly into the cavity. A blunt probe may be needed to manipulate the cotton into the lesion and, depending on the site, it may be necessary to carry out the procedure by means of indirect vision using a mouth mirror.

Precautions

Avoid touching the mucosa with the caustic oil of cloves.

Follow-up Care

Refer the patient to a dentist, preferably within 24 hours.

Acute Apical Infection

In this condition, the patient experiences toothache that is accurately localized to the affected tooth which will be sensitive to gentle percussion with an instrument. Again, caries is the common primary cause and is usually evident. If the infection has extended through the alveolar bone, there may be inflammation of the mucosa overlying the root apex, but this is a late development.

Treatment consists of establishing drainage by extracting the tooth or by opening the root canal to allow drainage through it into the mouth. Some symptomatic relief may be obtained from antibiotics and analgesics. The patient should be referred to a dentist as soon as possible. In all infections by mixed oral flora, penicillin is the antibiotic of choice until the results of culture and antibiotic sensitivity tests are received. For patients allergic to penicillin, erythromycin should be prescribed.

Periodontal Abscess

This condition results from a local exacerbation of chronic periodontitis. The toothache is accurately localized and, on examination, inflammation and swelling will be seen on the labial or lingual side of the affected tooth. Usually chronic periodontitis is evident elsewhere in the mouth.

Drainage of a Periodontal Abscess

Equipment

Blunt probe
Mouth mirror
Local anesthesia (if necessary)
Suction equipment

Method

Drainage may be obtained, often without the need for local anesthesia, by gently inserting a blunt probe, parallel to the long axis of the tooth, via the gingival sulcus into the abscess cavity, thereby allowing the pus to drain into the mouth.

Precaution

Probing for drainage should be done delicately to avoid spreading the infection.

Follow-up Care

Prescribe warm sodium bicarbonate ($NaHCO_3$) mouthwashes to be used for 5 minutes every 3 hours to encourage continued drainage and to keep the area clean. Antibiotics are only indicated in cases where evidence exists that the infection is spreading.

Pericoronitis

This condition develops when the potential space between the enamel and follicle of an erupting tooth becomes infected. This is the cause of teething pains in infants. When the eruption of the tooth is unimpeded, pericoronitis is self-correcting within a week or so. Pericoronitis causes more severe and continuing infections around impacted teeth and occurs in adolescents and adults, most frequently around mandibular third molars. The patient complains of accurately localized pain and sometimes of discharge, swelling, and trismus; the last symptom is caused by inflammation of the masseter muscle. On examination, swelling of the mucosa and discharge may be seen overlying the impacted tooth, which is often hidden by swollen soft tissues.

Irrigation of Pericoronitis

Procedures

Simple irrigation will produce temporary relief of symptoms but antibiotics and warm mouthwashes should also be prescribed.

Equipment

Irrigation syringe
Mouth mirror
Supply of warm isotonic solution of NaHCO$_3$
Suction equipment

Method

Introduce the tip of the irrigation syringe under the flap of the inflamed soft tissue (operculum) overlying the affected tooth and gently flush the area with about 50 ml of warm solution. Continuous suction of excess solution is necessary.

Follow-up Care

Prescribe antibiotics and warm NaHCO$_3$ mouthwashes to be used vigorously for 5 minutes every 3 hours.

TOOTH EXTRACTION

The extraction of teeth is an art that can only be mastered by repeated practice. When performed by a skilled dentist, tooth extraction is simple and relatively atraumatic, but when performed by a novice, it can spread infection, lacerate tissues, fracture bone, and cause the patient great mental stress. Therefore, it is not ordinarily a procedure that should be performed by the inexperienced. There are, however, occasions when a dentist is unavailable and the procedure must be done by a physician because it is the only means to effectively relieve pain and control infection. In the majority of cases, tooth extraction will be done because of acute apical abscesses. Inexperienced operators should only attempt to remove erupted teeth. A severely decayed or carious crown is not in itself a contraindication

Dentistry

to extraction. The removal of impacted teeth or buried roots should not be attempted.

Radiographs should always be available prior to attempting a tooth extraction so that the physician may see the configuration of the roots and thereby avoid complications (Fig. 3–3).

Several techniques are available for tooth extraction, but only Guy's technique will be described here.

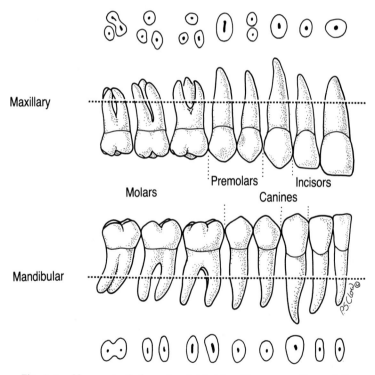

Fig. 3–3. Human teeth from the right side with cross sections of the roots.

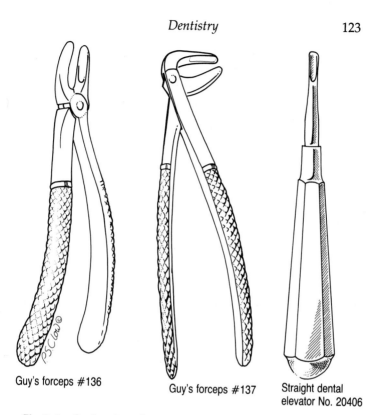

Guy's forceps #136

Guy's forceps #137

Straight dental elevator No. 20406

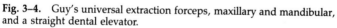

Fig. 3–4. Guy's universal extraction forceps, maxillary and mandibular, and a straight dental elevator.

Equipment

Local anesthesia equipment
Suction equipment
Guy's universal forceps, No. 136 and No. 137 (Fig. 3–4)
Straight dental elevator, No. 20406 (Fig. 3–4)
Needle drivers
Scissors
000 silk or catgut suture
Sharp probe

Method

The tooth should be anesthetized as described earlier in this chapter. Test for the adequacy of the local anesthesia by pushing a sharp probe firmly into the periodontal ligament via the gingival sulcus. Both the surgeon and the patient should be satisfied with the anesthesia. Pressure will be perceived by the patient during this test and during the extraction, presumably felt in the adjacent unanesthetized tissues, but no pain should be felt.

Position of the Patient. The patient should be seated in a chair with a solid headrest and placed in a comfortable and easy position with the head and trunk in the same line.

Position of the Operator. For maxillary teeth the operator stands on the right of the chair opposite the patient's pelvis and turns his upper body toward the patient's head. For the mandibular anterior teeth, the same position may be used or the operator may stand behind the patient. For the right mandibular cheek teeth (premolars and molars), the operator stands directly behind the patient, bending over the patient's head to see the operative area. Standing on a stool about 8 inches high makes this approach easier, particularly for shorter operators. For the left mandibular cheek teeth, the operator stands on the patient's left side opposite the trunk. (The above directions are for right-handed operators and must be reversed for left-handed people.)

Support of the Head, Jaws, and Alveolar Processes. The alveolar bone around the tooth to be extracted should always be firmly held and supported between the left thumb and forefinger (Fig. 3–5). In so doing, the lip or cheek is also displaced and protected. Grasping the alveolar ridge around the tooth supports the labial bone and prevents excessive displacement if the bone fractures (as it fre-

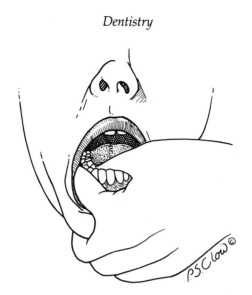

Fig. 3–5. Supporting the mandible and the alveolar bone with the left hand, prior to forceps extraction of a molar.

quently does), while accidental slippage of the forceps' beaks results in their running into the operator's fingers rather than into the patient's soft tissues. When mandibular teeth are being extracted, the mandible should be supported by the other three fingers of the left hand placed beneath the lower border.

Forceps Extraction

The butt of the left handle of the forceps rests in the middle of the palm and is held firmly in this position by the thumb and forefinger (Fig. 3–6). The middle and fourth finger close the right handle, while the little finger placed on the inside of the right handle, opens the beaks. Upper and lower forceps are held in the same way. Using this grip, with the wrist kept rigid, the force required to dis-

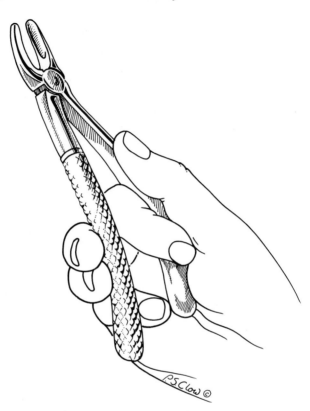

Fig. 3–6. Method of gripping extraction forceps.

lodge the tooth is applied by the whole arm; the forceps serve as a functional extension.

Holding the forceps in this way, the beaks are applied to the neck of the tooth and pushed up the root as far as possible. Always try to extract the root; the crown will come with the root, although the converse is not true. In those teeth with conical roots, the blades act as a pair of wedges, and pressing them up the root surfaces may occasionally displace the tooth from its socket without applying additional leverage. In most instances, however, additional extractive force is needed. Whereas rotational or buccolingual movements are used for specific teeth, depending on their individual anatomy, the final extractive movement in all cases is toward the buccal side with a concomitant continued application of force in an apical direction up to the moment of delivery. It may be noted that when using this technique teeth are pushed out rather than pulled.

Maxillary Incisors

The roots of these teeth are nearly round in cross section; rotation of the tooth will disrupt the fibers of the periodontal membrane, thus facilitating extraction (Fig. 3–7).

Maxillary Canines

Although rotational movements are indicated for maxillary canines, this tooth is often firmly embedded and may require loosening with an elevator.

Maxillary Premolars

The first premolar usually has two roots, and one of these is often broken during extraction. These teeth may be moved palatally and buccally a few times to weaken the periodontal membrane, before finally pushing the teeth out to the buccal side.

Maxillary Molars

Usually these teeth have three roots, two buccal and one palatal. The forcep blades should be carefully positioned on the mesiobuccal and palatal roots before being pushed up into the periodontal space. Again some movements in the bucco-palatal plane (i.e., side to side motion) may be made first to loosen the attachment before finally carrying

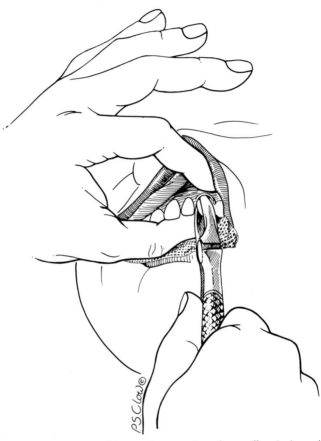

Fig. 3–7. Application of forceps for extraction of a maxillary incisor with the thumb and forefinger of the left hand supporting the alveolar process.

forceps and tooth outwards with continuing firm upward pressure maintained.

Mandibular Incisors

The roots are usually flattened laterally; thus the extractive force should only be directed downwards and outwards.

Mandibular Canines and Premolars

The roots of these teeth are usually conical enough for the teeth to be rotated slightly before the final downward and outward pressure is applied.

Mandibular Molars

These teeth have two roots, a mesial, which is usually the larger, and a distal. The forceps' blades should be applied carefully to the mesial root, then pressed downward (Fig. 3–8). Some movements may be made in the buccolingual plane to loosen the tooth prior to the final delivery toward the buccal aspect.

Use of Dental Elevators

Dental elevators can produce great pressure; they should be applied cautiously. The straight elevator is held with the handle in the palm and the forefinger extended along the blade, so that only 1 cm or so of blade protrudes. With the teeth and alveolar processes firmly supported by the thumb and forefinger as described above, the tip of the blade is placed at the mesiobuccal corner of the root and pressed apically as far as possible. The blade is then twisted, using the alveolar bone as a fulcrum, to put pressure on the tooth and to disrupt the periodontal membrane (Fig. 3–9). The blade of the elevator should bite into the cementum covering the root. If the tooth anterior to the one being extracted is absent, the elevator blade is better placed on the

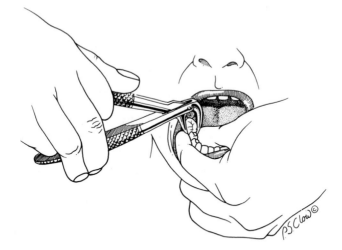

Fig. 3–8. Application of forceps for extraction of a right mandibular molar.

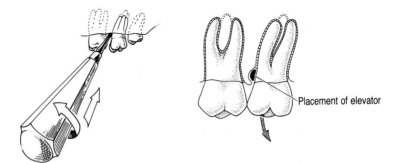

Fig. 3–9. Application of a dental elevator to loosen a maxillary molar.

medial side of the tooth root. In most cases, the elevator will loosen the tooth, but final removal has to be done by forceps.

CIRCUM-ORAL SPACE INFECTIONS

These infections commonly result from a spreading apical infection, but may also result from a spreading periodontal abscess or from acute pericoronitis. The infections are usually of mixed bacterial origin and contain many oral commensals. The only specific infections occasionally occurring from these primary causes are actinomycosis, and cellulitis (Ludwig's angina) owing to hemolytic streptococcal infection.

Vestibular Abscess

This lesion is formed when a periapical infection spreads buccally through the alveolar bone and a collection of pus forms above the reflection of the oral mucosa in the buccal sulcus, that is, in the vestibule of the mouth. Such abscesses forming on molar or premolar teeth lie on the oral side of the attachment of the buccinator. They are readily visualized, tender and inflamed, and the swelling reduces or obliterates the sulcus. The causative tooth is usually carious or heavily filled and is tender on gentle percussion.

Incision and Drainage of a Vestibular Abscess

Equipment

Local anesthetic equipment
Scalpel with No. 15 blade
Curved mosquito forceps
Suction equipment

Method

Anesthetize the mucosa over the abscess. Make a shallow incision parallel to the long axis of the sulcus from 1 to 2 cm long over the highest point of the swelling. If drainage of pus does not occur immediately, open the incision into the abscess cavity by pushing the forceps into it with the jaws closed and then by opening the blades. Drainage may be aided by gently pressing a finger on the overlying skin. Leave the incision open. Suction must always be available.

Precautions

Too deep an incision severs small blood vessels and causes excessive bleeding. If required, deepening of the wound to reach the pus should always be done by blunt dissection with forceps. If a small blood vessel is cut, it should be picked up in the forceps and tied off with 000 catgut.

Follow-up Care

Warm $NaHCO_3$ mouthwashes should be prescribed and used vigorously every 3 hours. Prescribe antibiotics and refer the patient to a dentist as soon as possible.

Palatal Abscess

Occasionally an apical infection on a maxillary tooth will spread medially to produce a palatal abscess. The palatal mucosa is tightly bound to bone; thus the infection often tracks posteriorly to the looser tissue at the junction of the hard and soft palates before localizing and producing a pus-filled swelling. This abscess most often originates from apical infection on the lateral incisor tooth. Incision and drainage are exactly as described for a vestibular abscess.

Precautions

Avoid damage to the greater palatine vessels by incising

only through the epithelium and deepening the incision by blunt dissection.

Infraorbital Space Abscess

This sausage-shaped space lies on the anterior surface of the maxilla and is enclosed superiorly by skin, laterally by the levator muscle of angle and medially by the levator muscle of the upper lip and ala of nose. Left untreated the abscess usually points through the skin just inferior to the medial canthus of the eye. Infection gains access to this space from the apical infections on any maxillary tooth from the central incisor to the first molar.

The clinical presentation is a red, tender swelling lateral to the nose and beneath the eye. Both upper and lower eye lids are often swollen due to lymphedema. The causative tooth is either grossly carious or heavily filled and tender to pressure.

Incision and Drainage of Infraorbital Space Abscess

Equipment

Same as for incision and drainage of vestibular abscess.

Method

Anesthetize the mucosa at its reflection over the canine tooth. Make a 2-cm incision through the mucosa parallel to the sulcus at its highest point over the canine. By blunt dissection, using closed mosquito forceps kept in contact with the bone, introduce the forceps into the abscess sac and allow drainage into the mouth. Suture a drain in the wound (made from a piece of sterile surgical glove about 3×1 cm). This should be removed in 48 hours. Leave the incision open.

Precautions

During the blunt dissection to locate the pus, keep the forceps in contact with the bone to avoid damage to the anterior facial blood vessels.

Follow-up Care

Warm $NaHCO_3$ mouthwash should be prescribed and used vigorously every 3 hours. Prescribe antibiotics and refer the patient to a dentist as soon as possible.

Pterygomandibular Space Abscess

This space is bounded laterally by the vertical ramus of the mandible, medially by the medial pterygoid muscle with its lower point being the insertion of this muscle, superiorly by the lateral pterygoid, posteriorly by the parotid gland (deep portion) and anteriorly by the buccinator/ superior constrictor. It is infected by direct spread from pericoronitis on the mandibular third molar or from an apical infection on this tooth that breaks through the bone on its lingual aspect.

The clinical features are trismus due to involvement of the medial pterygoid in the infection, swelling of the soft tissues posterior to the third molar and of the soft palate with displacement of the uvula to the opposite side. In severe cases, the swelling causes respiratory obstruction and the patient carries the head in a characteristic anterior posture.

When the trismus prevents access to the mouth, the abscess has to be incised and drained under general anesthesia or under a mandibular nerve block achieved via an extraoral approach. If the trismus is less severe, it may be drained via the mouth. Only this last procedure will be described.

Incision and Drainage of Pterygomandibular Space Abscess

Equipment

Same as for incision and drainage of a vestibular abscess.

Method

Anesthetize the mucosa at the junction of buccinator and superior constrictor by infiltration. Make a 2-cm incision vertically along the line of the pterygomandibular raphe at the level of the occlusal plane. Pass mosquito forceps through the incision, keeping the tips in contact with the medial surface of the mandibular ramus, until drainage is obtained. Suture a rubber drain in place. Leave the wound open.

Precautions

Avoid damage to the lingual and inferior dental nerves by keeping the scalpel incision shallow and maintaining contact between the forceps tips and the bone.

Follow-up Care

Antibiotics and warm $NaHCO_3$ mouthwashes should be prescribed just as in an infraorbital space infection. Remove the drain in 48 hours, and refer the patient to a dentist.

Submandibular Abscess

This cigar-shaped space is bounded by the deep fascia of the neck, which splits to enclose the submandibular salivary gland and lymph nodes, and is attached to the lower border of the mandible and to the mylohyoid ridge. Infection may gain access to the space by direct spread from a mandibular molar apical infection penetrating the lingual cortex of the mandible inferior to the mylohyoid attachment or by lymphatic spread from a primary focus in the facial skin or anywhere else in the mouth. Formation of an abscess in a case of submandibular lymphadenitis is indicated by the development of a superficial erythematous spot on the skin over a submandibular space that is swollen and fluctuant to bimanual palpation. Needle aspiration may be used to confirm the presence of pus and to provide a specimen for bacterial examination of antibiotic sensitivity.

Incision and Drainage of Submandibular Abscess

Equipment

Same as for incision and drainage of vestibular abscess plus swabs and antiseptics for skin preparation.

Method

Prepare the skin for a surgical incision and inject local anesthetic as described above. Make a 2 cm incision just through skin 2 cm inferior to the lower border of the mandible and parallel to the crease lines of the skin. Pass closed mosquito forceps into the wound and open the jaws to allow adequate drainage of pus. Suture a rubber drain into the wound. Cover the wound with a loose dressing.

Precautions

Keep the incision 2 cm clear of the inferior border of the mandible to avoid trauma to the facial artery and vein.

Follow-up Care

Prescribe appropriate antibiotics. Remove the drain in 48 hours, and refer the patient to a dentist.

Submental Abscess

Abscesss may form on either the deep or superficial aspects of the mylohyoid muscle in the midline. If on the deep aspect, they produce a swelling in the floor of the mouth between the sublingual salivary glands and may be incised and drained as for a vestibular abscess. If located on the superficial aspect, the abscess forms between the anterior bellies of the digastric muscle with the skin forming the roof and the mylohyoid the floor. Submental abscesses arise from lingual spread of periapical infection on mandibular incisors. Incision and drainage is carried out exactly as for a submandibular abscess, the incision is made in a skin crease 1 to 2 cm posterior to the symphysis menti.

CONTROL OF POST-EXTRACTION HEMORRHAGE

Patients presenting with post-dental extraction hemorrhage are generally experiencing secondary hemorrhage, bleeding starting from several hours up to 48 hours after the surgery. Such bleeding is usually from local causes, but when it is caused by systemic bleeding diathesis, in addition to the appropriate medical treatment, the direct measures described under method to control the hemorrhage should also be employed. Local causes that may result in secondary hemorrhage in the mouth include traumatic displacement of the clot, which can occur during mastication, transient increases in blood pressure from various causes, which may reopen a severed small vessel, and infection, which may give rise to bleeding up to a week or so after the surgery.

It is difficult to estimate the volume of blood lost from intraoral hemorrhage because blood is invariably diluted by saliva. A history must be taken with particular reference to previous bleeding experience; if this suggests the possibility of a systemic abnormality, appropriate hematologic tests should be ordered.

Equipment

> Suction equipment
> Swabs
> Saline
> Local anesthetic equipment
> Mosquito forceps
> Needle holders
> Scissors
> Tweezers
> Silk 000 sutures
> Gelatin sponge

Method

The face and lips should first be cleansed using swabs moistened with normal saline, and the patient should be firmly reassured that the bleeding will be controlled and no permanent damage will ensue. The mouth should be then thoroughly cleansed of blood, clot, and saliva by means of moist swabs and gentle suction. This will enable the bleeding points or areas to be clearly visualized. Temporary control of the bleeding may be obtained by having the patient close the mouth firmly on packs of saline moistened gauze placed over the site of bleeding.

The mucosa around the bleeding area should then be anesthetized using 2% lidocaine with 1:100,000 epinephrine, both the lingual and labial mucosa are injected at a distance of at least 1 cm from the wound margins. Any bleeding vessels large enough to be recognized should be picked by tissue forceps and tied off; these vessels are uncommon.

The mucoperiosteum surrounding the bleeding socket should then be sutured, ideally using a single horizontal mattress suture to act as a purse-string (Fig. 3–10). If the local tissue relationships preclude this, then several single

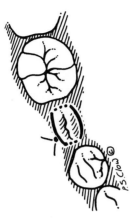

Fig. 3–10. Horizontal mattress suture placed to close an extraction wound.

interrupted sutures should be placed buccolingually across the bleeding socket. In many instances, suturing in itself is sufficient to control bleeding. If oozing continues, small pieces of gelatin sponge should be packed into the socket beneath the sutures. A moistened gauze pack is placed over the wound, and the patient is asked to bite firmly on it for 30 minutes.

Follow-up Care

The sutures should be removed in 4 days.

TRAUMATIC INJURIES TO THE TEETH AND ALVEOLAR PROCESSES

Traumatic injuries of this type are common, frequently occurring during sporting activities and usually affecting the incisor teeth. The procedures described below are for use only where the injuries are confined to the teeth and alveolar process; it is *always* necessary to have objective radiological evidence that no other fractures of the facial bones are present before carrying out this procedure.

The conditions in this category include subluxation or partial dislocation of teeth, and avulsion or total dislocation, both of which are almost invariably accompanied by fractures of the alveolar bone and sometimes by mucosal lacerations. Treatment is seldom needed for the small bone fractures, but the mucosal lacerations may require suturing.

Clinical examination must include digital palpation of the traumatized teeth and visual examination of the occlusion, which often provides the most obvious evidence of tooth displacement. Any avulsed teeth should be washed gently, ideally with sterile normal saline; if not, they should be kept moist under tap water preparatory to replacement. A complete radiographic examination of the jaws, including the mandibular condylar necks, must be obtained.

Equipment

Local anesthesia equipment
Erich arch bars
0.018-inch stainless steel fracture wire
Tissue forceps
Wire cutters
Swabs
Suction equipment

Method

The traumatized teeth sockets should be anesthetized and the mouth gently cleansed of blood and debris, using damp swabs and suction. Any suturing of mucosal lacerations should be done at this stage. Subluxated teeth should be repositioned in their sockets by firm pressure of the finger, and the accuracy of the repositioning checked by examining the occlusion. Avulsed teeth should be re-

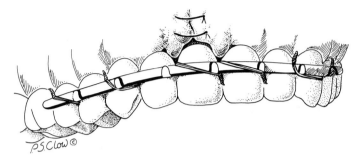

Fig. 3–11. Erich arch bar wired to maxillary teeth for the purpose of splinting the right central incisor.

placed in their sockets if they have been out for less than 3 hours. It is necessary first to remove the blood clot from the socket, usually by suction.

The displaced teeth are then splinted by wiring them to the Erich arch bar. This bar is made of a metal that is easily malleable by finger pressure. A suitable length of wire should be cut, and the arch bar should be molded to lie in contact with the necks of the teeth on the labial aspect extending from a first molar or second premolar to one or other of the same teeth on the opposite side. With the bar cut to length and molded to shape, several 8- to 10-cm lengths of the fracture wire should be cut. One wire should be passed around the neck of a sound tooth; canines are ideal if available. The arch bar is laid in position and by using locked tissue forceps is tied to the tooth neck by twisting the free ends of the fracture wire around it into a spiral. Considerable pressure can be generated in twisting fracture wire in this way, so care should be exercised. A second circumferential wire should then be placed to attach the bar to a sound tooth on the opposite side of the mouth. Minor adaptions to fitting of the arch bar may be made at this stage. The bar should be tied to two more teeth, one on either side of the subluxated or avulsed tooth and lastly the damaged tooth should be tied to the bar (Fig. 3–11). The occlusion should be checked again to make sure that the teeth are correctly positioned. The unnecesary lengths of tie wires should then be cut off and the ends tucked between the teeth to avoid irritation of the lips and buccal mucosa.

Follow-up Care

The patient should be instructed to maintain good oral hygiene by using a toothbrush and $NaHCO_3$ mouthwashes. Prescribe antibiotics and refer the patient to a dentist for further care.

4
Dermatology

M.G. Lester

ELECTROSURGERY

Clinical Uses

1. Cosmetic and Therapeutic
2. Therapeutic
   a. Destruction of benign superficial lesions such as verrucae (warts), molluscum contagiosum, and small growths such as seborrheic keratoses, small skin tags, benign nevi, etc.
   b. Epilation of small sebaceous and epidermoid cysts.
   c. Removal of small malignant skin tumors such as basal cell epitheliomas (less than 1 cm in diameter), small areas of Bowen's disease, and premalignant lesions such as small actinic keratoses.

Precautions

This method should not be used in a patient who has an implanted cardiac pacemaker since alterations in the pacemaker's electronic control may result. Alcohol should never be used to prepare the skin for injection of the local anesthetic since the spark from the Hyfrecator may cause the alcohol to ignite.

Equipment

1- or 2-ml syringe with short 25- or 27-gauge needle
Local anesthetic (e.g., 1% lidocaine)
Hyfrecator with needle-type electrode
Sterile thumb forceps

Method

Following sterile preparation of the skin with an aqueous antiseptic solution, a wheal of local anesthetic is raised directly under the lesion to be desiccated. The needle electrode wire is plugged into "LO" on the Hyfrecator and the dial set at about 25. It is best to begin with a low current and increase it as necessary. Lesions with cystic contents will require a higher setting on the dial (40 to 50). Desiccate the lesion gently until it appears charred or dry. The dry lesion may then be gently scraped or pulled off with a pair of sterile thumb forceps. Further mild burning of the base for a moment or two should destroy the lesion. *Note:* A variety of minor variations to the above procedure can be made as the operator gains experience in the use of the equipment.

Results

This procedure will destroy most superficial lesions, leaving only a flat, perhaps slightly depressed, hypopigmented area of scarring. This is a minor problem, but the patient must be warned prior to performing the procedure.

CRYOTHERAPY

Superficial skin lesions can also be destroyed by severe cold. Either carbon dioxide snow (-79°C) or liquid nitrogen (-196°C) can be used. These agents act by causing cell injury and death due to a combination of extracellular ice formation and resultant hypertonic damage to the cells. Depending on the temperature of the material used, the pressure applied, and the time that the agent is in contact with the skin, the result can vary from a slight superficial peeling (such as with a moderate sunburn) to actual bulla formation with very deep damage to the underlying tissue. The variety of skin conditions that can be treated with cryotherapy is similar to those that can be treated with electrodesiccation (Hyfrecator). The major drawback of this method is that carbon dioxide snow or liquid nitrogen are not always available.

Clinical Uses

Cryotherapy is used effectively in the treatment of:
1. Small, superficial skin lesions such as actinic keratoses, seborrheic keratoses, superficial basal cell cancers, and verrucae (vulgaris and plantaris). These latter do especially well when treated with liquid nitrogen.
2. Keloid scars can be treated with cryotherapy (with or without intralesional steroid infiltration at the same time).
3. Minor conditions such as comedonal acne or papular pustular acne can benefit by the drying and peeling action of carbon dioxide snow.

Carbon Dioxide Snow

Method

A piece of solid carbon dioxide snow is wrapped in enough layers of dry gauze to protect the operator's hands.

A knife is used to shape the dry ice to fit the lesion. The piece is then dipped briefly into a small beaker containing acetone and then applied to the lesion. Gentle pressure should be applied directly on the lesion, leaving the dry ice in contact for a few seconds until blanching of the lesion occurs.

For use on acne vulgaris, the dry ice can be crushed into a slush, with the addition of a small amount of acetone. The slush is then placed into 2 or 3 layers of dry, ordinary gauze and applied to the face for a few seconds. This will cause superficial peeling. For acne vulgaris, the whole face can be treated at one sitting.

Liquid Nitrogen

This chemical is usually transported and stored in a thermos bottle that is capped with loose gauze to allow the gas to escape as nitrogen returns from a liquid to a gaseous state. Obviously, storage and cost are a problem if this mode is used only occasionally.

Cotton swabs of a size suiting the lesion are dipped in liquid nitrogen. The swabs are then applied to the lesion, using moderate pressure for a few seconds. The pressure applied and time allotted must be enough to get a distinct whitening of the lesion that extends a millimeter or two around the rim of the treated area. This causes a frozen depression that will flatten as thawing takes place, causing a small blister which will form a hard, dry crust. The crust will fall off in 10 to 14 days and eliminate all or most of the lesion. A slightly hypopigmented flat scar may result.

Precautions

Pain is the major problem with cryotherapy. Since no local anesthetic is used, some pain occurs with application of the material. This pain may persist for a few hours and is followed by the development of unpleasant looking large bullae, often hemorrhagic, which will quickly dry up and eventually fall off. A second application may be necessary 2 to 3 weeks later to completely eradicate the lesion. After healing has taken place, there is frequently a change in the pigmentation of the skin, with hyper- or hypopigmentation or a mixture of both. This condition usually improves with time but may be distressing to the patient in the interim.

Care must be exercised so that important tissues deep to the treated lesion are not damaged by the freezing. This damage results when too much pressure is applied for too long a time. This pertains especially to digital nerves, which could be damaged if warts on the fingers were treated with liquid nitrogen. Freezing of these nerves would result in postoperative hypoesthesia. Usually this disappears in time.

BIOPSY

Punch Biopsy

Equipment

Biopsy punch (available from most surgical supply houses). Disposable punches are available, varying in size from 2 mm to 7 mm)

Local anesthetic (e.g., 1% lidocaine with or without epinephrine)

70% isopropyl alcohol

Sterile small, curved scissors

Method

After local anesthesia, the appropriate sized punch is selected (Fig. 4–1). The cutting edge is then applied to the lesion, and with a twisting or rotating motion between the thumb and index finger, pressure is exerted against the

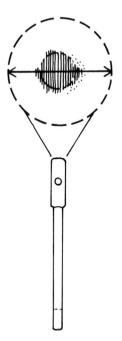

Fig. 4–1.   Punch biopsy.

lesion until the depth required for biopsy is attained. The punch is then discarded. The lesion is made to bulge slightly by squeezing it between the thumb and index finger. The circular biopsy can then be cut and removed with a pair of small, curved scissors. The biopsy is then placed in formalin and submitted for pathological examination.

A small, bleeding hole is left in the lesion. This defect can be treated with an electrocautery unit (Hyfrecator); a larger defect will require one or two dermal sutures.

Scalpel Biopsy

Minor surgical procedures are described in Chapter 17 under Minor Surgery. Scalpel biopsies can be performed when the area is desensitized by means of a suitable anesthetic. (Caution: never use a solution containing epinephrine to infiltrate digits.) A piece of tissue can be removed that includes both the lesion and the nearby normal skin. This should be submitted in formalin for testing. The skin defect is sutured to minimize scarring. Usually 4-0 dermalon skin suture is used.

PATCH TESTS

When any form of allergic contact dermatitis is suspected, patch tests are useful in helping to confirm the diagnosis and in identifying the causative agent.

Equipment

Patch test materials are obtainable from medical laboratories and contain the majority of topical agents known to cause sensitization. Special bandages can be obtained to simplify the application.

Method

When the appropriate materials have been selected, for example, cosmetics and materials from industry or hobbies, the appropriate material is placed on the pad and applied to the skin. These pads are taped in place and left there for 48 hours (Fig. 4–2). Take care to number the patch tests accurately and to keep the copy of the distribution in the patient's chart so that positive reactions may be properly identified.

Note: After the patient returns following the 48-hour application, the patches should be removed and the patient

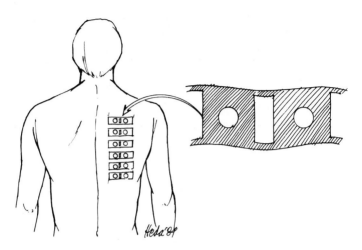

Fig. 4–2. Patch testing.

should be allowed to sit in a quiet room for at least an hour to allow all tape reactions to subside and to eliminate any chance of false positive reactions. The patch tests are then read, starting at zero, then $1+$, $2+$, or $4+$, depending on the intensity of the reaction. Now the patient can be told what tests have been positive and can opt either to return in 96 hours or to have a family member take further readings at home to see if there are any delayed positive reactions.

It is important to know how to read the patch tests in order to get a proper interpretation. It is also important to check that the materials applied were properly diluted and not in a strong enough concentration to produce a primary irritant reaction, which is nonallergic and cannot be counted as a positive allergic reaction. Do not apply materials as they are supplied by the patient. No one would walk around with a piece of soap on the skin for 48 hours under an occlusive bandage: this would obviously cause a primary irritant reaction. If you are uncertain about what concentration should be applied or how the material should be diluted, consulting a dermatologist or one of the numerous textbooks containing such information will clarify the problem. A reaction occurring within a few hours, especially if it is severe, probably indicates a primary irritant reaction rather than true allergy. This kind of situation is difficult to interpret and the expertise of a dermatologist should be sought.

INTRALESIONAL THERAPY

The use of intralesional medications is growing rapidly in dermatology practice. Dermatologists have been using intralesional steroids for several years for a variety of reasons and, more recently, intralesional bleomycin has been introduced for the treatment of large verrucae, resistant to other forms of therapy.

Equipment

Sterile syringe
27 or 30 gauge needle
Intralesional steroid (I most frequently use 10 mg per ml triamcinolone, and depending on the number of injections and the severity of the problem, I will dilute this with local anesthetic or sterile water to either 1/2 or 1/3 of the original concentration)

Method

The lesions to be injected are prepared by wiping them with alcohol and injecting material directly under the periphery of the lesion, working around the border of the lesion (Fig. 4–3). If a lesion is relatively large, I will inject material 12, 3, 6 and 9 o'clock, and wait for approximately a month to assess the results, and then reinject at 2, 4, 8

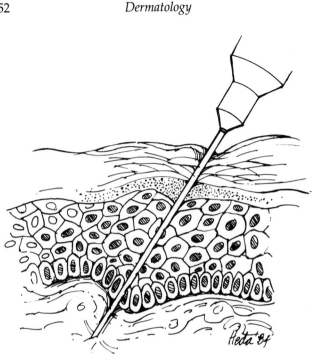

Fig. 4–3. Intralesional therapy.

and 10 o'clock. If a lesion is small, one or two injections can infiltrate the entire lesion.

Clinical Uses

Intralesional steroids are effective in treating a variety of skin diseases including inflammatory cystic acne, psoriasis, discoid lupus erythematosus, isolated patches of neuro-dermatitis or other eczematous dermatitides occurring on fingers, palms, or elsewhere on the body, alopecia areata, localized areas of lichen planus, lymphocytoma cutis and granuloma annulare. Almost any inflammatory skin disease that is localized into small, isolated areas can be treated successfully with this method. The greater the number of lesions that I plan to inject at any one sitting, the more dilute I make the solution; this avoids side effects. If there are too many lesions to inject in one visit, I will inject a dozen or more, wait for 3 or 4 weeks, and then repeat the process until all of the lesions have been successfully treated.

Results

Results can be seen within a matter of days and may persist for weeks or even months after the patient has been injected. Injections may be repeated as required but try to wait at least 3 or 4 weeks between visits.

The injections should not be given too superficially or too deeply. The former may result in ulceration and the latter in dermal atrophy, leaving a depressed area, often with hypopigmentation at the site of the original lesion. Fortunately, both the atrophy and hypopigmentation are self-limited but may take 3 to 4 months before resuming a more normal appearance; warn the patient about this possibility.

Systemic side effects after the administration of intralesional steroids usually do not develop, but when steroids are injected in fairly large quantities, it causes alteration of the menstrual cycle in some women. Local side effects include steroid atrophy, hypopigmentation, ulceration, secondary infection, or sterile abscess.

There are three preparations currently available: triamcinolone acetonide (Kenalog), triamcinolone (Aristocort parenteral), and betamethasone suspension (Celestone). The material that I have had the most experience with is Kenalog, 10 mg per ml, either in full strength or in a range of dilutions from 2 mg to 5 mg per ml by dilution with sterile water.

Special Situations for Intralesional Steroid Therapy

1. Injection of the base of a psoriatic nail can sometimes greatly improve the appearance of the nail. This procedure is painful and a digital block may be required.
2. Oral lesions of aphthous stomatitis can be injected, especially if only one or two lesions exist. This method produces excellent results.
3. Herpes simplex on any location of the body (excluding ocular herpes) responds dramatically to intralesional steroids, especially if injected soon after the appearance of the lesion. It was found that the recurrence rate can also be reduced by these injections, but I have had no experience with recurrence rates responding in this fashion.
4. Inflammatory acne cysts of the face, back, and chest respond excellently. It is common to inject 8 to 12 lesions at one sitting.
5. *Keloids.* The younger the keloid, the more effective the treatment. It is noted that injection within 1 year may flatten a keloid; but I have experienced good results with lesions that are 3 or 4 years old. With keloids, I attempt to inject both into and under the lesion. If the lesion is too old and too firm to be injected directly, I inject under it for the first couple of sittings in an attempt to soften it, and usually by the second or third approach, the keloid itself is soft enough to accept the intralesional therapy. Injections are repeated at monthly intervals, until the keloid is flat enough to satisfy the patient. Usually the pruritus of keloids will disappear after the first injection. Be careful to avoid atrophy of the tissues around the keloid, which results when material is injected too widely. Not all keloids will respond to this therapy, but it is worth attempting because no other procedure

is known to be consistently beneficial. Although the procedure may be rather painful, no local anesthesia is used for these injections.

HYPERBARIC OXYGEN

This method has been used for years to avoid the bends in deep sea divers. It has also been used in cardiac surgery. I think it is not truly hyperbaric; but generally, a high enough concentration of oxygen can be forced over the lesion being treated to make a significant difference.

Equipment

Nasal catheter
Supply of oxygen
Plastic bag with elastic bands

Method

This procedure is chiefly used for ischemic ulcerations on the legs. The plastic bag is placed over the foot and lower leg (wherever the ulceration may be located), and the top is sealed around the leg, with either scotch tape or an elastic band. The nasal catheter is then introduced under the cellulose tape so that it is lying within the confines of the bag, and the oxygen is run in at 4 liters per minute, for approximately 3 to 4 hours a day, either continuously, or divided into 2 hours in the morning and 2 hours in the afternoon. The bag generally will inflate like a balloon with this flow, and any excess will escape around the loosely applied elastic band or scotch tape (Fig. 4–4).

Precautions

Prohibit smoking in the room when oxygen is being used. Make certain that the cellulose tape or elastic band is not constrictive.

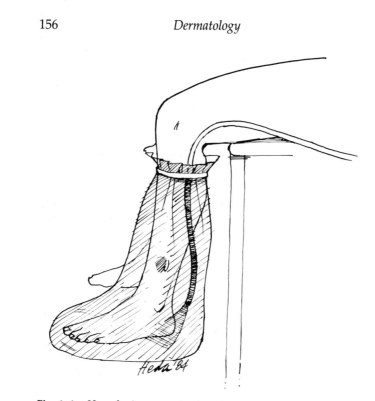

Fig. 4–4. Hyperbaric oxygen treatment.

TOPICAL THERAPY WITH CYTOTOXIC AGENTS

This method of treatment is excellent for people with marked and diffuse actinic degeneration of the bald portion of the scalp, forehead, face, or exposed "V" of the neck, and arms. In diffuse situations, it is impossible to treat the individual lesions with either electrosurgery or liquid nitrogen.

Equipment

Topical 5-fluorouracil in concentrations ranging from 1% to 2% to 5%. Personal preference is for 2% in polyethylene glycol or 5% in an ointment base.

Method

The patient should be told to apply the material sparingly with the fingertips to the affected areas daily at bedtime. The hands should then be thoroughly washed. If there is no response in 10 to 15 days, increase applications to twice daily. Generally, within a few days the patient will exhibit a marked inflammatory reaction characterized by erythema, increased scaling of the lesions, and almost a burn-like appearance. Note that the therapy usually spares clinically normal skin, even though it is applied to unaffected areas. Always warn the patient that there will be a marked inflammatory reaction and the severity of the reaction will usually correlate to the skin's response to the material. Usually 2 weeks are sufficient to treat the average patient's scalp, face, or "V" of neck. The patient is examined at the end of 2 weeks to assess the extent of the inflammatory reaction. If it is severe enough to indicate that an appropriate reaction has occurred, a topical corticosteroid cream is then applied once or twice daily to reduce the inflammatory reaction and return the skin to normal appearance. This process usually requires 2 to 3 more weeks. Thicker lesions and lesions on the hands and arms usually require longer forms of treatment with a stronger concentration.

When the skin clears, it will appear much cleaner and younger. The patient must then be warned either to apply topical sun screens or wear a hat, depending on the areas exposed to sunlight.

Individual lesions may begin to recur within 6 to 12 months. Instruct the patient to return immediately for elimination of these lesions, either with electrosurgery or liquid nitrogen, as they are usually smaller and less numerous, and thus more easily treated by localized therapy.

ACNE SURGERY

This method of opening and draining cysts, and removing comedones is still of use in the treatment of acne, although, with the advent of many more topical and systemic agents, acne surgery is becoming less frequently used.

Equipment

26-gauge needle
Comedone extractor (Fig. 4–5)
Small, pointed scalpel blade

Method

Comedones. The skin is carefully cleansed, usually with alcohol. Then, with the 26-gauge needle or with the small tip of the scalpel blade, any closed lesions are carefully opened just by pricking the top of the area to be treated. The contents can then be easily expressed with the comedone extractor. Open comedones can be treated as such. Any lesions that require excessive pressure to evacuate are left alone. Explain the reason for this to the patient.

Cysts. Acne cysts can be emptied by using a small syringe and 30- or 27-gauge needle, or by opening with a scalpel and draining through the opening made. With the advent of intralesional steroids, however, I open cysts less frequently and find that healing is improved with intralesional steroids and less scarring is produced.

NONSURGICAL REMOVAL OF FUNGAL AND DYSTROPHIC NAILS

Nails have been surgically removed for decades. More recently, a new technique for chemical removal of nails was discovered in the Soviet Union. This method uses a

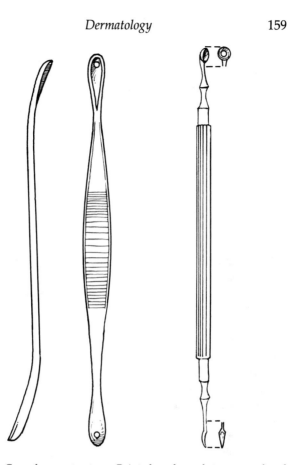

Fig. 4–5. Comedone extractors. Pointed end used to open closed comedones.

urea ointment, which has been used there successfully to remove fungal and dystrophic nails.

Equipment

Urea paste, either in a 40% or 20% concentration
Tincture of benzoin

Dermatology

1 inch adhesive tape
Plastic film wrap

Method

Tincture of benzoin is applied to the skin immediately around the sides and base of the nail and the remainder of the distal portion of the digit (Fig. 4–6A). Following this, 1-inch adhesive tape is applied to the skin directly up to the border of the nail to surround the nail plate completely (Fig. 4–6B). The ointment is then applied to the nail and occluded with a piece of plastic film wrap, which is wrapped around the entire toe (Fig. 4–6C). This is then covered with 1-inch elastic adhesive tape that is left in place for 1 week, and the patient is instructed to keep the foot completely dry (Fig. 4–6D).

After 7 days, the dressing is removed and the nail is either avulsed completely or debrided back as far as possible, without causing any discomfort. If any significant portion of the nail remains, and if the periungual skin is not irritated, the urea is reapplied in the same fashion for another 7 days. After removal of the dystrophic nail, the nail bed is either permitted to dry normally or treated with appropriate topical medication, depending on any signs of fungus infection or irritation from the material that would require a topical steroid.

Formulation of Urea 40% Ointment

Apparatus:

      Hot plate
      Metal container
      Torsion balance
      Mortar and pestle

Ingredients:

      Urea 40 g
      Anhydrous lanolin 20 g
      White beeswax 5 g
      White petrolatum 35 g

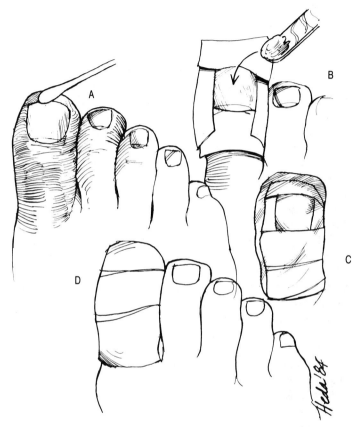

Fig. 4–6. Application of urea paste to fungal or dystrophic toe nail.
A. Application of tincture of benzoin. **B.** 1 inch adhesive applied to skin around nail to protect skin. Urea ointment then applied to nail. **C.** Plastic film wrapped around nail over ointment. **D.** Final covering with 1 inch adhesive.

Procedure:
1. Grind urea to a fine powder in mortar.
2. Melt white beeswax, then add anhydrous lanolin and white petrolatum and heat until all ingredients are liquified. Remove from heat.
3. Slowly incorporate urea into the liquid mixture.
4. Stir until the preparation starts to congeal.
5. Pour into 100-g ointment jars.

Label:
100 g
Urea 40%
White beeswax 5%
White petrolatum 35%
Lot No.   Date
For External Use Only

In avulsing nondystrophic nails that are causing the patient pain and discomfort, 10% salicylic acid added to the 20% urea preparation has been found to be more effective than the urea alone.

FUNGUS EXAMINATION

When a superficial fungus infection is suspected (skin, nails or hair) a test to confirm the presence of the fungus should always be done.

Equipment

Sterile scalpel
KOH (potassium hydroxide) 10% solution
Glass microscope slides
Microscope

Method

Skin. Using the blunt rather than the sharp edge of the scalpel, the superficial surface scales of the advancing border of the lesion are taken and placed on a slide. A drop of KOH solution is placed on the slide and the preparation examined under the lower power of the microscope. Typical mycelia will be seen if a fungus is present.

Nails. The scrapings should be taken from the undersurface of the nail. The surface of the nail is rarely infected; the subungual debris contains the fungus.

If the nail has not been cut for a long period of time, the more superficial layers of the debris should be discarded and a deeper specimen sought. Similarly, if the infected nail is long, it should first be cut and trimmed and then specimens taken for fungus examination.

Note: If suitable laboratory facilities are available, the specimen obtained by this method can be sent to the laboratory for examination and culture. Culture reports may take 4 to 6 weeks to receive. Antifungal treatment may be started as soon as the specimen has been obtained, but the patient should be warned that the outcome of the laboratory test may indicate that a fungus was not present and another treatment may be necessary.

Unna's Paste Boot

by Norma MacLeod, R.N.
Division of Dermatology,
Sunnybrook Medical Centre

The boot is fashioned from a commercially prepared roller-type gauze bandage, 4 inches wide and impregnated with paste. It may be used to treat lower extremity ulcerations of varying etiology, but its primary usefulness lies in long-term management of the chronic and recurrent ulcers of circulatory deficiencies.

Clinical Use

Uses vary from superficial erosions in already compromised tissue, to extensive, deep, crater-like ulcerations. A relatively clean ulcer base is desirable, therefore debridement and local cleansing treatment (for a few days or weeks) should precede application of the boot.

Equipment

Dome paste bandages (commercially available), or prepared according to formula

Tube gauze and Scholl's applicator, or elasticized bandages

Leg rest allowing elevation of limb for easy application

Large sized bandage scissors (7½ inches)

Method (Fig. 4–7)

The bandage is applied directly to the skin and extends from the tarsometatarsal junction to the tibial tubercle. Keep the patient's foot at a right angle while applying. Make a circular turn around the foot then direct the bandage obliquely over the heel; repeat until adequately covered. Progress up the leg, cutting the bandage frequently to avoid folds and overlapping each preceding turn by a good margin. Smooth the bandage with hands as would be done if applying a plaster cast. Apply in a pressure gradient manner, i.e., adequate pressure to ankle area, lessening as it reaches the calf. Two to four layers are sufficient. The boot eventually hardens to the consistency of a soft cast. Apply four or more layers of tube gauze using Scholl's applicator to maintain gradient pressure. Alternatively, use elasticized bandages as an outside cover.

Contraindications

These include ulcers that appear badly infected with heavy exudate, and the presence of phlebitis, cellulitis, and

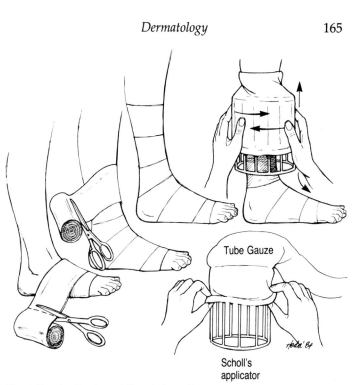

Tube Gauze

Scholl's
applicator

Fig. 4–7. Application of Unna's Paste Boot.

gross edema. There may be low a tolerance to the boot if atrophy blanche is demonstrated around the ulcer, particularly over the malleoli.

Disadvantages

1. A relatively slow method of treatment.
2. Occasional acute allergic reactions to ingredients of boot.

Points for Patient Information

1. Explain the importance of noting hindrance to circulation.

2. The boot should not cause undue discomfort.
3. Normal walking shoes (low heeled, comfortable) should be worn.
4. If pruritus occurs under boot, have boot removed.
5. Exudate will penetrate through bandage.
6. Keep boot dry.

Follow-Up Care

Change the boot on a weekly basis until healing is well established, then change every 2 weeks; continue until skin is completely healed. Cut off boot with heavy bandage scissors, avoiding ulcer area.

Preparation of Paste

If commercially prepared Dome paste bandages are unavailable, Unna's paste may be prepared with the following composition:

Zinc oxide—100 g
Gelatin—150 g
Glycerin—400 g
Calamine—100 g (optional)
Water—300 ml

Gradually add gelatin to cold water, stirring constantly. Allow to stand 10 minutes, then heat over steam until gelatin dissolves. Combine zinc oxide, glycerin, and calamine to make a smooth paste. Add to gelatin and water, stirring carefully until the mixture becomes a smooth jelly. Before application, allow mixture to cool until just warm.

Application

Cleanse leg thoroughly, and apply talcum powder. Using a soft brush, apply paste to leg. Cover paste with gauze bandage. Repeat procedure until 4 layers each of paste and bandage are applied. Leave bandage in place up to 2 weeks.

Remove by soaking it in warm water if necessary, or by using heavy bandage scissors.

Note: A correctly applied boot will provide good gradient support to the lower leg, thus helping to reduce venous hypertension and to control edema. The boot allows the patient to be ambulatory and, if properly applied, is comfortable. The patient is relieved of the responsibility of maintaining dressings, and the cost of community health services is reduced, e.g., the cost of a daily visiting nurse.

5
Emergency

Peter L. Lane

CHIN LIFT (Fig. 5–1)

Clinical Uses

1. Noninvasive technique used to displace posterior tongue anteriorly to improve airway patency.
2. Most useful in unconscious or semiconscious patients.

Method

With the patient in the supine position, the anterior aspect of the mandible is grasped between the operator's thumb and fingers. The mandible is displaced anteriorly, bringing the posterior tongue forward off of the posterior pharynx. An acceptable alternative to this is to insert the thumb into the mouth and grasp the lower incisors. This should not be attempted in any patient with the potential to bite the operator's thumb.

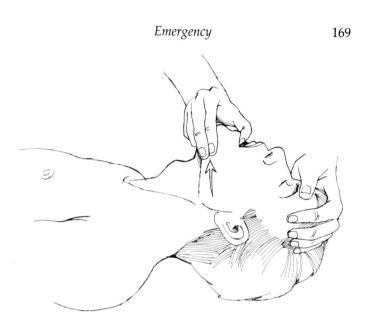

Fig. 5–1. Chin lift to open airway.

Precautions

Care should be taken in treating a patient who may have a cervical spine injury. Because of the direction of the force employed to lift the mandible, care must be taken not to deviate the head and neck. This is a noninvasive technique to temporarily improve airway patency. More definitive control of the airway should be achieved as soon as possible.

JAW THRUST PROCEDURE (Fig. 5–2)

Clinical Uses

1. Useful as a preliminary technique to improve airway patency by lifting the base of the tongue off the posterior pharynx.

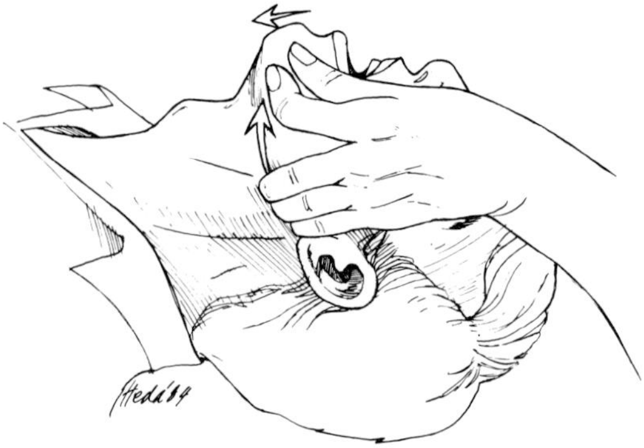

Fig. 5–2. Jaw-thrust maneuver.

2. An acceptable alternative to the chin lift, particularly
when used on an injured patient.

Method

With the patient either supine or seated, the physician
positions himself at the head of the patient if supine or
behind the patient, if seated. With both hands on either
side of the patient's head and neck, inline traction can be
applied to the cervical spine to stabilize potential injury,
while the jaw-thrust technique is employed to open the
airway. In the jaw-thrust technique, the hands are placed
on either side of the face with the fourth and fifth fingers
of each hand on the mandibular rami, proximal to the angle
of the jaw. At the same time, the thumb and index fingers
of each hand are used to grasp the mandible more anteriorly. The mandible is then opened with the thumb and
index fingers, while the fourth and fifth fingers are used
to deviate the mandible anteriorly. The palms and forearms
stabilize the head and neck, while the procedure is performed.

Precautions

This is a noninvasive technique to temporarily improve airway patency. More definitive control of the airway should be achieved as soon as possible.

OROPHARYNGEAL AIRWAY INSERTION

Clinical Uses

An airway adjunct that is useful on a temporary basis to maintain the airway patency between the posterior tongue and the posterior pharynx.

Equipment

The oropharyngeal airway is a curved ovoid tube made of plastic or rubber. The correct size is premeasured using the surface anatomy of the patient. When measured against the lateral aspect of the patient's face, the oropharyngeal airway should extend from the lips to just beyond the angle of the mandible.

Method

Two equally effective techniques exist.
1. In the inverted technique, the oropharyngeal airway is inserted in the inverted position until the tip reaches the soft palate, at which point it is rotated 180° into the correct position and advanced to its final resting position (Fig. 5–3).
2. In the direct vision technique, a tongue depressor is used to lift the tongue off the posterior wall of the pharynx, and the oropharyngeal airway is inserted under direct vision (Fig. 5–4).

Precautions

If incorrectly inserted, the oropharyngeal airway can push the tongue farther back against the posterior wall of

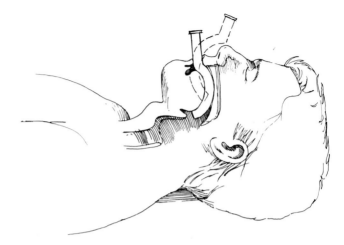

Fig. 5–3. Oropharyngeal airway insertion (inverted technique).

the pharynx and aggravate the airway obstruction (Fig. 5–5). In addition, in patients with an intact gag reflex, the insertion of the oropharyngeal airway can precipitate gagging and vomiting. The oropharyngeal airway does not provide definitive airway protection against aspiration; if this risk exists (i.e., no gag reflex) more definitive control should be instituted as soon as possible. Suction equipment should be available.

NASOPHARYNGEAL AIRWAY INSERTION
(Fig. 5–6)

Clinical Uses

The nasopharyngeal airway is useful in temporarily maintaining airway patency in a patient who may not tolerate insertion of the oropharyngeal airway, e.g., the head

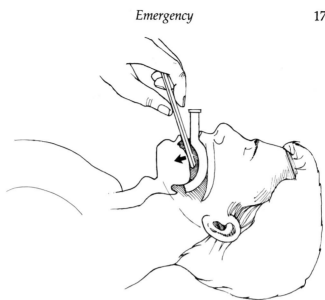

Fig. 5–4. Oropharyngeal airway insertion (direct-vision technique).

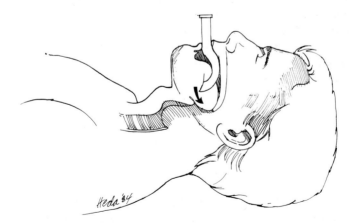

Fig. 5–5. Incorrectly inserted oropharyngeal airway.

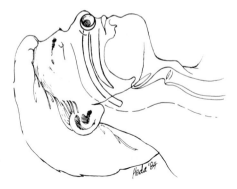

Fig. 5–6. Nasopharyngeal airway in place.

injured patient with clenched jaws or the seizing patient with clonus.

Equipment

The correct size nasopharyngeal airway is required. These are constructed of soft rubber or plastic tube and extend from the nose to the posterior pharynx behind the tongue. The correct size of the nasopharyngeal airway is important and can be estimated prior to insertion by placing the airway against the lateral aspect of the patient's face. The nasopharyngeal airway should extend from the nasal ala to the angle of the mandible.

Method

The airway is lubricated with water soluble jelly lubricant prior to insertion to facilitate sliding through the nose. It is inserted close to the midline along the inferior aspect of the nostril and gently advanced into the posterior pharynx behind the tongue.

Precautions

Insertion may be difficult in some patients because of peculiarities of anatomy, polyps, previous trauma, etc. If significant resistance exists during the attempted insertion, force should not be used and the other nostril should be attempted. In addition, some patients tolerate the procedure better if a lubricant containing a local anesthetic such as lidocaine is chosen. This procedure may cause epistaxis; suction should be ready. The nasopharyngeal airway does not provide definitive airway protection against aspiration. If this risk exists (i.e., no gag reflex), more definitive control should be instituted as soon as possible.

ENDOTRACHEAL INTUBATION

Clinical Uses

For definitive airway control and/or the institution of mechanical ventilation, endotracheal intubation is necessary in a variety of clinical settings, including the following:

1. The comatose patient with no gag reflex.
2. The patient in respiratory failure requiring ventilation.
3. The critically head-injured patient requiring hyperventilation to reduce intracranial pressure.
4. The anesthetized patient who cannot control his/her secretions.
5. The patient with major maxillofacial injury and bleeding into the airway.
6. The patient with a respiratory burn who is in danger of developing acute airway obstruction.
7. The patient with neck trauma who may develop airway obstruction.
8. The patient with impending airway obstruction as a result of local infection.

Equipment

Suction with tonsil-tip and endotracheal suction attachments

Oxygen source

Bag-valve-mask equipment

Water soluble jelly lubricant

Lidocaine anesthetic spray

Flexible stylet

Laryngoscope with curved and straight blades

10-ml syringe

Cuffed endotracheal tube of the appropriate size

Choosing the correct size tube need not be a complicated process. The following guidelines may help:

Adults:

males require 7.5- to 9-mm internal diameter and females 6.5- to 8-mm internal diameter.

Children

premature infants require 1.5- to 2.5-mm internal diameter (noncuffed).

full-term newborns need 3-mm internal diameter (noncuffed).

5-year-olds require 5-mm internal diameter.

10-year-olds require 6-mm internal diameter.

A general rule that may help in estimating size is that the tube should be slightly larger than an estimate of the size of the nares or the fifth finger of the patient.

Method

Once the decision has been made to intubate the patient, adequate preparation is key to success. All equipment should be assembled at the bedside within easy reach of the physician. The correct sized endotracheal tube should be chosen and the cuff inflated briefly, prior to intubation to check that it does not leak. The tube should then be

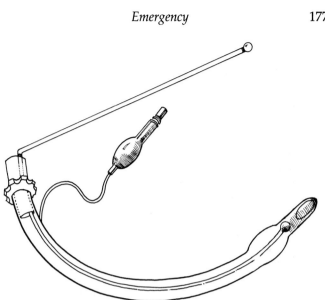

Fig. 5–7. Endotracheal tube with stylet in position.

lubricated. If oral intubation is to be performed, the tube should be cut prior to insertion. For most adult patients, a tube cut between 24 and 26 cms will mean that the hub of the tube is in correct position once it is fully inserted. Tonsil-tip suction should be within easy reach and activated at this point. If the flexible stylet is to be used, it should be inserted during the preparatory stage so that the tip of the stylet is not protruding beyond the tip of the tube (Fig. 5–7). The stylet should be bent to facilitate insertion into the trachea. In an awake or semiconscious patient, it is usually wise to insert the laryngoscope initially into the mouth to visualize the vocal cords and to spray the posterior pharynx and, if possible, the vocal cords, with the lidocaine spray. This will help to extinguish the gag and cough reflexes and facilitate successful intubation.

Positioning is an important part of the preparatory

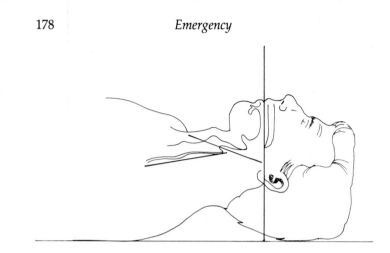

Fig. 5–8. Head in neutral position.

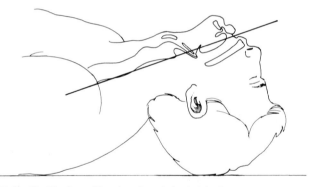

Fig. 5–9. Positioning of head and neck for intubation.

phase. In order to align the axes of the oral cavity, pharynx, and trachea as much as possible, the sniffing position is preferred; i.e., the head should be extended on the neck, and the neck should be flexed on the thorax (Figs. 5–8, 5–9, 5–10). A folded towel beneath the patient's head will often facilitate this. The head should be held extended either by the physician's elbow or by another operator's

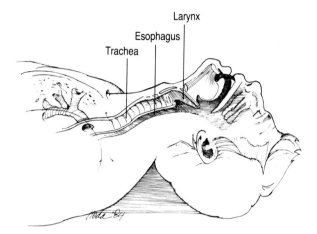

Larynx

Esophagus

Trachea

Fig. 5–10. Orotracheal intubation: anatomy.

hand. The final part of the preparatory phase is to super-oxygenate the patient by using the bag-valve mask and hyperventilating the patient with high flow oxygen just prior to attempted intubation.

Insertion Phase. With the patient correctly positioned, the laryngoscope blade is inserted along the right side of the mouth to deviate the tongue to the left. If the curved blade is used, the tip should be advanced to the vallecular (Fig. 5–11). If the straight blade is used, the tip should be advanced just past the epiglottis (Fig. 5–12). The laryngoscope should now be lifted along the longitudinal axis of the handle (not levered on the upper incisors). This should serve to lift the epiglottis up out of the line of vision and expose at least the posterior one-half of the larynx and vocal cords (Fig. 5–13). If this is unsuccessful in exposing the vocal cords, pressure applied over the cricoid cartilage by an assistant can serve to deviate the trachea posteriorly and bring the larynx into view.

Emergency

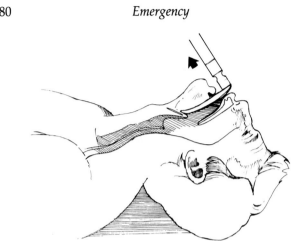

Fig. 5–11. Orotracheal intubation: curved blade laryngoscope.

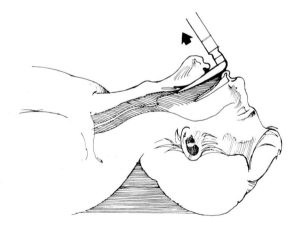

Fig. 5–12. Orotracheal intubation: straight blade laryngoscope.

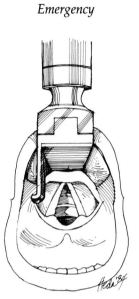

Fig. 5–13. Orotracheal intubation: direct view of vocal cords.

Once the vocal cords are visualized, the endotracheal tube should be taken in the right hand, advanced along the right side of the oral cavity and pharynx and between the vocal cords into the trachea. The tube should be advanced such that the cuff lies just inferior to the vocal cords. If the stylet is used, it should now be removed. Now the position of the tube should be checked by attempting a few quick ventilations, while auscultating the lung fields and epigastrium. If air entry is heard in both lung fields and not in the epigastrium, the cuff of the tube should be inflated with enough air to prevent leakage (5 to 10 ml). Once the cuff has been inflated, lung fields and the epigastric area should again be auscultated during inflation with the bag-valve apparatus. If air entry is heard in both lung fields and not in the epigastrium, successful placement is inferred. If air entry on the left is less than that on the right, endobronchial intubation in the right main-stem bronchus is suspected. The cuff is deflated, withdrawn 1 or 2 cm, and then reinflated with air as before.

As soon as possible after insertion, a chest radiograph should be performed to check tube placement. The tip of the tube should be seen on the radiograph at least 1 to 2 cms above the carina. If it appears to be in the right main-stem bronchus, the tube should be withdrawn the appropriate distance and the cuff reinflated. The tube should now be securely taped into place. With most patients, this can be effectively achieved with one or two long strips of adhesive or plastic tape. In some patients, however, tape will be inappropriate because of facial hair or facial injury. An acceptable alternative for these patients is to tie the tube in place with either tracheostomy tube ties or firmly tied gauze bandage.

Precautions

In the conscious or semiconscious patient, insertion of the laryngoscope and/or the tube may give rise to a significant gag and cough reflex. In some patients, this may result in vomiting; thus, tonsil-tip suction must always be available and in good working order. Care must be taken during insertion of a laryngoscope, particularly in the area of the epiglottis as pharyngeal and glottic injury is a potential complication. Bleeding from such injuries can be profuse and lead to aspiration and airway obstruction.

As above, care should be taken when lifting the laryngoscope. The line of force should be in the long axis of the laryngoscope handle. Levering of the laryngoscope blade on the upper incisors can result in broken central incisors. Inappropriate or rough insertion of an endotracheal tube can result in damage and more spasm of the vocal cords. Remember that spraying the vocal cords with local anesthetic can help to prevent some problems.

The initial and subsequent checking of tube placement and position is critical. Even though securely taped, tubes can become dislodged from the trachea as a result of a severe cough or movement during transfer of the patient. Frequent assessment of air entry and lung compliance is essential.

NASOTRACHEAL INTUBATION (Fig. 5–14)

Clinical Use

1. Primarily of use in potential cervical spine injured patients (head injured patients, facial injury patients, etc).
2. Of some use in children or other patients who may be inclined to bite a tube inserted through the mouth.

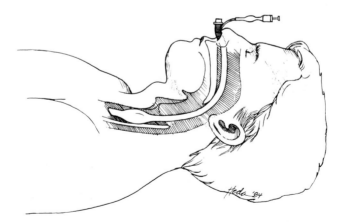

Fig. 5–14. Nasotracheal intubation.

3. Of use when unimpaired access to the oral cavity is necessary, such as for dental surgery.
4. Of some use in patients with prominent gag reflex.

Equipment

A functioning suctioning device with tonsil-tip and endotracheal-tube suction catheter attachments
Oxygen source
Bag-valve-mask ventilation apparatus
Water soluble jelly lubricant
Local anesthetic spray (lidocaine)
Vasoconstrictor spray for nasal mucosa
Stethoscope
Endotracheal tube

Method

Preparation. As with endotracheal intubation, preparation is key to successful intubation. Choosing the correct tube size is important. Tube size should be approximately a half millimeter smaller than for oral endotracheal intubation. As a result, most adult males will require between 7 and 8.5 mm internal diameter and most adult females between 6 and 7.5 mm internal diameter tube.

Because the procedure often results in bleeding from the nasal mucosa, spray it first with a topical vasoconstrictor such as 5% cocaine solution or Neo-Synephrine. In addition, because the procedure can lead to considerable pain, the use of a topical anesthetic spray, such as lidocaine, is important.

Positioning of the patient is significantly different for nasotracheal intubation. The technique is a blind technique. The patient should be maintained with the head and neck in the neutral position, preferably with an assistant stabilizing the head and neck with in-line traction applied.

Insertion Phase. After preparation of the nose and superoxygenation of the patient, the cuff of the endotracheal tube is checked and lubricant applied. The larger nostril is chosen after initial visual check to rule out major obstructions as a result of polyps, trauma, etc. The tube is advanced along the floor of the nasal cavity into the nasopharynx. At this stage, some resistance is often encountered. If this is significant and the tube cannot be advanced, force should not be applied, and the other nostril should be attempted.

The tube should be advanced along the curve of the nasopharynx into the hypopharynx. Here the tube should be observed for the presence of water vapor that develops with each breath. Alternatively, the operator's ear can be placed beside the hub of the tube to listen for air movements along the tube.

The tube should now be advanced slowly as the patient inspires. If it appears that air movement has ceased, it is likely that the esophagus has been intubated and the tube should be withdrawn until air movement is again observed. Now pressure may be applied to the cricoid cartilage, in order to occlude the esophagus and deviate the trachea posteriorly. This will more likely result in successful intubation. Once the tube has been advanced and air movement continues, or a good cough ensues, a few attempts at ventilation should be performed to assess tube position. As with endotracheal intubation, both lung fields and the epigastrium should be auscultated to ensure correct tube placement. Once appropriate tube placement has been confirmed, the tube should be securely taped into place.

Precautions

This technique should not be employed in patients with major maxillofacial trauma where the possibility of a cribriform plate fracture exists. Similarly, because the technique is a blind one and dependent upon the movement of air, it cannot be used on a patient who has suffered respiratory arrest.

The nasotracheal route can, and often does, give rise to significant epistaxis. This is usually not problematic once definitive airway control has been obtained with a cuffed tube, but suction should be available during the procedure to cope with any blood in the airway.

A potential complication of the procedure, particularly if roughly done, is that of laceration and subsequent infection of the retropharyngeal area. The use of soft tubes and a gentle technique can avoid this complication. Because the procedure is uncomfortable, it is important for all but the deeply unconscious patient that the head and neck be secured by an assistant applying in-line traction.

ENDOTRACHEAL TUBE SUCTIONING

Clinical Uses

To remove secretions from endotracheal tubes and lower trachea; it forms a necessary part of tracheal toilet in the intubated patient.

Equipment

Suction apparatus with low and high suction capabilities
Flexible suction catheters with side port (Fig. 5–15)
Mask
Sterile gloves
Bowl with sterile water

Method

With the operator masked and gloved, the sterile catheter should be attached to the suction tube. With the side port open and no suction applied, the catheter should be ad-

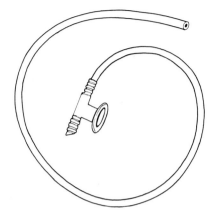

Fig. 5–15. Intratracheal suction catheter.

vanced into the tube rapidly with one hand while the other hand secures the tube. The side port of the suction catheter is then occluded to produce suction at the tip, and the catheter is withdrawn. Twisting the catheter during withdrawal can facilitate suctioning of secretions adhering to the side of the tube. After each advancement and withdrawal of the catheter, the patient should be given a few full breaths with the ventilator device to reoxygenate. Secretions should be removed from the inside of the suction catheter by the suctioning of the sterile water in between insertions into the endotracheal tube.

Occasionally, with adhering secretions or blood, instillation of 5 to 10 ml of sterile water through the endotracheal tube can dilute secretions and facilitate more effective tracheal toilet.

Precautions

Sterile technique should always be maintained to prevent infection, a significant complication of the introduction of the catheter through the endotracheal tube.

Repeated attempts at suctioning without interposed ventilations can result in significant hypoxia and hypercarbia. This can be detrimental to head-injured and/or respiratory failure patients.

Insertion of the suction catheter into the tube and then into the trachea can result in significant vagal stimulation. This can result in significant bradycardia or even sinus arrest in some patients. It usually results in a brisk coughing episode if the cough reflex is present. The ECG should be monitored during this procedure.

NEEDLE CRICOTHYROTOMY

Indications

Inability to intubate.

Clinical Uses

Needle cricothyrotomy is a temporary measure used only when surgical cricothyrotomy is unavailable. This is primarily of use in the prehospital setting, but may occasionally be of value in hospitals.

Anatomy (Fig. 5–16)

The cricothyroid membrane is easily identifiable in most patients and is now recognized as the most accessible route to emergency surgical management of the airway. The cricothyroid membrane, an avascular structure, extends from the cricoid cartilage inferiorly to the thyroid cartilage superiorly and forms the anterior border of the larynx in this area. It can be palpated in most patients as the transverse

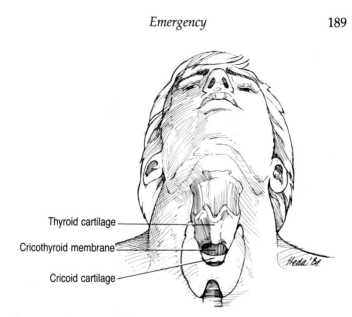

Fig. 5–16. Anatomy of the cricothyroid membrane.

indentation between the thyroid cartilage superiorly and the cricoid cartilage inferiorly.

Equipment

A large bore plastic cannula (No. 12 or No. 14 gauge)
Appropriate 'Y' connector oxygen tubing and high flow oxygen source or an adapter (e.g., hub from a No. 3 pediatric endotracheal tube)
Bag-valve ventilation apparatus

Method

Once the cricothyroid membrane has been identified by palpation with the patient in the supine position, the anterior neck is prepared. The catheter over needle device is then inserted at an angle of approximately 60° to the horizontal, in the sagittal plane in the midline (Fig. 5–17). Once

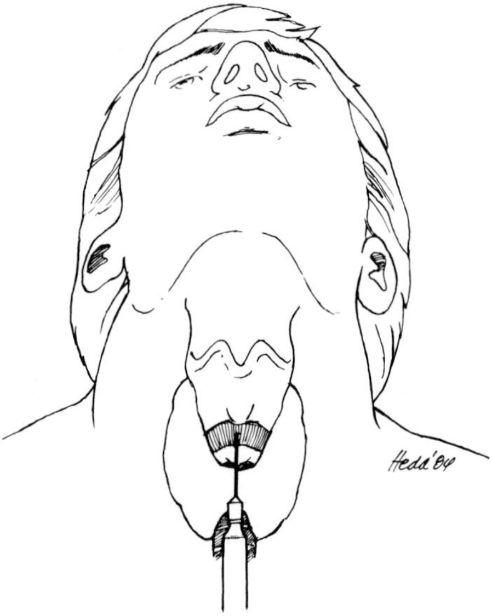

Fig. 5–17. Needle cricothyrotomy.

it is through the membrane and air is heard to move
through the catheter, the catheter is advanced and the
needle is withdrawn. The hub of the catheter is then attached to the Y connector, if the jet insufflation technique
is to be used, or attached to the adapter and bag-valve
device, if positive pressure ventilation is to be attempted.
The catheter should be held in place manually, until more
definitive airway control can be gained.

Precautions

Care must be taken not to advance the needle too far or
potential damage of the posterior wall of the trachea may
result. This can cause significant bleeding as well as insertion of the catheter into the mediastinal structures or even
the esophagus.

Ventilation through the needle cricothyrotomy can be achieved through the two techniques: jet insufflation with a high flow oxygen source and intermittent occlusion of the Y connector, or positive pressure ventilation using a bag-valve device. With either technique, the needle cricothyrotomy provides a temporary method for the introduction of oxygenated air into the lungs. Resistance to flow is high and expiration of gases is limited; as a result, hypercarbia persists. Definitive control of the airway should be effected as rapidly as possible.

Particularly, care should be taken in children because the cricoid cartilage provides the only anterior support to the upper trachea. If damaged during attempts of cricothyrotomy, this may preclude an effective surgical cricothyrotomy or even effective surgical tracheostomy.

SURGICAL CRICOTHYROTOMY

Indications

Failure to intubate.

Clinical Uses

Now accepted generally as the appropriate surgical technique for emergency management of the airway.

Anatomy

See discussion under needle cricothyrotomy and Fig. 5–16.

Equipment

Sterile prep and drapes
No. 10 scalpel blade and handle
Hemostats or Jackson tracheostomy forceps
Tracheostomy tapes

Tracheostomy tube size No. 5 or No. 6
Bag-valve ventilator device
Tracheostomy dressing

Method

With the patient in a supine position, the cricothyroid
membrane is identified by palpation. The area is prepared
and draped. A vertical or transverse incision is made
quickly but carefully through the skin and the cricothyroid
membrane (Fig. 5–18). The blunt end of the scalpel or the
tracheostomy forceps is inserted to spread the incision, and
the tube is inserted through the opening and advanced
(Fig. 5–19). A few ventilations are attempted with the bag-
valve apparatus to insure correct placement, and the cuff

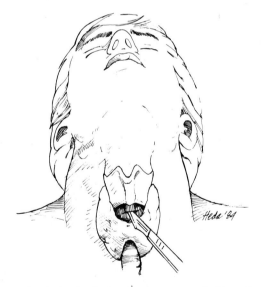

Fig. 5–18. Surgical cricothyrotomy (transverse incision through the
membrane).

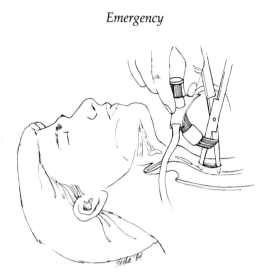

Fig. 5–19. Surgical cricothyrotomy (insertion of the cuffed tracheostomy tube).

of the tube is inflated. The tracheostomy dressing is applied and the tapes attached to secure the tube in place.

Precautions

While in most patients the cricothyroid membrane is an avascular structure, occasionally a small vessel is encountered that can lead to some bleeding. Care must be taken not to injure the posterior wall of the trachea in the region with either the scalpel or other instruments employed. If time permits, sterile suction apparatus should be available to deal with any bleeding encountered. A few patients may develop a late complication of subglottic stenosis, but complication rates are comparable with other surgical methods of airway control.

The cricothyroid approach is inappropriate for small children because the cricoid cartilage represents the only rigid support of the anterior wall of the upper trachea. If intubation is impossible, an emergency tracheostomy is the only technique available.

PROCEDURES TO CLEAR THE AIRWAY IN A CHOKING VICTIM

Upper airway obstruction is most commonly a result of impaired consciousness arising from cardiac arrest, head injury, or trauma. Upper airway obstruction can itself lead to inadequate oxygenation and subsequent unconsciousness. A variety of procedures may be employed by the rescuer in assisting a patient with partial or complete upper airway obstruction. The procedures will be described initially, and subsequently the sequence of the use of these procedures for different types of airway obstruction will be outlined.

Back Blows

Method

With the victim standing or sitting, the rescuer positions himself behind or beside the victim. The left hand is placed anteriorly over the victim's sternum to support the victim, and with the heel of the right hand, four sharp blows are delivered to the victim's spine between the scapulae. The direction of the blow should be in the posterior-anterior direction, directed slightly cephalad (Fig. 5–20).

With the victim lying, the rescuer kneels beside the victim and rolls him onto his side so he is facing the rescuer with his chest against the rescuer's knees. Four sharp blows are delivered to the back with the heel of the palm, striking the thoracic spine between the scapulae. The direction of the blows should be in the posterior-anterior direction, directed slightly cephalad (Fig. 5–21).

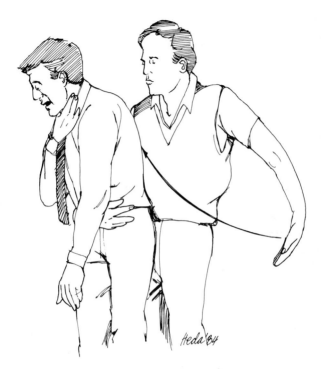

Fig. 5–20. Back blows (standing position).

Back Blows in the Infant or Small Child. The child should be lifted and placed prone on the rescuer's left forearm, with the head and face supported by the left hand. The child's head should be tilted slightly downwards to use gravity. Four sharp blows should be delivered with the heel of the palm to the upper thoracic spine between the scapulae, directed slightly cephalad.

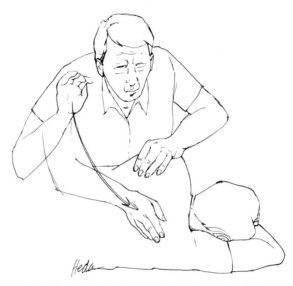

Fig. 5–21. Position for back blows when the victim is found lying on the ground (he is rolled to face the rescuer).

Precautions

Back blows should only be attempted in cases of complete airway obstruction. If used in the situation of incomplete airway obstruction, blows may convert an incomplete obstruction to a complete obstruction in both adults and children.

Manual Thrust Techniques

Victim Standing or Sitting. As in cardiopulmonary resuscitation (CPR), the victim is positioned supine with the rescuer kneeling at the side of the patient. The rescuer reaches both arms around the victim and grasps one fist with the other hand in front of the victim at the level of the xiphisternum. The rescuer turns sideways to place the hip against the victim's back (Fig. 5–22). The rescuer

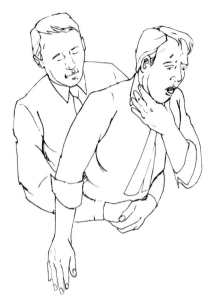

Fig. 5–22. Abdominal thrust.

squeezes the fist into the epigastric area four times with a quick upward thrusting motion.

Victim Supine. As in CPR, the victim is positioned supine with the rescuer kneeling at the side of the patient. The rescuer establishes the landmarks for chest compressions as with CPR by defining the costal margin and the xiphisternum. The heel of the cephalad hand is placed on the sternum, two finger breadths above the xiphisternal junction, and the other hand is placed on top thus on the sternum and delivers four chest compressions. As with the chest compressions in CPR, these should be sharp, downward thrusts, depressing the sternum 3 to 5 cm with each thrust (see Figs. 5–31, 5–32, 5–33).

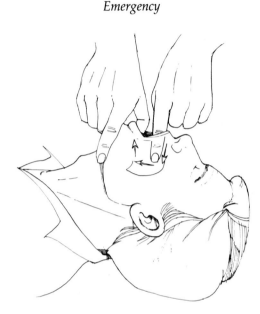

Fig. 5–23. The finger sweep for oropharyngeal foreign bodies.

Finger Sweep

Method

The airway should be opened with a chin lift or jaw thrust maneuver, as previously described. The index finger of the dominant hand of the rescuer is introduced along the side wall of the oral cavity and advanced as far as possible into the pharynx. The finger is then swept across the oropharyngeal area to the opposite side of the pharynx, and any foreign body encountered is retrieved, using a hooking action to sweep it anteriorly and out of the mouth (Fig. 5–23).

Precaution

Be careful not to push any foreign body farther into the airway and impact it.

Sequence of Procedures in Different Settings

Conscious: Partial Airway Obstruction

With a conscious patient who is still moving some air, i.e., phonating or demonstrating stridor, the rescuer should not attempt any active techniques to dislodge the obstruction. Instead, the rescuer should encourage the victim to lean forward and cough as forcefully as possible, in an attempt to expel the foreign body. If the patient is ventilating well enough to remain conscious, it is dangerous to interfere with the airway unless the rescuer is prepared to proceed immediately to surgical cricothyrotomy.

Conscious: Complete Airway Obstruction

Indications

The victim cannot phonate or cough and no stridor is heard.

Sequence

1. Four back blows.
2. Four manual thrusts.
3. Repeat four back blows and four manual thrusts until the foreign body is dislodged. If the patient becomes unconscious, lay the patient down and proceed to the sequence for the unconscious victim.

Unconscious: Complete Airway Obstruction

Indications

Complete obstruction of the airway in an unconscious victim. Cleaning the airway in a victim with complete airway obstruction who has become unconscious takes priority over all other interventions, whatever the clinical setting.

Sequence

1. Attempt mouth-to-mouth ventilation or bag-valve-mask to mouth ventilation.
2. Check for pulse; if none found, proceed with CPR.
3. Call for help.
4. Reposition the head and attempt to clear the airway.
5. Four back blows.
6. Four chest thrusts.
7. Finger sweep. At this stage it may be necessary to remove the victim's dentures, if present.
8. Attempt to ventilate. If successful, continue ventilation; if unsuccessful, repeat sequence of four back blows, four chest thrusts and finger sweep.
9. If obstruction persists, consider immediate laryngoscopy and foreign body removal with forceps, and/or surgical cricothyrotomy (p. 191).

Follow-Up Care

The patient who has sustained a temporary complete airway obstruction, particularly if it has caused unconsciousness, needs follow-up care. Some or all of the foreign body may well have been aspirated farther into the tracheobronchial tree. A chest x-ray radiograph is indicated and bronchoscopy may be required.

BAG-VALVE-MASK VENTILATION

Indications

Respiratory failure, impaired consciousness leading to hypoventilation, and major head injury necessitating hyperventilation.

Equipment

Oxygen source
Bag-valve-mask device (Fig. 5–24)

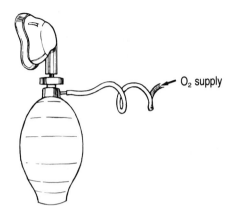

Fig. 5–24. Bag-valve-mask device.

Selection of mask size (preferably clear plastic to facilitate viewing the airway)
Functioning suction apparatus

Method

1. An oropharyngeal and/or nasopharyngeal airway should be inserted prior to attempted ventilation.
2. An appropriate sized mask should be chosen so that a good seal is formed from above the nose to below the lower lips.
3. The mask attached to the bag is applied to the face with the narrow portion placed superiorly over the nose and the broader flare of the mask portion placed inferiorly over the mouth.
4. The operator's thumb and index finger should be placed above and below the central port of the mask (Fig. 5–25).
5. The third, fourth, and fifth fingers should be applied along the mandible, effecting a tight seal between the mask and face (Fig. 5–25).

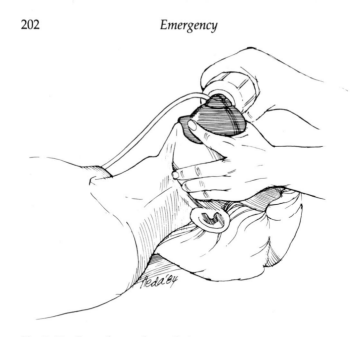

Fig. 5–25. Bag-valve-mask ventilation.

6. With the other hand, the bag is compressed firmly to provide the desired tidal volume. Maintenance ventilation for most patients should involve a tidal volume of approximately 10 cc's per kilogram. Hyperventilation for head injured patients should involve a total volume of between 12 and 15 cc's per kilogram.
7. The seal of the mask should be checked with each ventilation to detect a hissing sound indicative of a poor seal.
8. The chest and the abdomen should be observed for movement with inflation. Both sides of the chest should rise symmetrically with inflation.

Precautions

Inflation of the lungs in the normal patient should require only 15 to 20 cm water of inflation pressure. The operator should develop a feel for lung compliance by the degree of resistance encountered with inflation. If inflation pressures of over 25 to 30 cm of water are required, there is a significant risk that the stomach will be inflated. During ventilation with a bag-valve-mask system, the abdomen should be observed for gastric distention. Distention of the stomach can quickly lead to vomiting and aspiration. Functioning suction apparatus must be available at all times while bag-valve-mask ventilation is employed. In addition, if the airway is not adequately opened, particularly if the head is flexed, gastric distention may also occur.

BAG-VALVE-TUBE VENTILATION

Indication

Ventilation of the patient with tracheal tube in place.

Method

The mask should be removed from the bag-valve-mask system and the universal connector port attached to the adapter of the endotracheal tube. Ventilation can then proceed in the same fashion as described above for bag-valve-mask ventilation. Again, the chest wall should be observed for symmetrical movement and the lung fields auscultated for air entry.

Precautions

Positive pressure ventilation via bag-valve-mask or bag-valve-tube techniques can aggravate an existing pneumothorax. In addition, particularly in the presence of a bleb on the lung surface or fractured ribs, positive pressure ventilation can create a pneumothorax. It is essential to auscultate both lung fields periodically during ventilation. In addition, a change in the degree of airway resistance encountered by the operator compressing the bag should be a clue that pneumothorax may be developing. As a result of this above complication, any patient with documented rib fractures who must undergo positive pressure ventilation should have chest tubes placed prophylactically on the side of the rib fractures.

NEEDLE THORACOSTOMY

Clinical Uses

Needle thoracostomy technique represents a rapid emergency technique to both diagnose and temporarily alleviate a pneumothorax. It is not definitive management, but provides a brief respite while the necessary equipment can be assembled to insert a chest tube.

Equipment

Sterile swab
Flexible plastic cannula over needle

Method

The second intercostal space is identified by palpation, at the level of the sternomanubrial junction. The appropriate site for insertion is in the midclavicular line anteriorly. The area is quickly prepared. The large bore catheter over needle apparatus (No. 14 or No. 16 gauge) is inserted perpendicular to the chest wall into the second intercostal space in the midclavicular line. The catheter is inserted through the chest wall into the chest cavity and the needle is removed (Fig. 5–26).

If a hissing sound is heard, it indicates the presence of

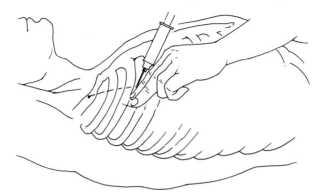

Fig. 5–26. Needle thoracostomy.

a pneumothorax with some element of tension; if blood is recovered, it indicates a significant hemothorax. In either instance, chest tube thoracostomy should be undertaken as soon as possible. In the interim, the hub of the needle can be left open to air or a sterile finger cot with the end off can be attached to act as a one-way valve device.

Precautions

This technique can, of course, produce a pneumothorax as a needle is being introduced directly into the chest cavity. It should therefore only be attempted if a significant suspicion of pneumothorax exists, i.e., decreased or absent breathing sounds on the side involved, in conjunction with increased airway resistance. A second potential complication, depending on the site of insertion, is laceration of the intercostal or internal mammary artery. This risk is minimal, if the procedure is correctly performed. Therefore, a follow-up chest radiograph is essential after needle thoracostomy.

CARDIOPULMONARY RESUSCITATION

Indications

Cardiac arrest with absent pulse and absent spontaneous respirations.

Equipment

None

Method

With the patient supine, the rescuer should kneel at the side of the patient at the level of the thorax. If the patient is unresponsive as established by shouting at him and/or providing a painful stimulus, the airway should be opened. If there is no question of trauma, this can be accomplished by head tilt and chin lift techniques. The head should be extended and the neck lifted (Fig. 5–27). The chin lift maneuver as described previously should be employed.

Absence of breathing should be established via the look-listen-feel technique. The rescuer should place his ear over

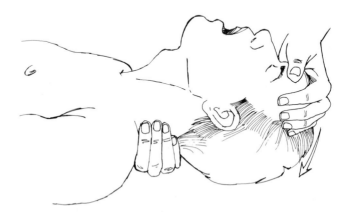

Fig. 5–27. Head tilt to open the airway.

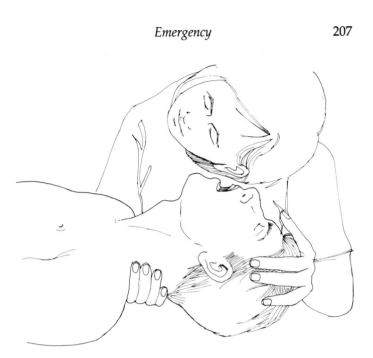

Fig. 5–28. Assessing for respiration: look, listen, feel.

the mouth and nose of the patient, listening and feeling for air movements, while observing the anterior chest wall for expansion (Fig. 5–28).

Having established the absence of a breathing beat, four quick ventilations should be attempted using the cephalad hand to pinch the nose shut while the caudad hand is kept beneath the neck to elevate it. The rescuer's mouth is placed over the victim's mouth, and four quick full breaths are given without allowing time for full lung deflation between breaths (Fig. 5–29). This maintains positive pressure in the airway and helps to fully inflate the lungs. Absence of a pulse should now be established. The rescuer places his second and third fingers over the carotid artery, just lateral to the larynx, to palpate for a pulse. This should be

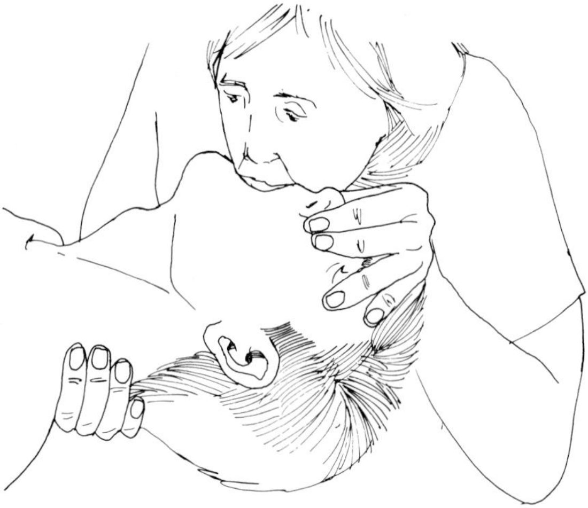

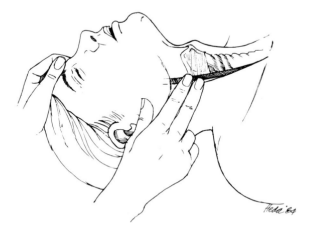

Fig. 5–29.　Mouth-to-mouth ventilation.

Fig. 5–30.　Palpation of carotid pulse at larynx.

done on the near side of the patient (Fig. 5–30). If a pulse is present, rescue breathing should continue with one breath every 5 seconds. If the pulse is absent, the rescuer shall immediately call for an ambulance.

Chest compression should now begin. With the caudad hand, the rescuer feels for the near costal margin and palpates the xiphisternum (Fig. 5–31). The heel of the cephalad hand is placed two finger breadths above the xiphisternal junction, and the caudad hand is placed on top (Fig. 5–32). The rescuer, still kneeling at the side of the patient, should now lean forward so that his shoulders are directly over the victim's sternum.

The elbows should remain straight by locking them, and chest compression should be effected by a quick downward

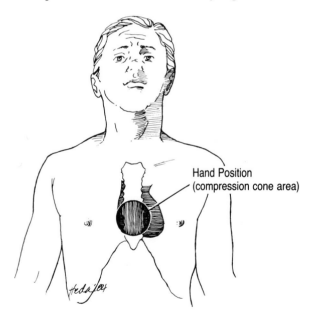

Fig. 5–31. Hand positioning for manual chest compressions.

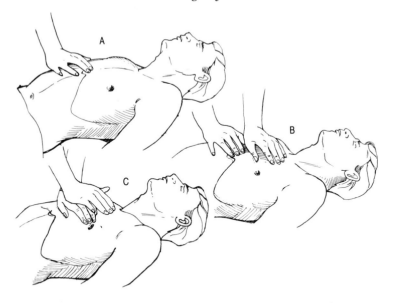

Fig. 5–32. Method of locating correct site for sternal chest compression. **A.** Caudad hand identifies xiphisternum. **B.** With the fourth digit of the caudad hand placed on the xiphisternum, a space of two finger breadths is noted proximally on the sternum. **C.** The heel of the cephalad hand is placed just proximal to the identified two finger breadths. The caudad hand is placed on top for compression.

thrust with sufficient force to depress the sternum 3 to 5 cm (Fig. 5–33). The pressure should be released to allow for venous return. The time allowed for release should be equal to the time taken for compression. There should be no pause between compressions, and the rescuer's hands should not be lifted off the chest between compressions. Compression should be performed at a rate equal to 80 compressions per minute, i.e., just more than 1 compression per second.

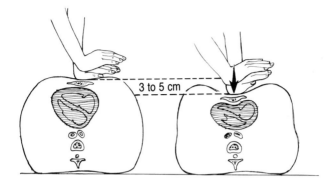

3 to 5 cm

Fig. 5–33. Chest compressions.

Sequence for One-Man Cardiopulmonary Resuscitation

The ratio of compressions to ventilations should be 15 to 2. Compressions should be performed at a rate equal to 80 per minute. The 2 ventilations following 15 compressions should not interrupt compressions for more than 5 seconds. As a result of this rate, a total of 60 compressions and 8 ventilations should be delivered during each minute of CPR (Fig. 5–34).

After the first 1-minute cycle of 15 compressions alternating with 2 ventilations, the rescuer should check for breathing and pulse; subsequently this check should be performed every 4 to 5 minutes.

Sequence for Two-Man Cardiopulmonary Resuscitation

If a second rescuer is present (who has identified to the satisfaction of the first rescuer that he is knowledgeable of the sequence and procedures for cardiopulmonary resuscitation), the two-man sequence may be used.

The ratio for the two-man sequence of compressions to ventilations is 5 to 1, i.e., the second rescuer should provide 1 breath for every 5 compressions performed by the first

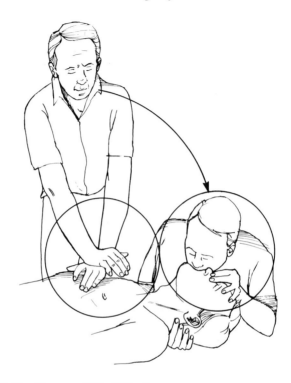

Fig. 5–34. One man CPR—15:2 ratio.

rescuer (Fig. 5–35). As a result, the rate of chest compressions should be slowed from 80 to 60 per minute. A useful mnemonic device is the following:

1-1000, 2-1000, 3-1000, 4-1000, 5-1000, (breath), 1-1000. . .

Ventilations during the two-man sequence should be interposed between the fifth and first compressions of the cycles involved. As such, inflation should begin at the start of the relaxation phase of the fifth compression, and lung deflation will occur with the compression phase of the fol-

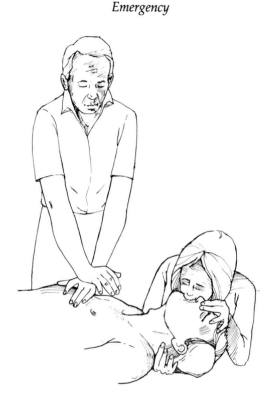

Fig. 5–35. Two man CPR—5:1 ratio.

lowing first compression. The ventilator-rescuer should feel frequently for the carotid pulse to ensure the effectiveness of compression.

Precautions

CPR poses a variety of potential complications. Gastric distention is a frequent hazard and should be anticipated. Vomiting and aspiration commonly occur even with effective CPR. Fractures of the bony and cartilaginous structures of the chest wall occur, particularly with overly vigorous chest compressions or in elderly or disabled patients; this is unfortunate because the effectiveness of chest compressions in the presence of a disrupted chest wall is minimal. Similarly, as previously noted, positive pressure ventilation in the presence of rib fractures can result in tension pneumothorax.

DEFIBRILLATION

Indications

Ventricular fibrillation; ventricular tachycardia with no output resistant to synchronized cardioversion.

Clinical Uses

Electrical defibrillation is the technique of choice to attempt to restore an effective cardiac rhythm in ventricular fibrillation.

Equipment

Cardiac monitor–defibrillator apparatus
ECG leads and electrodes
Conductive gel for defibrillator paddles

Method

1. The conductive gel or cream should be applied to the paddles.
2. Defibrillator power should be turned on and the synchronization mode disengaged.
3. An energy level should be established between 200 to 300 Joules delivered energy.
4. The defibrillator should be charged.
5. Once fully charged, the paddles should be placed on the chest. One paddle should be applied to the right chest at the right sternal border below the clavicle.

The second paddle should be placed in the area of the apex of the heart in the left lower lateral chest. Firm pressure should be applied to ensure conduction (Fig. 5–36).

6. The rhythm on the monitor should be rechecked to confirm continued ventricular fibrillation or tachycardia.

7. The operator should shout "all clear" to ensure that

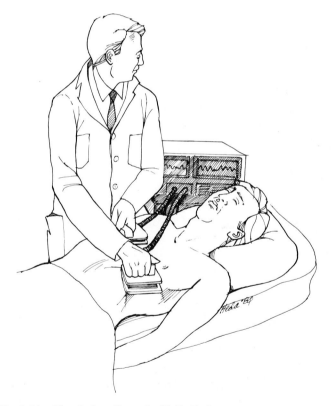

Fig. 5–36. Electrical cardioversion/defibrillation.

no person is in direct contact with either the patient or the stretcher.

8. Both buttons of the defibrillator apparatus should be pressed simultaneously while firm pressure is applied to the paddles to deliver the shock.

9. The rhythm on the monitor should be rechecked. Unless complexes are immediately seen, CPR should be continued for at least 15 seconds before again ceasing and rechecking the rhythm.

10. If ventricular fibrillation persists, a second defibrillation should be attempted as soon as possible while CPR is continued during the charging phase.

11. If an organized rhythm has been restored, CPR should be discontinued and the pulse checked. If a pulse is absent, CPR should continue.

12. If the second countershock is unsuccessful, CPR should continue while further treatment ensues; i.e., endotracheal intubation, commencement of I.V. therapy: I.V. sodium bicarbonate, epinephrine, etc. At least 2 to 3 minutes should be allowed between successive cycles of 2 countershocks to allow for circulation of drugs, improved oxygenation, and to avoid myocardial muscle damage as a result of rapid, successive shocks.

VAGOTONIC MANEUVERS

Clinical Uses

1. To increase vagal tone.
2. Particularly useful to convert a supraventricular tachycardia.
3. May also be of diagnostic use to slow ventricular response in cases of atrial fibrillation or flutter.

Method

Several methods have been employed and reported; those considered potentially useful are described. All methods described can only be performed in a setting with full resuscitation capabilities, with an intravenous line in place, and with ECG monitoring devices in place.

Valsalva Maneuver. The Valsalva Maneuver is perhaps the simplest technique and one that many patients will have tried themselves if they have experienced episodes of tachycardia. The maneuver is performed by attempting forced expiration against a closed glottis. This is often best described to the patient as an effort similar to bearing down during childbirth (Fig. 5–37). The maneuver should not be attempted by patients who are significantly short of breath or unable to control their airway well.

Gag Reflex. Stimulation of the gag reflex by depressing

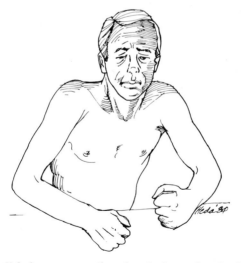

Fig. 5–37. Valsalva maneuver (forced expiration against the closed glottis).

the root or base of the tongue with a tongue depressor also increases vagal tone. Again, it should not be attempted in any patient with impaired consciousness, impaired airway control, or impaired breathing. Suction should be available.

Diving Reflex. Immersing the patient's face in cold water increases vagal tone. This is often logistically impossible, but the technique may be used as an option for some patients.

Carotid Sinus Massage (CSM). Of the methods described, carotid sinus massage is the most practical vagotonic maneuver and usually the most successful. The patient should be placed on a stretcher in a semi-sitting position at 45°. Both carotids should be auscultated for the presence of carotid bruits.

The maneuver is contraindicated if bruits are present or if the patient has a history of transient ischemic attacks (TIA) or cerebral vascular accidents. The carotid artery is palpated between the larynx and the medial border of the

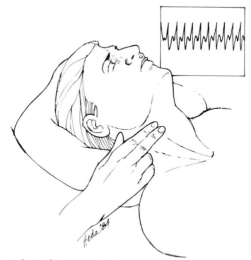

Fig. 5–38. Carotid sinus massage.

sternocleidomastoid. Firm massage is applied to compress the carotid artery and carotid sinus body between the fingers and the vertebral column (Fig. 5–38). (The procedure is a painful one, and the patient should be forewarned.) Massage without releasing the pressure. Massage should not be performed on both carotid arteries at the same time. If unsuccessful on one side, the contralateral carotid may be massaged after a sufficient period of 10 to 15 seconds between massages. Usually the technique is effective after one to two massages; if ineffective there is little point in persisting.

Massage should be discontinued if the patient experiences any neurologic symptoms such as visual disturbances, changes in the level of consciousness, transient paresthesia, or weakness, etc. TIAs and cerebral vascular accidents have been associated with CSM on rare occasions but are recognized as potential complications.

Precautions

Vagotonic maneuvers are indicated in patients suffering uncomplicated supraventricular tachydysrhythmias, but contraindicated in complicated tachydysrhythmias, i.e., those associated with chest pain, shortness of breath or impairment of consciousness. As described under cardioversion, such patients should be cardioverted immediately either chemically or electrically.

INTRACARDIAC INJECTION

Indications

Injection of medication directly into the heart when no other access route is appropriate.

Clinical Uses

There are few, if any, uses for intracardiac injection. It has now been documented that most medications that are of value in the cardiac arrest situation can be effectively administered through the endotracheal tube. Thus, if venous access is a problem, intratracheal administration as described below should be employed. Intracardiac injection is associated with significant morbidity and mortality and is rarely, if ever, indicated.

Method

Two potential routes exist:

The Xiphisternal Approach. The technique here is much the same as that for pericardiocentesis. The xiphisternal junction is identified, prepared, and draped. The needle is inserted at the left xiphisternal junction and aimed for

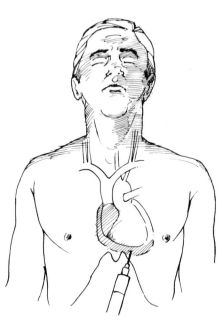

Fig. 5–39.   Intracardiac injection: xiphisternal approach.

the left scapular tip (Fig. 5–39). For intracardiac injection, there is no need to monitor the V_1 lead. The needle is advanced with syringe in place aspirating until blood is returned. The medication is then injected and the needle withdrawn.

The Anterior Approach. The landmarks of the fourth intercostal space at the left sternal border are identified. The area is prepared and draped. The needle, with syringe attached, is directed posteriorly. The needle is advanced while aspirating on the syringe until blood is returned (Fig. 5–40). Medication is then injected and the needle withdrawn.

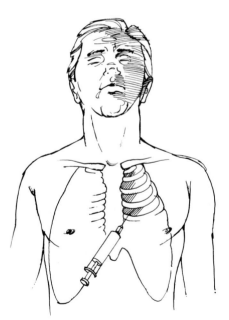

Fig. 5–40. Intracardiac injection: the anterior approach.

Precautions

Intracardiac injection is associated with a number of serious and potentially lethal complications including ventricular dysrhythmias, laceration of coronary arteries, pericardial tamponade, pneumothorax, pneumopericardium, infection, and sepsis.

INTRATRACHEAL ADMINISTRATION OF MEDICATIONS

Clinical Uses

Administration of certain medications via the endotracheal tube when venous access is a problem has been shown to be of comparable effectiveness to administration by the I.V. route. Hence, particularly in the cardiac arrest situation, administration of medication by the tube represents an effective, accessible route. Drugs which have been shown to provide acceptable serum levels following administration via the endotracheal tube include: epinephrine, lidocaine, atropine, naloxone, and diazepam.

Equipment

Desired medication and dose drawn up in a syringe and
    diluted with sterile water to 5 to 10 ml of solution
Endotracheal tube correctly positioned
Bag-valve ventilation apparatus

Method

The medication is drawn up in a syringe and diluted to 5 to 10 ml of liquid. Prior to its instillation, the patient is hyperventilated for 4 or 5 breaths. The bag-valve device is then disconnected from the endotracheal tube. The medication is injected quickly into the tube with sufficient force to deliver it to the trachea (Fig. 5–41). The bag-valve is

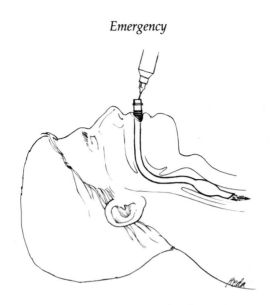

Fig. 5–41. Intratracheal administration of medications.

again connected to the adapter of the tube, and several quick ventilations are given at a rate of approximately 1 per second.

Precautions

Not all medications can be delivered by this route. In particular, it would appear that lipophobic drugs such as bretylium tosylate are poorly absorbed by the endotracheal route and should be avoided.

PNEUMATIC ANTI-SHOCK GARMENT (PASG)

Clinical Uses

The PASG is of particular value in cases of hypovolemia caused by trauma, pelvic fractures, abdominal aortic aneurysms, gastrointestinal (G.I.) bleeding, or postpartum hemorrhage. The garment is of less value in the management of shock from other causes: anaphylactic, neurogenic, septic, or addisonian crisis. It is absolutely contraindicated in the presence of congestive heart failure with pulmonary edema.

Equipment

Appropriately sized pediatric or adult pneumatic antishock garment complete with foot pump (Fig. 5–42). Some brands of the garment include pressure gauges for the individual compartments. These are not essential for routine use but may be helpful, particularly if used in air evacuation situations to monitor the garment pressure.

Method

Application. Three methods for application of the garment exist. By far the safest and easiest method is to have the garment placed on the stretcher or fracture board prior to transferring the patient onto it. If this is not possible,

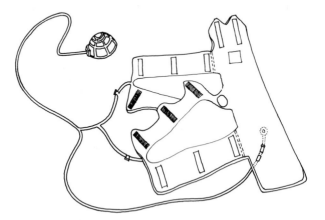

Fig. 5–42. Pneumatic anti-shock garment.

the garment can be applied by lifting the patient's legs and pelvis and sliding the garment up beneath the patient. This is contraindicated in most trauma situations because of the potential of a thoracic or lumbar spine injury. Hence, in these situations, the garment should be rolled and applied under the patient by log-rolling the patient. This technique requires at least three people; one to stabilize the head and neck and apply inline traction to the neck; a second to apply gentle traction to both legs and a third to roll the patient towards himself so that the garment can be placed beneath the patient, and then to roll the patient back, pulling the garment through the other side.

With the above considerations, the following procedures for application of the garment should be followed:

The patient's vital signs should be assessed and the indications for the garment confirmed. The garment should be unfolded and applied according to one of the techniques described above. The top of the garment should not be above the costal margin; this avoids impairment of respiration (Fig. 5–43). The two leg compartments and abdominal compartments should then be wrapped around the

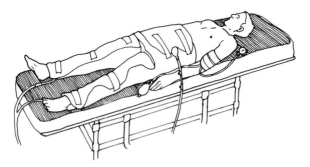

Fig. 5–43. Pneumatic anti-shock garment (positioned up to the lower costal margin).

patient with the Velcro straps applied firmly. The hoses should be connected to the appropriate compartments. The stopcock of both leg compartments should be placed in the open position and the stopcock of the abdominal compartment closed.

The leg compartments of the garment should be inflated to the desired pressure using the foot pump. Usually this means that they are fully inflated until the Velcro strips start to snap, or until the pop-off valve starts to hiss (104 mm Hg internal garment pressure).

Vital signs should again be checked. If the abdominal compartment is required and not contraindicated (i.e., no evisceration or impalement injuries; no third trimester pregnancy) the abdominal compartment should then be inflated as well.

Deflation. The garment must be deflated *slowly*. Rapid

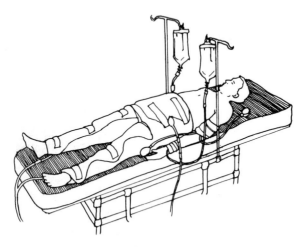

Fig. 5–44. Pneumatic anti-shock garment. (Removal of garment should not be attempted until fluid volume and blood pressure have both been restored.)

deflation can result in a sudder major reduction in cardiac after load and consequent asystolic arrest. Complete deflation should take a full 15 to 20 minutes (Fig. 5–44).

The stopcocks of all compartments are in the closed position. The hoses of all compartments are disconnected. The operator's thumb is placed over the end of the spigot of the abdominal compartment, and the stopcock is moved to the open position. Blood pressure is taken. I.V. lines are checked to ensure that they are all operating well. Preferably, ECG leads should be placed on the patient and the cardiogram monitored during deflation. A small amount of air is let out of the garment, using the operator's thumb, and the blood pressure is checked continuously during deflation. Should the blood pressure drop more than 5 to 10 mm of mercury systolic pressure, deflation ceases and I.V. infusion rate is increased. If the blood pressure does not return, the garment is reinflated. If the blood pressure holds during deflation of the abdominal compartment, the leg compartments are slowly deflated in turn, using the same procedure with continuous blood pressure monitoring. After full deflation, the garment is unwrapped to allow examination and access to the lower torso and lower extremities.

Precautions

By far the major complication associated with the use of the pneumatic anti-shock garment is rapid or premature deflation. The garment must not be unwrapped until fully deflated. A deflation procedure involving slow deflation and continuous blood pressure monitoring must be followed. The garment, of course, should not be cut with scissors. If the patient's blood pressure remains unstable, the garment can remain in place, inflated, until the surgeon is ready to open the chest for a thoracotomy to cross-clamp the aorta, or to prepare and open the abdomen for a formal laparotomy. In such cases, of course, anesthesia should be induced prior to deflation.

The garment causes a variety of dystrophic skin changes because of the pressure phenomena. This is particularly the case if the garment is applied over clothing; if time permits, clothing should be removed prior to its application.

The garment causes venous congestion in the lower limbs, and the feet may appear blue during appropriate application and inflation of the garment.

Inflation of the abdominal compartment causes significant increase in intra-abdominal pressure. This can result in defecation, urination, vomiting, and aspiration. All of these potential sequelae should be anticipated. If time permits prior to inflation, a Foley catheter should be inserted into the bladder and a nasogastric tube inserted to decompress the stomach. Meticulous attention should be paid to the airway during inflation of the abdominal compartment and, if possible, the airway should be protected with a cuffed endotracheal tube or at least, functioning suctioning apparatus should be available.

Some reports exist suggesting the garment may contribute to compartment syndromes in the legs. With this in mind, the garment should be inflated to the lowest possible pressure necessary to stabilize the patient's blood pressure. Similarly, the garment should not be worn any longer than is absolutely necessary.

As stated above, the only absolute contraindication to the use of the garment is the presence of pulmonary edema. In such patients, the increase in both pre-load and afterload is seriously detrimental to cardiac function and potentially lethal.

NITROUS OXIDE/OXYGEN INHALATION ANALGESIA

Indications

Short-term self-administered inhalation analgesia.

Clinical Uses.

This is particularly of value in the prehospital and emergency department settings for pain relief from orthopedic injuries to allow for manipulation and/or examination. In addition, some patients with other forms of abdominal or chest pain may benefit from inhalation analgesia. A final and important clinical use is for the patient in labor. Considerable experience exists, particularly in the United Kingdom, with the use of self-administered nitrous oxide for patients in active labor.

Because nitrous oxide comes out of solution much more readily than other gases, its use in clinical situations where gas exists in a closed space is contraindicated. Hence, it should not be used where there is a potential for pneumothorax, bowel obstruction, venous air embolism, etc.

Equipment

Two varieties of appropriate nitrous oxide oxygen equipment exist. Each involves the use of a demand-valve mask, such that gas only flows when the patient applies the mask to the face, producing a negative seal. One system involves the use of a cylinder of premixed 50% oxygen and 50% nitrous oxide. The other system involves a cylinder of each gas fed through a regulator valve to ensure a constant 50-50 mixture.

Method

If the gas is self-administered, the patient should be instructed prior to its use. In particular, the patient should be told to expect some mild nausea, giddiness, etc.

The valve or valves of the cylinders are turned on. The mask is tested to ensure appropriate flow of the gas. The patient then applies the mask directly over the nose and face. The patient must apply some pressure to ensure a good seal and then should be encouraged to take deep

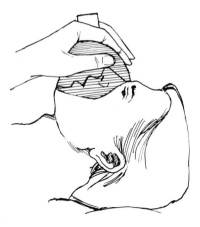

Fig. 5–45. Nitrous oxide/oxygen inhalation analgesia (self-administered via demand-valve mask).

breaths so as to create enough negative pressure to result in gas flow (Fig. 5–45).

Precautions

As noted above, the use of nitrous oxide in patients with closed space gas can result in rapid expansion of the gas in the closed space. This can occur after only one or two inspirations and hence the gas should not be used in any patient with potential chest trauma, abdominal pain NYD, vomiting, bowel obstruction or gastric distention, etc.

With the gas, most patients experience some mild nausea, dizziness, light-headedness, and euphoria. Appropriate functioning suction apparatus should be available in case the patient vomits. A few patients are particularly sensitive to nitrous oxide and may become unconscious with the use of the gas. Because the gas is self-administered, the hand simply falls away and the flow of gas ceases. For this reason, the gas should always be self-administered, and the mask should not be held on by another person.

The premixed cylinders of 50% oxygen and 50% nitrous oxide should not be used or stored for extended periods of time in cold climates. The gases tend to separate at cold temperatures (i.e., below 0°C). As a consequence, the administration of high concentrations of nitrous oxide may result. If the cylinder has been stored for an extended period of time or has been exposed to a cold climate, it should be inverted three or four times to ensure mixture prior to use.

6
Ear, Nose, and Throat

J.M. Nedzelski

USE OF HEAD MIRROR

The small orifices of the head and neck cannot be properly examined or treated without adequate illumination. A hand held light source is useful for making a diagnosis (e.g., foreign body), but it frequently precludes these objectives. Excellent fiberoptic source lights mounted on a head band are also available and virtually no practice is required to successfully illuminate the area under study. Unfortunately these are expensive and therefore not commonly found in the average practitioner's office. The head mirror as a light source, however, is inexpensive and portable, and if the following principles are followed, successful use of a head mirror can easily be achieved.

Position the mirror such that the back of it almost touches the forehead and cheek (Fig. 6–1). Ensure that a bright light source (i.e., naked light bulb) is beside and slightly behind the patient who is seated facing you. The light is on the examiner's "mirror-eye" side, (Fig. 6–2). Do not move your head to position the light, rather move the patient's head. *Note:* the light source is fixed.

EAR

Cerumen/Foreign Body Removal

Adult patients present with a complaint of aural fullness, slight hearing loss, and rarely, distinct discomfort or vague balance-related symptoms. Typically with an impacted foreign body, a child will have no specific complaint initially but may be distressed as a result of attempted object removal by a family member or ill-prepared medical personnel. Otoscopy readily reveals a plug of cerumen or the lateral edge of a foreign body. Before treatment is initiated, inquire whether the child has, or has had, a history of tympanic membrane perforation or otorrhea.

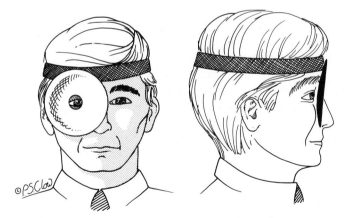

Fig. 6–1. The head mirror.

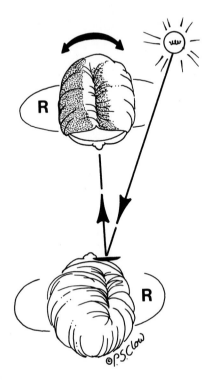

Fig. 6–2. Positioning the light source.

Precaution

If tympanic membrane perforation is suspected, irrigation is not to be used because of the possibility of causing an otitis media.

Equipment

Otoscope
Irrigating syringe
Plastic drape for protecting patient

K-basin for collecting irrigating fluid. This should be held
  below the external auditory meatus
Head mirror
Fine forceps (alligator, Hartmann)
Right-angled hook

Method

Cerumen Removal

Pull pinna posterosuperiorly to straighten cartilaginous
canal (lateral one third of external auditory canal) (Fig. 6–3).
With the other hand, direct the nozzle of the irrigating
syringe along the posterior cartilaginous wall to be sure
that the stream of water enters the canal, but at the same
time, make sure that the canal is not blocked by the nozzle.

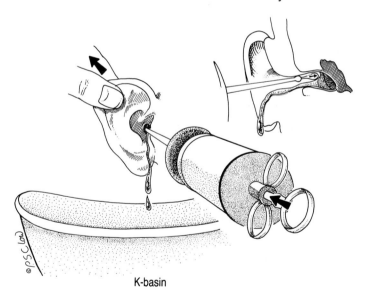

K-basin

Fig. 6–3. Cerumen removal.

This allows the return stream of water to escape from the canal without significantly increasing pressure against the tympanum. For patient comfort, it is helpful to first gently direct the water at the entrance of the external canal, and ask the patient if the temperature is comfortable. Irrigation may then proceed.

Irrigate briskly and repeatedly until cerumen floats free and out of the meatus. Mop the ear and inspect to ensure that all cerumen is removed and water drained. If the cerumen is extremely hard, and despite repeated efforts removal is unsuccessful, or if the patient becomes uncomfortable, *stop* irrigation. Advise the patient to insert baby oil or olive oil with an eyedropper twice daily to soften cerumen and suggest a repeat visit in one week when the attempt to remove cerumen should be repeated.

Foreign Body Removal

If patient is a child, it is imperative that he/she be properly restrained prior to attempted removal to prevent displacing the object medially through the tympanic membrane or lacerating the skin of the ear canal wall.

If the object is a live insect, drown it using mineral oil then irrigate as for cerumen removal.

If patient is a child, place him/her supine, and restrain the head. If on otoscopy the object appears irregular, removal may be effected by use of forceps. Use an aural speculum that is of the largest diameter that can be comfortably accommodated by the meatus. Carefully grasp the edge of the object with forceps and gently withdraw.

If the object is spherical and fills canal lumen or is organic (i.e., a pea), irrigation is definitely contraindicated. Removal is effected by use of a right-angled hook under direct vision (Fig. 6–4A). The right-angled pick is slid parallel to the skin of the floor and under the edge of the foreign body, turned 90° to impale the object (Fig. 6–4B) and then

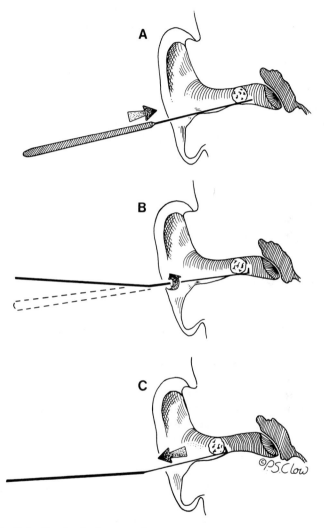

Fig. 6–4. Foreign body removal.

pulled gently laterally in an effort to dislodge (Fig. 6–4C). The maneuver is repeated, if necessary.

If, in spite of best effort, the foreign body has migrated medially beyond the cartilaginous-bony junction, or the child cannot be properly immobilized, stop the procedure. Patient referral is recommended, or attempt the procedure with the child anesthetized.

Severe Otitis Externa

Presentation

Patient presents with excruciating pain in the ear, exacerbated by any manipulation of the tragus or cartilaginous meatus. Frequently, the condition is associated with a history of ear manipulation (e.g., cotton swab) or swimming. Examination reveals marked edema of the meatus walls such that the lumen of the canal is completely or almost completely obliterated.

Equipment

Head mirror
Aural speculum
Suction (No. 5 ear suction) or fine cotton wipes (self-made)
$\frac{1}{4}$ inch iodoform strip-gauze packing approximately 6-cm long, cut along length to achieve $\frac{1}{8}$ inch width
1:20 aluminum acetate (Burrow's solution)

Method

If pain is severe, administer analgesia (i.e., meperidine or morphine) prior to initiating treatment. Under direct vision using the head mirror, aspirate or dry wipe exudate or debris from skin of lumen. Soak entire length of $\frac{1}{8}$ inch gauze in aluminum acetate solution and gently insert into narrowed lumen of external auditory meatus using bayonet forceps (Fig. 6–5). Instruct the patient to instill aluminum acetate solution drops (4 or 5) on the end of the wick every 4 hours. Remove wick in 36 to 48 hours. Dry wipe canal wall skin under direct vision. If the tympanic membrane is visible, discontinue wick and start on an antibiotic ear drop solution. If the tympanic membrane is not visible due to continued canal wall skin edema, reinsert a similar wick and review in 36 to 48 hours.

Myringotomy

Clinical Uses

Relief of severe pain associated with a closed space infection (middle ear) due to suppurative otitis media. Because of modern antibiotics, this procedure is not often necessary.

Equipment

Aural speculum
Head mirror or otoscope
Myringotomy knife
Bonain's solution (cocaine anesthetic mixture): Equal parts of cocaine hydrochloride, phenol, and menthol are mixed, grinding the crystals together to form a liquid mixture. This can be used as a local, topical anesthetic for the tympanum.

Method

The injection of a local anesthetic to obtain appropriate analgesia is generally as painful or more so than a quickly carried out myringotomy using a sharp knife. If analgesia is used, a small pledget of cotton soaked in Bonain's solution and placed onto the anterior tympanic membrane is adequate. This is left in place for 5 minutes and then removed. If the patient is a child, ensure that the head is

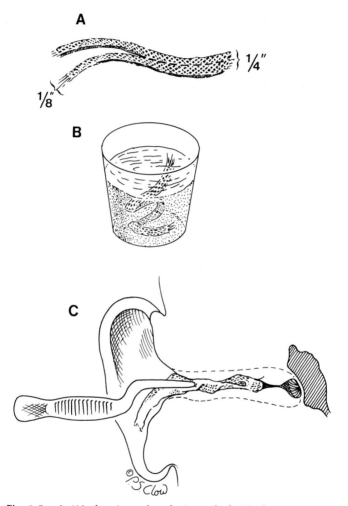

Fig. 6–5.   A. ¼ inch strip cut lengthwise to form ⅛ inch strip.
B. ⅛ inch gauze strip is soaked in aluminum acetate solution
C. ⅛ inch gauze strip, impregnated with aluminum acetate solution, gently inserted into external auditory meatus.

restrained. Perform myringotomy by a rapid thrust of the knife through the tympanic membrane (Fig. 6–6).

Precaution

Always perform myringotomy in the mid portion of the anterior one half of the tympanic membrane to prevent possible damage to the ossicles (posterior one half).

Hematoma of Auricle

Clinical Presentation

Swelling and obvious deformity of the pinna as a result of direct trauma. Aspiration is carried out to prevent subsequent development of an abscess as well as deformity of the pinna.

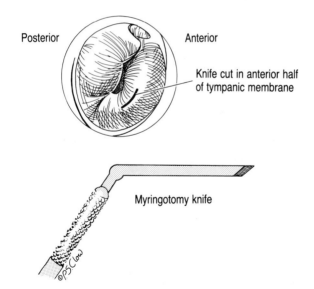

Fig. 6–6. Right tympanic membrane seen through otoscope.

Equipment

> One 2-ml syringe with ½-inch 27- or 25-gauge needle for local anesthetic
> One 5-ml syringe with 1-inch 18- or 20-gauge needle for aspiration
> Local anesthetic: 1% lidocaine with 1:200,000 epinephrine
> 4 × 4 inch surgical gauzes, iodoform strip gauze (½ inch)
> Cling or non elastic rolled gauze
> One red rubber catheter (No. 14) or equivalent
> 00 Nylon suture

Method

Under sterile conditions, the skin overlying the hematoma is infiltrated with local anesthetic. The aspirating needle (No. 18 or No. 20) is inserted and the hematoma aspirated (Fig. 6–7A).

If blood is clotted, use a scalpel and incise overlying skin and evacuate. Cut catheter into four or six pieces measuring approximately 1½ to 2 inches long (3 to 5 cm). Thread nylon suture through these and suture through skin of pinna such that one piece is applied to the front and another to the back of pinna. This is the most effective method to prevent hematoma reaccumulation (Fig. 6–7B).

A 4 × 4-inch gauze is placed behind the ear to provide a comfortable bed, and several 4 × 4 surgical gauzes are fluffed and placed over the pinna (Fig. 6–7C, D). The plain dressing is then wrapped around the head from the base of the occiput to the forehead to provide a pressure dressing (Fig. 6–7E). The dressing is removed 24 to 36 hours later to ensure that the hematoma has not reaccumulated. A similar dressing is reapplied for a further 48 to 72 hours.

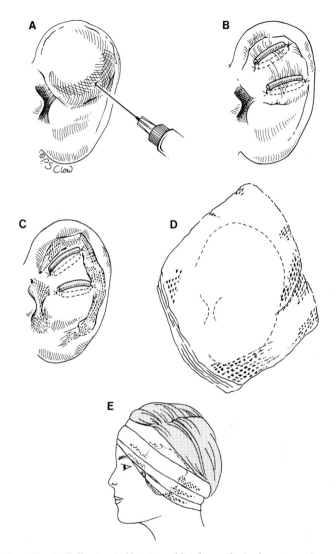

Fig. 6–7. **A.** Following infiltration of local anesthetic, hematoma is aspirated. **B.** Prevention of hematoma reaccumulation is achieved by threading nylon suture through pieces of catheter and suturing each pair through the pinna, thus providing local compression or tourniquet-effect. **C.** Positioning several pieces of fluffed gauze behind and over the pinna maintains it comfortably in its normal position. **D.** The final 4 × 4 inch gauze over the protected and supported pinna. **E.** Method of wrapping and bandaging head to stabilize bandage on pinna.

243

NOSE

Control of Epistaxis

Anterior Epistaxis

Clinical Presentation

In the majority of instances (greater than 80%), the bleeding site is anterior. This is generally from the nasal septum (Little's area or Kiesselbach's plexus) as a result of local dryness leading to ulceration (Fig. 6–8).

Equipment

Head mirror (head light)
Nasal suction
Cotton wipes
Topical decongestant-anesthetic (5% cocaine solution ideal)
$\frac{1}{4}$ inch petrolatum gauze strip
Surgicel
Silver nitrate cautery stick

Method

Have the patient sit up and lean forward to reduce venous pressure in the head and to prevent swallowing of an inordinate amount of blood. A small pledget of cotton moistened with 5% cocaine (well wrung out) is placed into each nasal fossa ensuring good contact with the nasal septum. The anterior cartilaginous nose is then compressed for 5 to 10 minutes (Fig. 6–9).

The cotton is removed and, if bleeding is stopped and the site of bleeding identified, silver nitrate cautery is judiciously applied along the length of responsible blood vessel (Fig. 6–10). It is important not to paint silver nitrate onto the nasal mucosa. Insert a small 1 × 1 cm-square of

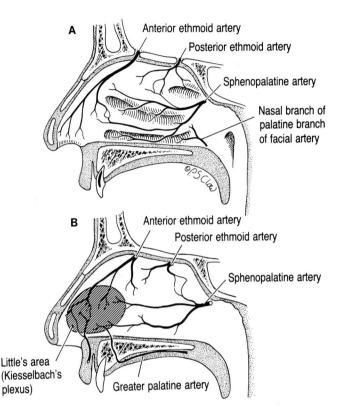

Fig. 6–8. **A.** Arteries to lateral wall. **B.** Arteries to septum.

Surgicel over the suspected site. Recommend the use of humidification as well as twice daily applications of petrolatum into the nasal fossae to reduce dryness.

If bleeding is brisk in spite of the preceding method, the patient requires insertion of an intranasal pack. Insert ¼-inch petrolatum-impregnated gauze strips; pack in layers beginning inferiorly, ensuring that the end of the strip is in the anterior portion of the floor of the nose (to prevent

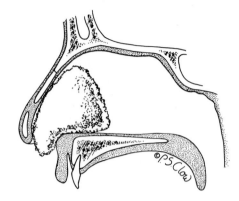

Fig. 6–9. Treated cotton is placed in each nasal fossa.

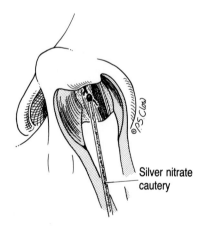

Silver nitrate
cautery

Fig. 6–10. Application of silver nitrate cautery.

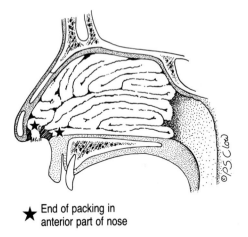

★ End of packing in
anterior part of nose

Fig. 6–11. Insertion of petrolatum saturated gauze.

this from falling into the nasopharynx), and pack firmly.
Pack side of bleeding site first, then pack contralateral side
slightly less firmly (to stabilize cartilaginous septum) (Fig.
6–11).

Precautions

Advise the patient to limit activities at home. Mild sedation is also advisable. Remove the packing in 36 to 48
hours. Recommend humidification and the intranasal insertion of petrolatum twice daily for 1 week as a moistening
agent.

Posterior Epistaxis

Clinical Presentation

If in spite of firm anterior nasal packing, the patient continues to bleed briskly into the nasopharynx, consider the
bleeding site to be posterior.

Equipment

In addition to the preceding, several 15-ml Foley catheters (No. 14) or manufactured posterior gauze packs are required.

Method

Cut tip off the Foley catheter just distal to the balloon cuff. Administer meperidine or morphine. Remove anterior nasal packs. Advance the catheter tip into the nasal fossa on bleeding side until the balloon is visible in the nasopharynx. Inflate 5 to 10 ml of air into ballon; pull back and hold firmly. Insert anterior packing as described previously. Ensure that the anterior pack insertion is such that the catheter is not pressed against the septum or lateral wall of the nasal fossa (Fig. 6–12). Anchor the catheter at the nasal vestibule using gauze as illustrated. The catheter

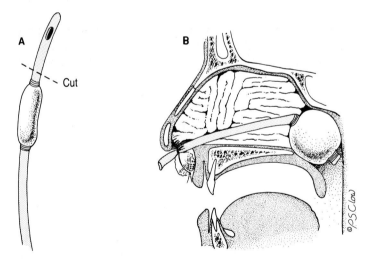

Fig. 6–12. **A.** Cut tip off of Foley catheter just distal to balloon cuff. **B.** Balloon visible in nasopharynx.

must not be applied against the skin of the nasal vestibule or nostril; this will lead to pressure necrosis.

Insert anterior packing *only* on the opposite side. Admit the patient to a hospital, and ensure that the hemoglobin and hematocrit are within normal limits. Type, cross-match, and administer blood as required. Remove packing only after the bleeding has stopped for at least 24 hours. Administer penicillin if posterior packing is used as this generally means the nose is to be packed for at least 48 to 72 hours. If bleeding is not stopped after firm anterior and posterior packing has been inserted, consultation is recommended.

Unfortunately, Foley catheters have a tendency to deflate after 24 to 36 hours. If bleeding recurs, a posterior nasal pack fashioned from a gauze square is recommended (Fig. 6–13). This is inserted into the nasopharynx using a catheter passed through the nose and pulled out the mouth (Fig. 6–14A). The strings attached are pulled firmly forward with the index finger of the opposite hand, positioning the gauze bolus into the nasopharynx (Fig. 6–14B). The anterior packing is inserted as previously described. The strings attached to the posterior gauze pack are tied over a gauze bolus (Fig. 6–15).

Septal Hematoma

Clinical Presentation

Following a blow to the nose, the patient presents with near total bilateral nasal airway obstruction. Remember: a nasal fracture never causes near total bilateral nasal airway obstruction. Examination reveals marked widening of the nasal septum with bulging of the mucosa into each nasal vault. Drainage of the hematoma prevents possible development of an abscess or ischemic necrosis of cartilage (saddle nose deformity).

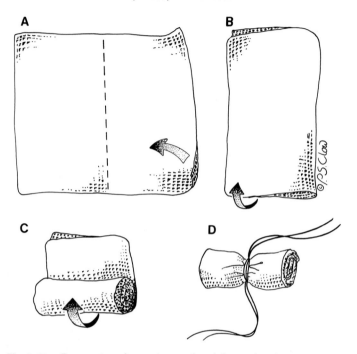

Fig. 6–13. Preparation of posterior nasal pack from a 4 × 4 gauze square.
A. 4 × 4 inch gauze square. **B.** Doubled over to make a 4 × 2 inch square.
C. Roll the doubled gauze. **D.** The roll of gauze is tied with string, leaving
the ends about a foot long.

Equipment

One 2-ml syringe with ½ inch 25- or 27-gauge needle
Local anesthetic (1.0% lidocaine); topical anesthetic (5%
cocaine)
Cotton strips, ¼ inch petrolatum impregnated gauze
packing
Bayonet forceps
Scalpel handle with No. 15 blade   (continued)

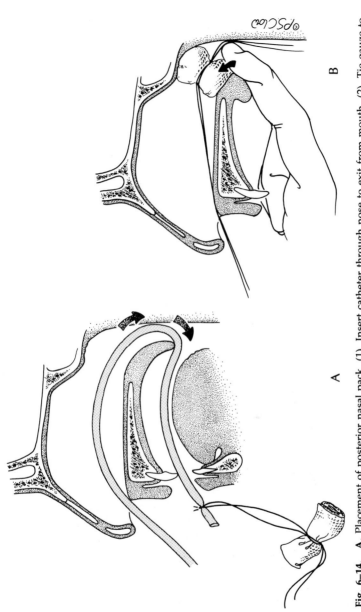

Fig. 6–14. **A.** Placement of posterior nasal pack. (1). Insert catheter through nose to exit from mouth. (2). Tie gauze to catheter to form a posterior pack. **B.** Pulling nasal catheter from nose places gauze in posterior nasal area.

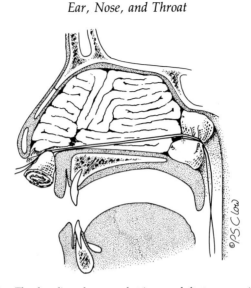

Fig. 6–15. The dangling pharyngeal strings are left at a convenient length for grasping for subsequent removal but not too long as to cause gagging.

Nasal suction
¼ inch Penrose drain or equivalent (e.g., elastic band)

Method

The nasal mucosa is topically anesthetized using cotton strips moistened with 5% cocaine (well wrung out). Then palpate septal hematoma with the end of the bayonet forceps to determine which side of the septum contains the hematoma (fluctuant), and which side is the displaced cartilage (Fig. 6–16A).

Infiltrate the septal mucosa on the hematoma side with local anesthetic. Using a scalpel, incise the mucosa vertically a distance of 1 cm. Aspirate or express hematoma, collapsing the mucosa onto the cartilage of the septum (Fig. 6–16B). Insert Penrose drain a distance of 3 to 5 cm (Fig. 6–16C).

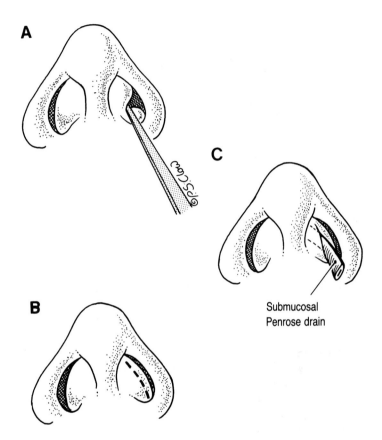

Fig. 6–16. **A.** Side with hematoma fluctuates when tested with bayonet forceps. **B.** Mucosal incision of 1 cm. **C.** Insert Penrose drain a distance of 3 to 5 cm.

Apply firm anterior nasal packing as described for control of anterior epistaxis. Pack the opposite nasal vault for purposes of counter pressure. Remove packs in 72 hours. Inspect to ensure that the hematoma has not reaccumulated.

Precautions

If the hematoma is of some duration, the blood may be coagulated and a longer incision required in order to evacuate the clot. Remember that an unrecognized hematoma which becomes an abscess is a potential life-threatening condition by virtue of drainage to the cavernous sinus.

Nasal Fracture

Clinical Presentation

Undisplaced fractures on clinical examination do not require reduction. Significant displaced fractures can be reduced in adults up to 7 to 10 days after injury versus 3 to 5 days in children.

Equipment

Cotton strips, 5% cocaine
2-ml syringe with ½ inch needle (25- or 27-gauge)
Local anesthetic
Blunt nasal elevator (i.e., Howarth)

Method

In children, reduction of nasal fracture requires a general anesthetic. In adults, premedication with meperidine or morphine may be sufficient. Intranasal anesthesia is obtained using cotton strips moistened with 5% cocaine. The root of the nose and lateral margin of nose are infiltrated with local anesthetic (Fig. 6–17A.)

A blunt nasal elevator is inserted medial to displaced nasal bone (Fig. 6–17B). Upward and lateral motions are

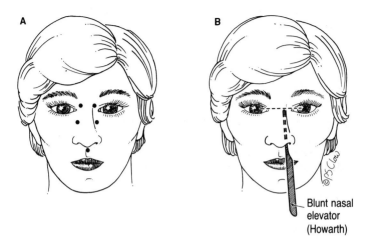

Fig. 6–17. **A.** Sites of infiltration with local anesthetic. **B.** Insertion of blunt nasal elevator.

carried out to dislodge bone. In the case of medial displacement of bone, this method usually results in satisfactory realignment. In instances of laterally displaced bone, reposition can be achieved by medial pressure using finger tips. If the fracture feels unstable, gently insert a small amount of intranasal iodoform gauze-strip packing under the bone for 2 days. If the fracture is more complex, i.e., involving torn nasal cartilages or the root of nose (nasal-frontal-ethmoid complex), immediate referral should be made.

Foreign Bodies

Clinical Presentation

Unilateral mucopurulent rhinorrhea in a child should always raise suspicion of the presence of a foreign body.

Equipment

  Head light
  Nasal speculum
  5% cocaine, cotton strips
  Right-angled hook
  Forceps (alligator or bayonet)

Method

Restrain child; apply local anesthetic using cotton strips moistened with 5% cocaine. Insert nasal speculum to visualize foreign body. If the object is irregular, grasp it with bayonet forceps and carefully remove (Fig. 6–18). If the object is smooth, use a right-angled hook, first passing the hook parallel to the floor of nose distal to the object. Turn

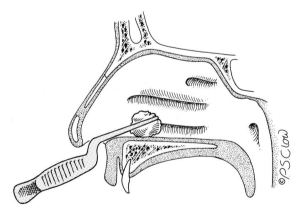

Fig. 6–18. Bayonet forceps used to grasp irregular foreign body.

the hook 90° and withdraw it such that the object is delivered into the anterior portion of the nose. If the child is cooperative, blowing the nose may deliver the object. If the foreign body is impaled into the posterior half of the nose and the child is uncooperative, general anesthesia is required for removal.

THROAT

Incision and Drainage of Peritonsillar Abscess (Quinsy)

Clinical Presentation

Severe sore throat, marked odynophagia, inability to fully open the mouth (trismus) as well as systemic upset. Examination reveals marked asymmetry of the tonsils, with the involved tonsil displaced medially and downward. There is definite swelling of the soft palate on the suspected abscess side, with displacement of the palate and uvula to the opposite side. In some instances, palpation will demonstrate fluctuation.

Equipment

Light source
Metal tongue depressor
Topical anesthetic (lidocaine spray)
2-ml syringe with ½ inch 25- or 28-gauge needle for local anesthetic (lidocaine)
No. 11 or No. 15 scalpel blade on a knife handle
Small curved hemostat
Meperidine or morphine
Suction equipment

Method

Have the patient sit up and lean forward. Premedicate with meperidine or morphine. Topically anesthetize throat using lidocaine spray. Infiltrate the upper lateral aspect with local anesthetic. Tape No. 11 blade or No. 15 blade such that only ¼ inch of tip is uncovered (Fig. 6–19A).

Incise area of pouting mucosa or fluctuance. If none is

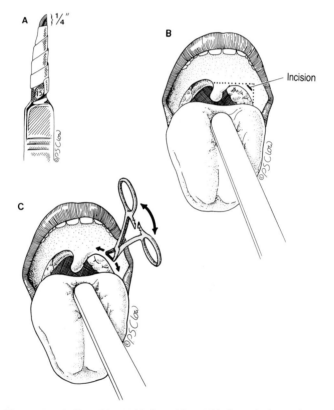

Fig. 6–19. **A.** Tape No. 11 blade or No. 15 blade such that only ¼ inch of tip is uncovered. **B.** Incise area of pouting mucosa or fluctuance. **C.** Insert closed hemostat. See text for more information.

noted, incise the soft palate at the upper pole of the tonsil directly above the anterior pillar and at the height of a line drawn horizontally through the root of the uvula (Fig. 6–19B). Have suction ready and use as needed.

Insert closed hemostat and spread in lateral and backward direction to get into the peritonsillar abscess cavity rather than into the substance of the tonsil (Fig. 6–19C).

Indirect Laryngoscopy

Indications

To examine for possible foreign body, i.e. fishbone, or visualize the larynx or hypopharynx in the instance of suspected associated neoplasm. *Never attempt indirect laryngoscopy if the patient has stridor.*

Equipment

  Head mirror
  Laryngeal mirror
  Gauze squares
  Topical lidocaine spray
  Heat source (hot water, light bulb)
  Forceps

Method

Anesthetize the posterior pharyngeal wall with topical lidocaine. Hold the protruding tongue tip with gauze, support the upper lip, have the patient breathe quietly through the mouth, and elevate the uvula with the back of the warmed mirror (Fig. 6–20A). Inspect the base of the tongue, epiglottis, arytenoids, vocal cords, and pyriform fossa. A foreign body such as a fishbone is frequently impaled in the base of the tongue (Fig. 6–20B).

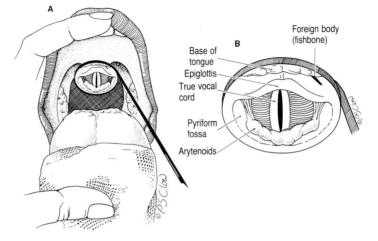

Fig. 6–20. **A.** Elevate the uvula with the back of a warmed mirror. **B.** Foreign bodies frequently lodge at the base of the tongue.

Precaution

It is important that the patient's head be stabilized or steadied for this procedure.

When holding the tongue with gauze, try not to hold the tongue too far downward or the lower teeth will cause pain as they impale the inferior surface of the protruding tongue.

The mirror should be warmed enough to prevent condensation of breath moisture, but not so hot that it burns the soft palate.

EAR PIERCING

Equipment

    2-ml syringe with 25- or 27-gauge needle

    Local anesthetic (1% lidocaine; 1:200,000 epinephrine)

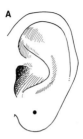

Mark desired position of earring

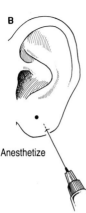

Anesthetize

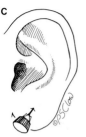

Pierce with 18-gauge needle and insert keeper

Fig. 6–21. Ear piercing.

No. 18 gauge needle
Alcohol swabs

Method

Ask the patient where the hole is to be made. Using a ballpoint pen, mark the proposed site of earring position. Check that both sides are at the same height.

Alcohol wipe both sides of lobule. Infiltrate site of proposed hole. Pass No. 18 gauge needle through lobule followed by the earring keeper. Advise the patient to keep the site clean with a daily alcohol wipe, suggest that keeper be turned daily. Earrings may be inserted in 2 weeks (Fig. 6–21A, B, and C).

$\overline{7}$
Gastroenterology

T.F. Shapero

PROCTOSCOPY

Indications

Hemorrhoids (piles), rectal bleeding, change in bowel habit, pain or difficulty in defecation, and anal lesions (fistula, pruritus).

Proctoscopy of the anorectal area in no way replaces sigmoidoscopy, but it is a simple office procedure for suitable cases of presumed local pathology, and may be done without preparation of the bowel.

Method

Following a rectal examination and with the patient in the left lateral position (Fig. 7–1), the buttocks are separated and the perianal area inspected.

The proctoscope, with obturator in place, is well lubricated and gently passed into the rectum; the instrument is pointed toward the umbilicus, thus lining it up with the

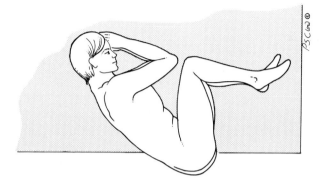

Fig. 7–1. Left lateral position.

anal canal. When the instrument has been fully inserted, the obturator is removed. Careful inspection is then made as the instrument is gently withdrawn, noting any local lesions such as hemorrhoids.

Precautions

Anal stenosis or severe pain on rectal digital examination dictates extreme caution when performing proctoscopy or sigmoidoscopy. Application of a topical anesthetic jelly may permit an otherwise unbearable examination.

SIGMOIDOSCOPY

Rigid Sigmoidoscopy

Rigid sigmoidoscopy provides a rapid and inexpensive assessment of the distal colon in patients with bowel-related complaints or in routine screening for bowel cancer. When disease of the colon is suspected, rigid sigmoidoscopy should be complemented by barium enema.

Indications

Rectal bleeding, anorectal symptoms such as tenesmus, fecal incontinence, and perianal pain; change in bowel habit (diarrhea or constipation). Surveillance for bowel neoplasia, especially in patients with previous colonic neoplasia, or in those with a strong family history of bowel cancer, or in inherited polyposis syndrome, or in screening patients with stool tests positive for occult blood. It is also used for evaluation and follow-up of inflammatory bowel disease.

Equipment

Sigmoidoscope (includes light source, barrel, obturator, and insufflation bellows)
Long swabs
Examining gloves
Lubricant
Source of electric current

Method

Preparation of the Patient. The lower bowel is often satisfactorily cleansed by advising a laxative the evening before and avoiding a solid breakfast on the morning of the procedure. A phosphate enema, administered shortly before the procedure, is usually adequate to enable good visualization of the rectum. Some physicians believe that insertion of a special rectal suppository such as bisacodyl (Dulcolax) 1 hour before the procedure is also a satisfactory preparation. If a barium enema is planned as part of the current investigation, the sigmoidoscopy may be done just prior to the radiograph, thus taking advantage of the already prepared bowel. If inflammatory disease is suspected, however, bowel preparation is unnecessary and may cause sufficient irritation to create the erroneous impression of inflammation at the time of sigmoidoscopy.

Take time to explain the procedure to the patient. Reassure him that the procedure, while uncomfortable, should not be painful. If pain is experienced, the procedure should be stopped or adjusted to relieve the pain.

Preparation of the Equipment and Setting. Check the function of the light bulb, air bag, and suction before the patient is placed in an uncomfortable position. Also prior to the procedure, lubricate the sigmoidoscope and place long swabs close by. A nurse or assistant nearby can be helpful to the operator and also serve to reassure an anxious patient.

Place the patient in the knee-chest position with the feet

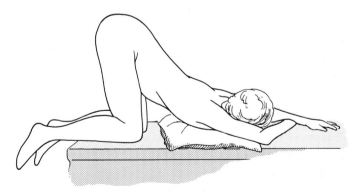

Fig. 7–2. Knee-chest position.

over the dropped end of the examining table (Fig. 7–2), with the head and shoulders comfortably settled into a large pillow. Frail patients should be examined in the left lateral position, although this posture decreases the likelihood of entering the sigmoid. Do a digital rectal examination to exclude palpable pathology, to check that the rectum is suitably prepared, and to note the direction of the long axis of the rectum along which you will blindly insert the sigmoidoscope. Digital examination will also serve to add extra lubricant to the anal margin prior to insertion of the instrument. Remove the examining glove.

Insert the sigmoidoscope, with its obturator in place, into the rectum. As this is done, keep thumb pressure on the distal end of the obturator. Otherwise the distal, sharp, and unprotected end of the instrument would be pushed blindly into the rectum. When gentle resistance occurs (at approximately 10 cm), remove the obturator.

With the lens cover closed, identify the lumen of the rectum. The sigmoidoscope should only be advanced under direct vision. Insufflation of a small amount of air by squeezing the attached bulb may be useful in locating the lumen. Use as little air as possible. If air is used several times, open the lens cover occasionally to allow decompression of the uncomfortably distended bowel.

After an initial anteriorly-directed segment, the rectum turns posteriorly following the curve of the sacrum. The examiner must, therefore, direct the external end of the sigmoidoscope anteriorly to permit the distal end to follow the posterior curve (Fig. 7–3). Three crescentic folds of mucosa (valves of Houston) will be encountered en route to the rectosigmoid junction (Fig. 7–4). The proximal aspect of these folds should be carefully examined to avoid missing hidden lesions.

At the rectosigmoid junction, encountered approximately 15 cm from the anus, the lumen bends sharply

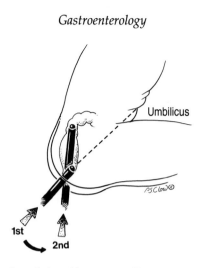

Fig. 7–3. Insertion of sigmoidoscope.

anteriorly and usually laterally to either side. Negotiation of this angulation may be difficult. Undue pressure exerted in an attempt to enter the sigmoid colon may produce considerable pain. Insufflation of a small amount of air may assist passage of the instrument at this point, but excess distention is uncomfortable and should be avoided. When the sigmoid is not entered with relative ease, it is unwise to persist because of the resulting marked discomfort and the risk of bowel perforation. If significant pain occurs, the instrument should be withdrawn until relief of pain is reported.

Assessment of the mucosa includes evaluation of the reflectivity (shininess) of the surface, the vascular pattern, and mucosal friability. Inflammation causes the lining to become finely irregular (granularity), resulting in a reduced reflection of light and a relatively dull appearance. Similarly, inflammatory processes obscure the submucosal vessels, which normally are clearly seen in an arborescent pattern. Friability of the mucosa, manifested as punctate

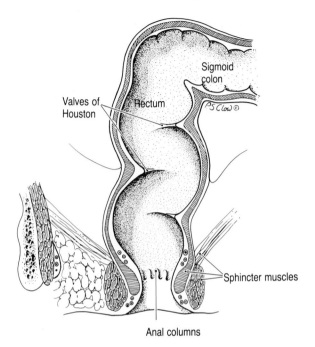

Fig. 7–4. Anatomy of the rectum.

bleeding on swabbing the surface, is a further sign of inflammation.

The bowel should be carefully inspected during withdrawal of the sigmoidoscope, since lesions may be missed during insertion. Particular attention should be paid to the distal rectum and anal canal, which are not generally visualized during introduction of the instrument. The presence of hemorrhoids or anal fissure should be noted. The sigmoidoscope is then removed. If the distal rectum and anal canal are not adequately visualized, such examination may be easier with the proctoscope.

Flexible Fiberoptic Sigmoidoscopy (FFS)

FFS, in comparison with rigid sigmoidoscopy, has the advantage of visualizing the colon to the splenic flexure. The detection rate in screening for colonic neoplasia is two to six times that of the rigid examination. FFS is considerably more expensive, more time consuming, and is not a substitute for total colonoscopy, which is mandatory whenever a neoplasm of the colon is detected. It is not recommended that FFS be attempted without familiarity with fiberoptic instruments and instruction from an experienced endoscopist.

Indications

Same as for the rigid sigmoidoscopy.

Equipment

Fiberoptic sigmoidoscope
Light source
Suction apparatus
Biopsy forceps
Examining gloves
Water soluble lubricating jelly

Method

The nature of the procedure, including the possibility of discomfort, should be explained to the patient.

The patient is prepared with one or two phosphate enemas. This regimen permits visualization proximal to the sigmoid in the majority of patients. With the patient in the left lateral position, a digital rectal examination is performed. If substantial amounts of formed stool are palpable, the preparation has been unsatisfactory and should be repeated.

After the light source and the air and suction channels

have been tested, the well-lubricated tip of the instrument is inserted through the anus with the gloved right hand. Thereafter, the endoscopist may advance the sigmoidoscope and rotate the directional cables himself, or may require an assistant to advance the instrument as he steers. After insertion into the rectum, the sigmoidoscope must usually be withdrawn slightly to identify the lumen. The instrument is advanced only when the direction of the passage is evident. Blindly pushing the sigmoidoscope leads to discomfort and to increased risk of perforation.

Frequently, the endoscope assumes a loop configuration, and introducing more of the instrument only increases the size of the loop without advancing the tip (Fig. 7–5). In this case, reducing the loop by withdrawing several centimeters may permit further progress. The instrument should be withdrawn as long as the tip is endoscopically

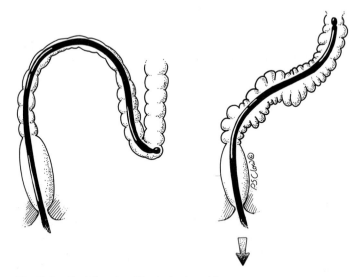

Fig. 7–5. Straightening fiberoptic sigmoidoscope.

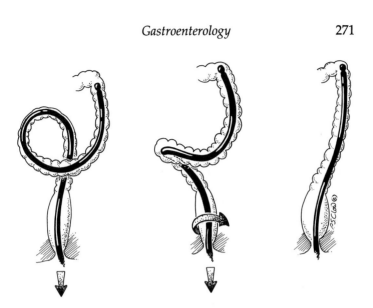

Fig. 7–6. Fiberoptic sigmoidoscopy reduction of sigmoid loop.

seen to remain at the same position. When the tip begins to withdraw, the instrument has likely assumed a satisfactory configuration. Sometimes, the reduction of the loop is assisted by rotating the instrument in a clockwise direction during withdrawal (Fig. 7–6). At other times, rotation of the endoscope can be useful to identify the lumen around sharp curvatures.

If pathology is encountered, biopsies can be taken with a biopsy forceps accessory. This requires an assistant, fixative solution, and access to a pathology laboratory. The location of any abnormality should be noted (distance from the anus). Endoscopes have centimeter markers on the exterior to indicate the length of instrument inserted. During insertion of the endoscope, stretching and looping of the bowel may produce an overestimate of the length of bowel traversed. It is preferable, therefore, to estimate distances during withdrawal, when the instrument is straighter. If a stricturing lesion is present, it is unwise to try to traverse the stricture unless the residual luminal diameter is clearly adequate to accommodate the instrument.

During insertion of the endoscope, the lumen is gently distended with air to facilitate passage. Liquid or semi-liquid stool or mucus can be aspirated through the suction channel. It is unwise to try to aspirate solid material. The usual result is blockage of the suction channel or soiling of the lens.

When the instrument has been inserted as far as possible, it is slowly withdrawn. The bowel should be carefully inspected during withdrawal as well as during insertion, since some areas of the bowel are better seen when traveling in one or the other direction. When withdrawing the instrument, some of the insufflated air should be removed.

DIAGNOSTIC PARACENTESIS

Indications

Ascites without a well-established diagnosis or an unexpected change in status of a patient with ascites of known etiology.

Clinical Uses

Aid to diagnosis of the etiology of ascites or of superimposed infection or neoplasia.

Equipment

22-gauge, 1½ inch needle
Disinfectant
Specimen containers
Adhesive bandage

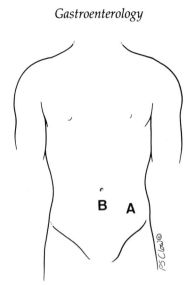

Fig. 7–7. Paracentesis puncture sites. **A.** Preferred site of diagnostic paracentesis. **B.** Preferred site of therapeutic paracentesis.

Method

The patient should be supine. If the volume of ascites is modest, he may be turned slightly toward the side of the intended puncture. Choose a site remote from palpable solid intra-abdominal organs, posterior to the level of dullness to percussion. The left lower quadrant is usually suitable (Fig. 7–7A)

Cleanse the area of puncture. There is no need for sterile drapes. Local anesthesia is unnecessary since its induction is no less uncomfortable than the procedure itself. Hold the syringe and needle in a dart-like fashion perpendicular to the skin. Advise the patient to anticipate a brief pin prick. With a quick jab, pass the needle into the peritoneal cavity.

Draw back on the syringe barrel to aspirate fluid. If none is forthcoming, advance the needle to the hub or angle the tip of the needle posteriorly. If this is unsuccessful, attempt to aspirate gently while slowly withdrawing the needle. If no fluid is obtained, the site should be abandoned and an alternative location selected.

The extracted ascitic fluid should be examined for cell count and white cell differential, malignant cells and organisms, and the content of amylase and protein. After removal of the needle, the site need be covered only with a plastic bandage. If ascites is suspected clinically but paracentesis fails, the presence of ascitic fluid can be assessed by an ultrasound examination.

THERAPEUTIC PARACENTESIS

Indications

Extreme abdominal discomfort, severely restricted mobility, or respiratory embarrassment arising from large amounts of ascitic fluid. This is often a recurrent problem when standard methods of diuresis are ineffective.

Precaution

This procedure should not be carried out if there is significant bowel distention or if there have been multiple previous abdominal operations. Cellulitis of the anterior abdominal wall is an absolute contraindication. Usually therapeutic paracentesis is done to make the patient more comfortable, so it would not be considered for an uncooperative or reluctant patient.

Equipment

Local anesthetic
10-ml syringe with 25-gauge needle
Trochar or plastic intravenous cannula (14 gauge)
Suitable agents for cleansing and sterilizing the skin

Mask and sterile gloves
Container to collect drained ascitic fluid

Method

Explain the procedure to the patient. Ask the patient to empty his bladder and then to lie relaxed in a supine position.

A site in the midline, some 2 to 5 cm below the umbilicus is chosen over the avascular linea alba (Fig. 7–7B). The skin is cleansed and locally infiltrated with a small amount of local anesthetic. When the anesthetic has taken effect, the trochar or plastic cannula is passed through the anterior abdominal wall. Entry into the peritoneum is felt by a give as this final resistance is passed.

Fluid should flow from the trochar or cannula, which is then connected to a suitable recipient container. The removal of two to three liters of fluid is well tolerated. Larger volumes have some risk of subsequent intravascular volume depletion as the ascites reaccumulates. If a patient requires repeated therapeutic paracentesis, consideration should be given to the insertion of a peritoneovenous shunt to provide more permanent relief.

After sufficient fluid has been removed, the trochar or cannula is removed and a firm, sterile gauze dressing is applied to cover the puncture site.

INSERTION OF NASOGASTRIC TUBE AND GASTRIC LAVAGE

Indications

Aspiration of gastric contents to prevent their entering the intestinal tract (e.g., gastrointestinal obstruction, selected cases of upper gastrointestinal bleeding).

Analysis of gastric contents for diagnostic purposes (e.g.,

assessment of gastric acid secretion, presence of blood, culture for mycobacteria tuberculosis).

Intragastric feeding.

Equipment

Standard nasogastric tube (No. 14 French usually adequate)

50-ml catheter-tip syringe

Cup of drinking water and a straw

Basin of ice

Water soluble lubricating jelly

Method

Cooling the tube in ice for a few minutes will render it stiffer and make it less likely to curl in the nasopharynx.

Insert the fenestrated end of the tube into either nostril and pass it through the internal nares into the nasopharynx. Continue to advance the tube through the pharynx, asking the patient to swallow. This can be facilitated by allowing the patient to gently sip and swallow water through a straw. As the patient swallows, the advancing tube will usually pass through the upper esophageal sphincter.

The tube can then be passed freely into the stomach, unless obstruction is present. Most tubes are marked externally at 18, 22, 26 and 30 inches from the distal tip. When the third marker passes the external nares, the tube is generally well-situated in the stomach (Fig. 7–8). The location of the tube in the stomach should be confirmed by aspiration of gastric contents through the tube and listening with the stethoscope placed over the epigastrium for gurgling when air is injected through the tube.

For gastric lavage, saline is injected through the tube and then aspirated after a short interval. It is preferable to inject 100 to 150 ml of fluid at a time to ensure some return.

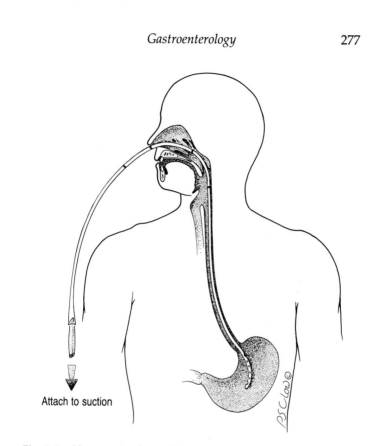

Attach to suction

Fig. 7–8. Nasogastric tube positioning.

Viscous gastric contents or blood clots are difficult to extract with standard tubes. A wider tube inserted through the mouth is preferable in such cases.

If the tube is to be left in place, it should be gently secured to the nose with taping, carefully avoiding undue pressure on the margin of the nares. The proximal end of the tube can be clamped or connected to a source of intermittent suction.

8
Hematology

John S. Senn

BONE MARROW ASPIRATION AND BIOPSY

Marrow Aspiration

Clinical Uses

Marrow tissue examination is used to evaluate marrow architecture, cellular morphology, abnormal components, and infectious agents.

Marrow aspiration obtains marrow for histologic and microbiologic study. Marrow biopsy preserves marrow architecture and is therefore more useful in evaluating neoplastic, granulomatous or other infiltrates. Aspiration may be done alone, but biopsy should always be accompanied by aspiration studies.

Anatomic Sites

Any bone containing bone marrow may be tested. Three sites are preferred: the sternum, anterior iliac spine, posterior iliac spine.

278

Sternal Marrow (Fig. 8–1)

Site. 1 cm inferior to the Angle of Louis (manubriosternal junction) and midway between the lateral edges of the sternum. The marrow cavity is shallow and bounded by bone under the skin and by bone anterior to the mediastinum.

Advantage. Easily accessible site, with ease of maintaining direct hemostatic pressure.

Disadvantage. Relatively thin bone close to the vital structures in the mediastinum. Rarely, shock syndrome occurs after vigorous marrow aspiration.

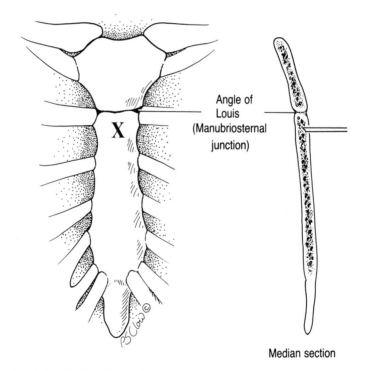

Angle of Louis (Manubriosternal junction)

Median section

Fig. 8–1. Testing of sternal marrow.

Iliac Crest Marrow—Anterior Iliac Spine (Fig. 8–2)

Site. 1 cm from the anterior limit of anterior iliac spine, and the cancellous bone is penetrated leading to a large marrow cavity.

Advantage. Easily identified site, not close to vital structures.

Disadvantage. If bleeding occurs after aspiration, direct hemostasis is difficult and tissues in the area are loose.

Iliac Crest Marrow—Posterior Iliac Spine (Fig. 8–3)

Site. 1 cm from the posterior limit of the posterior iliac spine: usually identifiable by a "dimple" seen directly over the area. This is usually 2 cm superior and 2 cm lateral to the cephalad end of the rectal crease in the prone position.

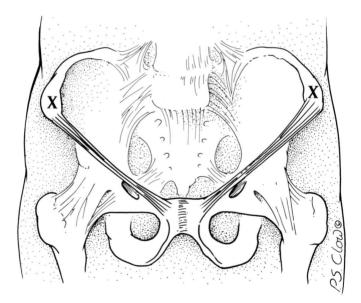

X - Anterior superior iliac spine

Fig. 8–2.   Iliac crest marrow: anterior iliac spine.

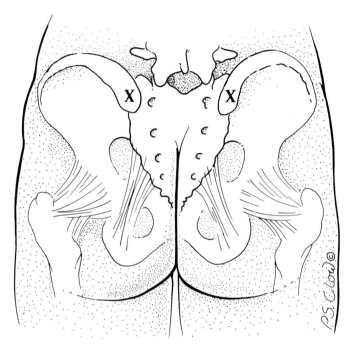

X - Posterior iliac spine

Fig. 8–3.   Iliac crest marrow: posterior iliac spine.

Advantage. Relatively insensitive site, with large marrow cavity, and cancellous bone to penetrate. Easy to maintain hemostatic pressure.

Disadvantage. Somewhat less easy to identify the site.

Equipment

Turkel needle (Fig. 8–4).

The outer needle is strong, and the shoulder prevents too deep insertion. The stylet should be fixed in place so

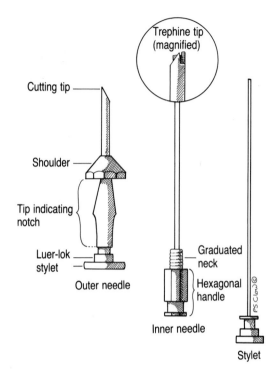

Fig. 8–4. Marrow aspiration needle (Turkel).

that it is flush with the cutting tip. The inner needle is less sturdy and is inserted after removal of the outer needle stylet. Insertion is possible to the graduated neck, and the inner needle is then turned clockwise and advanced with its cutting edge to remove a small bone and/or marrow core. The inner needle is then removed, and the core is extruded by the inner needle stylet.

Method

Using sterile gloves, the site of choice is cleansed with alcohol and povidone-iodine solution and then draped with sterile towels. 5 ml of 1% lidocaine is aspirated into a 5-ml syringe. Using a 25-gauge, ⅝ inch needle, lidocaine is injected intradermally, subcutaneously, and subperiosteally at the site for marrow aspiration. If necessary, a 22-gauge, 1½ inch needle may be used to reach the periosteum, after intradermal anesthesia. A 0.5 cm cut is made with a scalpel, penetrating to the periosteum at the site for marrow aspiration.

For sternal aspiration, the patient is supine. The outer needle is advanced to the bone and is introduced by a gentle clockwise-counterclockwise rotation method into the sternal cavity. After removal of the stylet, ½ to 1 ml of marrow is usually obtained using sharp suction by a 10-ml Luer-Lok syringe attached to the outer needle.

For iliac crest aspiration, the outer needle is advanced to bone and is introduced by gentle clockwise-counterclockwise rotation and pressure, until a yielding is felt, indicating entry into the marrow cavity. At this stage, the needle should be firmly embedded. The stylet is then removed, and the inner needle is inserted to its graduated neck, and then screwed for further penetration. The inner needle is then removed, and the contents (usually a small piece of bone) are expressed using the inner needle stylet.

Marrow is then aspirated through the outer needle, using sharp suction by a 10 ml Luer-Lok syringe: 3 to 10 ml of marrow can be obtained. Marrow is then flushed into a watch-glass containing a small amount of heparin. Spicules are retrieved, placed on a glass slide, and a film is prepared. The film is fixed and stained. When the marrow aspiration needle is removed, pressure is applied with sterile gauze, and a dry dressing is applied for 24 hours.

Marrow Biopsy

Clinical Uses

To obtain marrow with preserved architecture.

Equipment

Jamshidi needle (Fig. 8–5). The beveled obturator is locked in place prior to use of the Jamshidi needle. The blunt obturator is used after the biopsy has been obtained, and the needle has been removed from the biopsy site. It is used to express the biopsy from the needle.

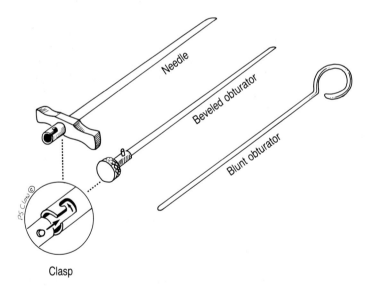

Clasp

Fig. 8–5. Marrow biopsy needle (Jamshidi).

Method

For skin preparation and anesthesia, see marrow aspiration. Biopsy is not done from the sternum; the posterior iliac crest is the preferred site.

Posterior iliac crest biopsy is done in the prone position. The beveled obturator is locked into the needle. The needle is advanced perpendicular to the bony site with the locked obturator in place. The needle hub is held in the palm, and the needle is advanced by forceful rotation through the bone. Entry into the marrow cavity is indicated by decreased resistance. The obturator is removed, and the needle is advanced farther 5 to 10 mm. The needle is then withdrawn 2 mm and rocked slightly to break off the marrow biopsy tissue.

A 10-ml Luer-Lok syringe is attached to the Jamshidi needle and suction is applied sharply and released. The needle is then removed with a rotating motion, and pressure is applied to the biopsy site. The biopsy tissue is removed from the needle by inserting the blunt obturator through the cutting end of the Jamshidi needle and expressing the specimen from the hub end into Zenker's solution. Biopsy imprints should be made prior to placing the tissue in Zenker's solution. A pressure dressing is applied to the biopsy site for 24 hours. The tissue is prepared by pathology for examination.

PHLEBOTOMY

Indications

Polycythemia, iron storage disease, pulmonary edema, porphyria cutanea tarda.

Method

Blood is removed using an 18-gauge, 1½ inch needle introduced into a large vein (usually the antecubital vein) of the reclining patient. Once secure venous access is achieved, the hub of the needle is taped in place.

Blood is collected into a plastic bag containing antico-agulant (ACD, Acid Citrate Dextrose) via plastic tubing which is connected to the needle already inserted into the patient's vein. The plastic container is placed below the level of the patient's venous access, and blood flows from the vein into the plastic bag. Increased rapidity of flow is encouraged by using a blood pressure cuff applied proxi-mal to the venous access and inflated above venous pres-sure but below arterial pressure.

Precautions

No more than 500 ml of blood should be removed at one time. If the patient develops light-headedness, tachycardia, or hypotension cease blood removal. The procedure should be completed in 30 to 60 minutes.

BLOOD TRANSFUSION

Clinical Uses

Blood or blood components are given to replace lacking blood elements. The use of the blood components needed is urged rather than the use of whole blood.

Method

Properly matched blood or blood components should be given within 30 minutes of leaving the hospital blood bank, so as to prevent contamination or inactivation of the blood products. The material to be transfused should be warm or cool, but it should not be heated (except in special cir-cumstances by the blood bank).

Blood should be given into a free-running intravenous line at a rate of 2 ml (30 to 50 drops) per minute. Slower administration may be required in cardiac decompensation, and an intravenous diuretic given 20 minutes prior to transfusion may be needed in this condition. More rapid transfusion may be required if intravascular blood volume is low.

Precautions

Be certain that the patient's name is on the unit to be given. The commonest reactions to transfusion are: fluid overload, febrile reactions, urticaria, and hemolysis.

Fluid Overload. Discontinue or slow transfusion and administer diuretic.

Chills and Fever. This common reaction (3% of transfusions) usually occurs late in the administration; other symptoms are absent, and urine is normal. It is usually due to leukoagglutinins. Check that the correct name is on the unit being transfused; check for previous similar reactions, and check urine and serum for hemoglobin. If there is no indication of hemolysis, continue transfusion more slowly and give antipyretic. If in doubt, discontinue the transfusion.

Urticaria Only. Give antihistamine and continue transfusion at a slower rate.

Hemolysis. This reaction is rare and produces chills, fever, pain in the chest, arms, and back, frequently with sweating and shock. It occurs shortly after starting transfusion and is often fatal. If in doubt about the reaction stop the tranfusion.

Any Reaction. Send blood for recrossmatching to the blood bank, and return any unused blood products to the blood bank.

BIBLIOGRAPHY

Turkel, H.: Trephine Technique of Bone Marrow Infusions and Tissue Biopsies. Consultant, Education and Training Division, Office of the Surgeon General, U.S.A. 14th Ed., 1963.

Jamshidi, K., and Swaim, W.R.: Bone marrow biopsy with unaltered architecture; A new biopsy device. J. Lab. Clin. Med., Series in Laboratory Medicine. 77(2):335, 1971.

Rywlin, A.M.: Histopathology of the Bone Marrow. Boston, Little, Brown, and Co., 1976.

Mollison, P.L.: Blood Transfusion in Clinical Medicine, 17th Ed. Oxford, Blackwell, 1985.

9
Neurosurgery

Michael L. Schwartz

MONITORING LEVEL OF CONSCIOUSNESS (GLASGOW COMA SCALE)

The concise description of a patient's state of consciousness has always been difficult because of confusion arising out of variance in the use of descriptive terms. With the advent of the Glasgow Scale and similar operational definitions of consciousness, it became possible to describe, on the basis of repeated, stereotyped, simple observations, a patient's level of consciousness and his progress.

Clinical Uses

The Glasgow Coma Scale may be used to follow a patient's improvement from a state of intoxication, his recovery from a concussion, or his decline with rising intracranial pressure.

Equipment

Pen and paper (preferably a sheet designed for the recording of neurologic observations)

Method

Three distinct observations are made each time the patient is examined. The interval between examinations may be as short as 15 minutes or as infrequent as every 4 to 8 hours. The observer is asked to record the patient's best response observed in the interval since the last observation and recording (see Fig. 9–4).

A patient's eyes may open spontaneously, in which case, a grade of 4 is assigned, or they may open in response to voice, not necessarily an instruction to open the eyes, as in the case of a drowsy but otherwise normal person. In this second case, a grade of 3 is assigned. If a painful stim-

Score		Stimulus	Response
Eyes open	4	Spontaneously	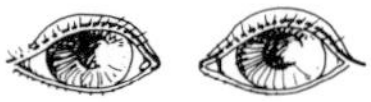
	3	To say, "Hello"	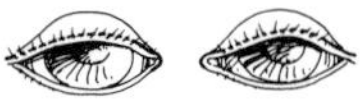
	2	To pain 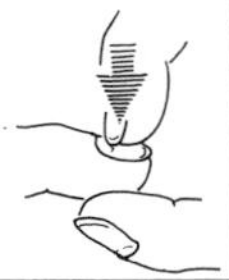	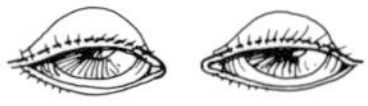
	1	None	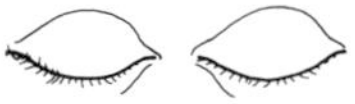
	C	Eyes closed by swelling	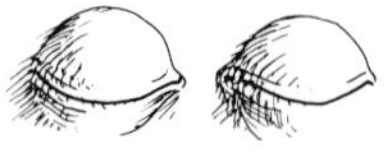

M.B. MACKAY©

Fig. 9–1. Glasgow coma scale—eye opening.

ulus is required to make the patient open his eyes, a score of 2 is recorded. If the patient's eyes remain closed regardless of external stimuli, a score of 1 is assigned. If the eyes are swollen shut, it is recorded by marking a "C" for closed on the chart (Fig. 9–1).

Best Motor Response (Fig. 9–2)

The patient is asked to comply with a simple command, for example, "raise your hand". If the patient is hemiparetic, the better side is considered. If there is a spinal cord injury that limits response, an appropriate instruction is devised. When the patient obeys the verbal command, a score of 6 is assigned.

A patient who is too obtunded to respond to a verbal command may still be tested by the administration of a painful stimulus, for example, pressure on the supraorbital margin. Such a stimulus is painful because the supraorbital nerve is compressed, but no harm is caused to the patient. A patient who is able to reach up and find such a stimulus is considered to have successfully localized it and achieves a score of 5.

When a painful stimulus is applied to a finger by compression of the nail bed of a patient who is unable to localize supraorbital pressure, the hand may be withdrawn by flexing the elbow. In such a case, a score of 4 is assigned.

Abnormal or spastic reflex flexion occurs when there is functional isolation of the intact thalamus from higher cortical centers. This decorticate posture is characterized by clenching of the fist and stiff flexion of the wrist and elbow with the hands applied to the trunk. A score of 3 is assigned to such a response.

Stereotyped, stiff extension of the elbows, often with clenching of the fists and pronation of the forearms, the so-called decerebrate posture indicates functional isolation of an intact pons and may be the patient's best response

Score		Stimulus	Response
	6	Obey commands, "Raise right arm"	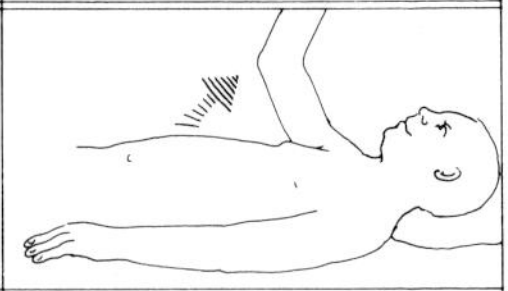
	5	Localized pain	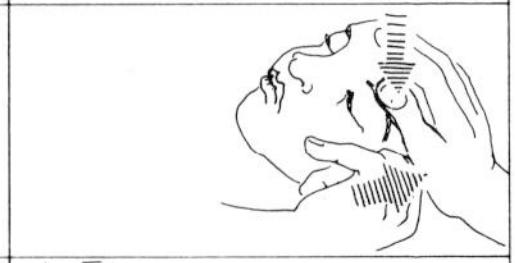
	4	Flexion to pain, "Withdrawal"	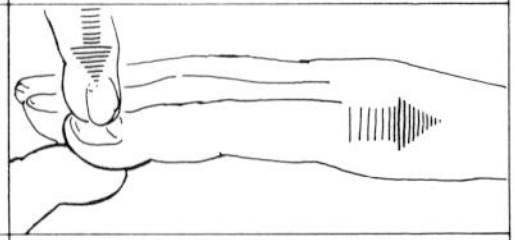
	3	Abnormal flexion to pain "Decorticate"	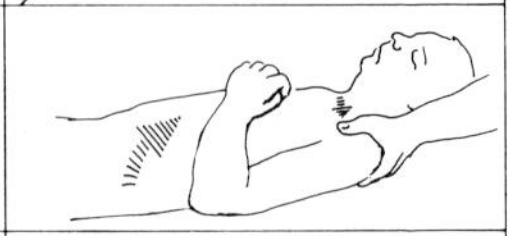
	2	Extension to pain "Decerebrate"	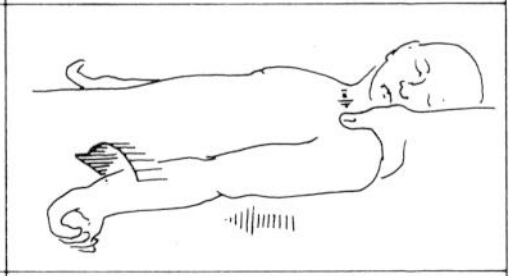
	1	None	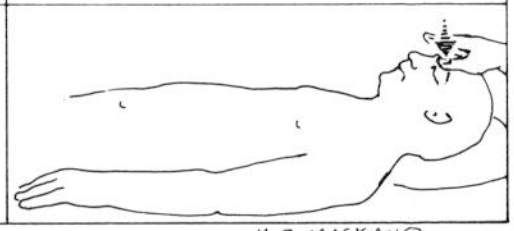

M.B. MACKAY ©

Fig. 9–2. Motor response.

to an external stimulus, in which case a score of 2 is given. Absence of motor response to external stimuli is scored as 1.

In a simplified version of the Glasgow Coma Scale both withdrawal by flexion of the elbow and spastic abnormal flexion are considered as a single category, and only five grades of motor response are considered.

Best Verbal Response (Fig. 9–3)

For the purposes of monitoring level of consciousness, no attempt is made to assess higher mental function. A full score of 5 is assigned if the patient is oriented to time, place, and person. If he is still able to converse but is disoriented, he is classified as confused and a score of 4 is given. Inappropriate single words, often uttered without relation to conversation, are scored as 3. Incomprehensible grunts and groans are scored as 2, and the absence of verbal

Score		Stimulus	Response
Best verbal	5	Orientated time, place, person	"It's Saturday." "I'm in hospital." "I'm John Doe."
	4	Confused	"Day?" "I don't know?"
	3	Inappropriate words	"* — — — !!" "Yesterday, Mummie."
	2	Incomprehensible sounds	"Groan."
	1	None	
	T	Endotracheal tube or tracheostomy	

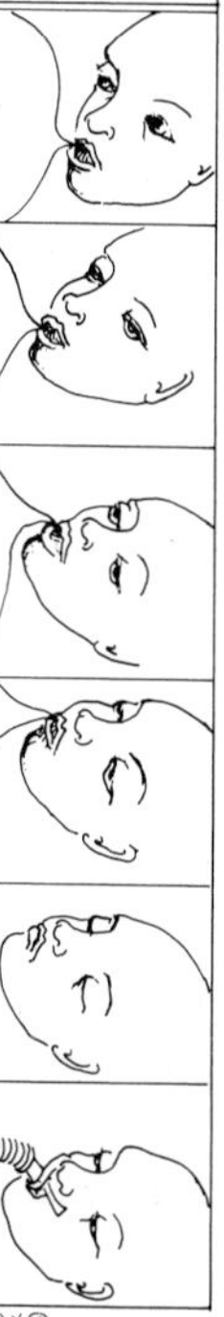

M.B. MACKAY ©

Fig. 9–3. Verbal response.

294 *Neurosurgery*

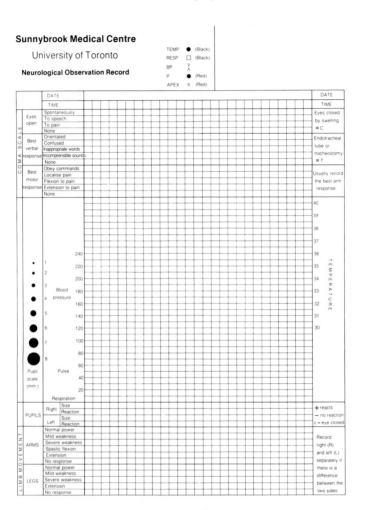

Fig. 9–4. Neurologic observation record.

response scores 1. The presence of an endotracheal tube or a tracheostomy is indicated by marking the letter "T" in lieu of the regular charting.

The Glasgow Coma Scale has been in use for 10 years. Although more complicated scales have been proposed, none is as widely used. By using a recording chart similar to the one illustrated, other indicators of the patient's status, such as pupillary size and reaction and vital signs may be recorded and followed. The graphic method permits rapid appreciation of decline or improvement in a patient's condition so the need for treatment or the efficacy of therapy in progress may be assessed (Fig. 9–4),

BIBLIOGRAPHY

Teasdale, G., and Jennett, B.: Assessment of coma and impaired consciousness. Lancet, 2:81, 1974.

Teasdale, G. Knill-Jones, R., and Van Der Sande J.: Observer variability in assessing impaired consciousness and coma. J. Neurol. Neurosurg. Psychiatry, 41:603, 1978.

LUMBAR PUNCTURE (SPINAL TAP)

Lumbar puncture is the simplest technique for obtaining a sample of cerebrospinal fluid (CSF). The pressure of the cerebrospinal fluid at the site of puncture is equal to intracranial pressure, provided that there is free communication between the ventricular system and the lumbar subarachnoid space. As many neurologic disorders are associated with changes in pressure and composition of the cerebrospinal fluid, the lumbar puncture is useful in the diagnosis of neurologic illness. Nevertheless, in the management of acute neurological disorders, there are only two indications for lumbar puncture; suspected bacterial or fungal meningitis and subarachnoid hemorrhage.

A relative contraindication to lumbar puncture is papilledema, but one may proceed if no intracranial mass such as hematoma, abscess, or tumor is suspected. When possible, CT scanning is advised prior to lumbar puncture. When the suspected diagnosis is bacterial meningitis, the necessity of obtaining CSF for culture and sensitivity overrides other considerations. An absolute contraindication to lumbar puncture is craniocerebral trauma, as the test adds no pertinent information and is potentially lethal should there be an intracranial hematoma.

The lumbar puncture needle must never be introduced through a region of suppuration because to do so would inoculate bacteria into the CSF.

Equipment

Surgeon's cap, mask, sterile gloves
Antiseptic solution
Fenestrated sterile drapes (where possible)
1% lidocaine solution, 20 ml
10-ml syringe, long needle 26-gauge
3 sterile centrifuge tubes with caps
No. 20- or No. 22-gauge lumbar puncture needle with stylet
3-way stopcock, 60-cm manometer (if CSF pressure is to be measured)

Method

Position the patient in the left lateral recumbent position with the craniospinal axis parallel to the floor and the posterior aspect of the pelvis perpendicular to the floor (Fig. 9–5). An assistant should help maintain the patient as flexed as possible. Palpate the spinous processes and the iliac crest. A line drawn between the iliac crests crosses the spine at approximately the level of L3 to L4 interspace. The sacrum is usually palpably convex, allowing positive identification of the L5 to S1 interspace.

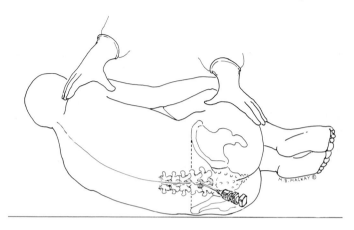

Fig. 9–5. Lumbar puncture.

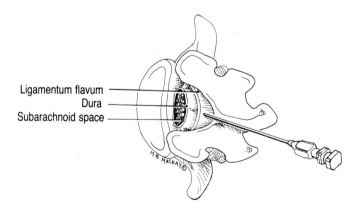

Ligamentum flavum ——
Dura ——
Subarachnoid space ——

Fig. 9–6. Lumbar puncture needle insertion process.

Prepare the skin with antiseptic solution; drape with the fenestration of the drape centered over the spine at the L4 to L5 and L5 to S1 level, and infiltrate with local anesthetic as deep as the interspinous ligament at the level selected (Fig. 9–6). Insert the lumbar puncture needle with the stylet in place between the spinous processes at the lowest possible interspace, directing the needle in the midline, parallel to the floor and approximately toward the umbilicus. If the needle impinges upon the lamina above or below the level of insertion, it may be partly withdrawn and redirected so that it passes cleanly into the spinal canal. As the ligamentum flavum is perforated, there is a slight "give". A second resistance is usually detectable as the needle punctures the dura. The patient often experiences a twinge of pain as the dura is broached. Any sensation should be felt in the midline posteriorly. Pain experienced to either side of the midline or referred to the leg indicates a lateral deflection of the needle and usually signals the need to redirect the needle more toward the midline for a successful entry into the subarachnoid space.

When it is suspected that the subarachnoid space has been entered (Fig. 9–7), the patient is allowed to extend the hips and knees so as to reduce intra-abdominal and hence cerebrospinal fluid pressure. The stylet is then withdrawn. The needle should be rotated slightly so as to ensure penetration of the arachnoid. If the cerebrospinal fluid pressure is low, the egress of fluid may be delayed. It may be necessary to have an assistant press on the abdomen of the patient or to elevate the patient's head slightly so as to increase the pressure.

When CSF is obtained (Fig. 9–8), the patient is positioned horizontal, and the stopcock and manometer are connected if the pressure is to be measured. Care should be taken to lose as little CSF as possible at this point so that CSF pres-

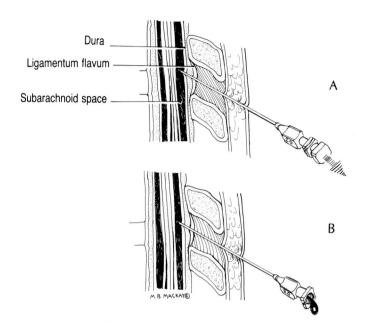

Dura

Ligamentum flavum

Subarachnoid space

A

B

M. B. MACKAY©

Fig. 9–7. Withdrawal of stylet after subarachnoid penetration. **A.** Subarachnoid space entered, stylet in place for insertion. **B.** Stylet is then removed to permit escape of cerebrospinal fluid.

sure, which tends to fall as CSF is withdrawn, will not be spuriously low.

A 5-ml aliquot of CSF should be obtained in each of the three centrifuge tubes (Fig. 9–9). In this way, CSF will be available for different laboratories, and the traumatic introduction of blood into the cerebrospinal fluid will be detected as the initial tube will be bloody, and the two subsequent tubes will be progressively clearer. The tubes should be labeled, and the clearest fluid sample sent for the cell count.

With the sample taken, the stopcock may be adjusted to

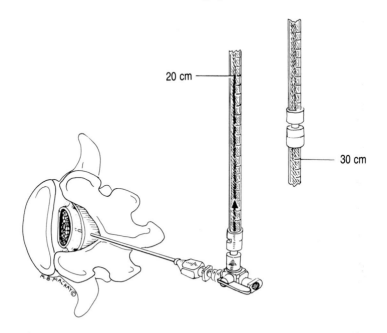

20 cm

30 cm

Fig. 9–8. After cerebrospinal fluid is obtained, the stopcock and manometer are connected to measure pressure.

measure the closing cerebrospinal fluid pressure, and the needle may then be withdrawn. The region of puncture should be massaged for a moment to break up the needle tract, thus rendering a persistent CSF fistula less likely. A small bandage should then be applied.

The cerebrospinal fluid should be examined for glucose, protein, and the number and type of cells should be counted. When meningitis is suspected, a culture and sensitivity of the fluid should also be obtained. For suspected subarachnoid hemorrhage, the fluid should be centrifuged and examined for xanthochromia (yellowish discoloration). When possible the opening and closing pressures should

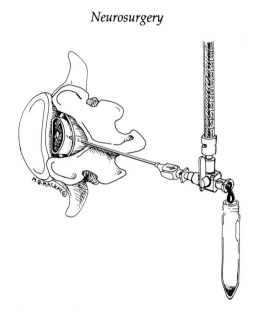

Fig. 9–9. Obtain a 5-ml aliquot of cerebrospinal fluid for each of the three centrifuge tubes.

be recorded along with a brief description of the clarity and color of the fluid. Following the procedure, the patient should be flat for 6 to 24 hours to prevent the development of "spinal headache".

EXPLORATORY BURR HOLES

It is unlikely that the average physician will have to make exploratory burr holes. The indication in virtually every case will be to diagnose and relieve rising intracranial pressure from an expanding epidural or subdural hematoma that fails to respond to nonoperative measures such as mechanical ventilation, the maintenance of an adequate systemic arterial blood pressure, and the intravenous administration of a 20 percent mannitol solution (1 g/kg body weight or 350 ml for a 70 kg person). An expanding intra-cranial clot on the surface of the brain is usually signaled by declining level of consciousness, worsening contralat-eral hemiparesis, and ipsilateral pupillary dilatation. When the entire brain shifts away from the clot, the cerebral pe-duncle may impinge on the contralateral sharp edge of the tentorium. This interrupts the contralateral corticospinal fibers above the motor decussation and produces a hemi-paresis ipsilateral to the hematoma. The dilating pupil is almost always ipsilateral to the lesion. Hence, it is the more reliable guide to burr hole placement. Always be prepared to place burr holes on both sides of the head in any case.

The burr hole serves as a means of diagnosis and pro-vides access to the cranial cavity so that a surface hematoma may be removed.

Equipment

This procedure should always be done under sterile con-ditions. With the use of hyperventilation and mannitol, the patient can almost always be sustained during transfer to the operating room, but on occasion the procedure may be performed in the emergency department. The entire head should be shaved, prepared, and draped in a sterile field. The physician should wear a surgeon's cap, mask, sterile gown, and gloves.

2 scalpels (one large and one small blade)
4 hemostats
Small self-retaining rake retractor
Fine-toothed tissue forcep
Non-toothed bayonet forcep
Periostial elevator
Brace, perforator, and burr
Leksell rongeur (6 mm)
Sharp right-angle neuro hook

Suction (In lieu of wall suction, large syringes, either of the plunger or rubber ball type, may be used.)

Cautery (although radio frequency generators of mono or bipolar type are usually used, cautery from small battery-powered devices may be adequate)

Bone wax

Gelatin foam (Gelfoam) (Absorbable gelatin sponge, USP)

Needle driver

3 to 0 braided nonabsorbable sutures on a round curved needle

3 to 0 monofilament suture material on a curved cutting needle

Method (Fig. 9–10, Fig. 9–11)

The first burr hole should be placed on the side of the suspected hematoma, one finger's breadth anterior to the tragus and one finger's breadth above the zygomatic process. A 3-cm incision is made perpendicular to the zygomatic process a finger's breadth anterior to the tragus. The superficial temporal artery will likely be transsected and should be cauterized or picked up with the hemostat and tied. If available, cutting cautery may be used to incise the galea and temporalis fascia and muscle so as to expose the underlying squamous temporal bone. A periostial elevator is used to strip the muscle off the bone. The handle of the scalpel may also be used. The self-retaining retractor is inserted and spread so that the temporalis muscle and the skin edges are retracted. Sufficient tension should be applied to stop bleeding of the skin edges. Uncontrolled bleeding from muscle or skin edges should be controlled before proceeding.

The perforator is mounted in the brace and the hole is produced. Characteristically, the squamous temporal bone is thin. The opening in the bone is enlarged using the burr.

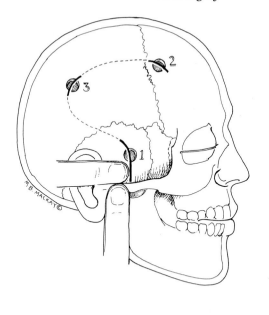

Perforator

Burr

Fig. 9–10. Placement of exploratory burr holes.

If the hematoma is epidural, it will be encountered at this point. To remove it adequately, it will be necessary to enlarge the burr hole using the Leksell rongeur. Epidural hematomas in the temporal region are usually caused by a laceration of the middle meningeal artery which runs in a groove in the temporal squama. The artery must be identified and either cauterized, waxed into the bone, or secured in some manner. The bone edges are waxed. Muscle, galea, and skin are reapproximated using the braided suture material in the muscle and galea, and the monofilament suture material in the skin.

Should no epidural hematoma be encountered, the dura at the site of the burr hole should be cauterized and cut in a cruciate manner using a small scalpel. The dura has two

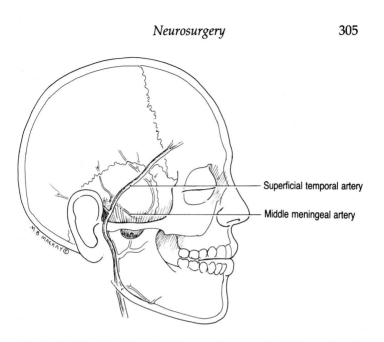

Fig. 9–11. Location of superficial temporal artery and middle meningeal artery.

distinct layers. If only the outer layer is incised initially, a sharp hook may be placed between the leaves of the dura to elevate it away from the brain.

The inner layer may then be cautiously cut with the operator taking care to avoid injury to the underlying brain. Cutting the dura in a cruciate manner produces four corners of dura that may be shrunk using the cautery to expose what lies beneath. If a subdural hematoma has been present for some time, there will be a membrane just deep to the dura that must also be incised carefully.

A second and third burr hole may be placed if nothing is found at the temporal burr hole or if additional points of access to the cranial cavity are required. The second burr hole should be placed 1 cm anterior to the coronal suture

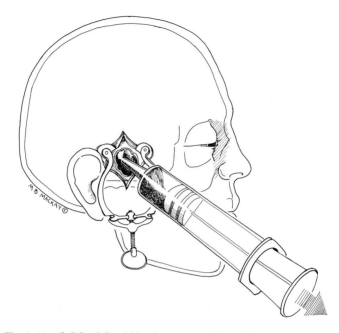

Fig. 9–12. Solid subdural blood is aspirated from the region of the burr hole.

(still behind the hairline) and 3 cm from the midline. The incision should be made parallel to the midline. No temporalis muscle will be encountered here, and the periosteum will be found directly beneath the galea. The procedure is the same as described above. A third burr hole may be placed at the parietal boss (the most prominent point in the parietal bone). Solid subdural blood should be cautiously aspirated from the region of the burr hole and liquid blood should be allowed to escape (Fig. 9–12). Cautious irrigation with saline is useful to rinse out blood pigment. A craniotomy is required to adequately remove fresh subdural blood (a description of craniotomy is beyond the scope of this book). The release of pressure via burr holes may suffice as primary treatment. A burr hole may be enlarged with the rongeur as described above, if a cranial opening larger than a burr hole is required.

Gelatin foam (Gelfoam) should be placed in the opening to prevent blood from the subgaleal space from entering the cranial cavity. The galea and skin are approximated as described above. If it is technically too difficult to approximate the galea, vertical mattress sutures through the skin will suffice.

The sequence may be repeated on the other side of the head.

Precautions

Meticulous sterile technique should always be used. Care to avoid injuring the brain is paramount.

Upon completion of the exploratory burr holes, ventilation and blood pressure support should be maintained, a voluminous sterile dressing should be applied to the wound and the patient should be transferred to a surgical unit.

The procedure described in this section is simplifed and is in no way a substitute for experience and practice under the direction of a trained surgeon. *The use of exploratory burr holes should be regarded strictly as a life-saving procedure when a patient will not survive transfer to the care of a trained surgeon.*

10
Obstetrics and Gynecology

W.H. Harris

OBSTETRICS

Dating of Pregnancy

The accurate dating of a pregnancy is important, particularly in high risk patients who have diabetes, Rh disease, high blood pressure, chronic renal disease, or a history of previous intrauterine growth retardation. It is also important to know the exact delivery date for a patient for whom an elective repeat cesarean section is necessary. Many times a physician cannot be sure whether or not a woman is postmature because of uncertain dates; this could lead to disastrous consequences if a postmature child were not delivered.

At the beginning of the pregnancy, the physician must determine from the patient the first day of the last menstrual period. The date is of no use when determined retrospectively. The length of pregnancy is 280 days from the first day of the last normal period; in order to calculate this add 10 days from the first day of the last normal period and subtract three months. Quickening is no use when the date is obtained retrospectively. The patient must be asked ahead of time to note the date that the fetus first moves. The date the fetal heart is first heard is not reliable because this depends on several factors including the thickness of the abdominal wall and the position of the fetus; however, it is usually heard with a fetoscope for the first time around the 20th week.

The uterus usually doubles in size at 8 weeks gestation, and it is 3 times the nonpregnancy state at 12 weeks. It may be just palpable suprapubically at this time.

At 18 weeks the uterus is usually about 2 cm below the umbilicus, at 20 weeks at the umbilicus, at 22 weeks 2 cm above the umbilicus, and at 28 weeks it is 28 cm from the height of the fundus to the symphysis pubis or halfway between the xiphoid process and the umbilicus. After 28 weeks, it is difficult to ascertain the gestational age of the fetus because this may depend on whether or not the fetus is engaged or what position the fetus is in. For example, in a transverse lie at 28 weeks, the uterus may be 24 to 26 cm above the symphysis pubis.

The symphysis-fundus height is another useful way of estimating gestational age. This test is of value only after 16 weeks, after which date the symphysis-fundus height in centimeters equals the gestational age in weeks. For accuracy, this measurement should be taken and recorded by the same observer on each occasion.

The prospective mother should be asked to note when she first feels fetal movement. A primipara first feels activity around 20 weeks, and this is reliable. A multipara may feel life earlier, making this method a less reliable way to determine gestational age.

Another method of documenting gestational age is to order ultrasound between 8 and 14 weeks. The crown-rump length is measured; this has a 95% accuracy limit within plus or minus 5 days. After that, the biparietal diameter can be measured between 16 and 24 weeks; this is accurate to within plus or minus 10 to 11 days. After the 24th week, ultrasound is a less reliable method of dating gestational age.

At 20 weeks, if the uterine size does not equal dates, ultrasound should be ordered. It should be ordered for all women having elective repeat cesarean sections and for women who are suspected of having intrauterine growth retardation.

Clinical Uses of Ultrasound

Ultrasound is used in obstetrics and gynecology in order to determine whether or not a threatened abortion is viable, to date a pregnancy, to locate the placenta, to verify the presence of a pelvic mass, to locate a "lost" intrauterine device, and to diagnose an ectopic pregnancy (in the presence of a positive pregnancy test the uterus is shown to be empty and an adnexal mass along with free fluid in the peritoneal cavity suggest an extrauterine pregnancy).

Bishop Score

This method of assessing the advisability of considering induction of labor in a patient believed to have prolonged or postdate pregnancy was described by Dr. E.H. Bishop in 1964.

BISHOP SCORE TABLE			
	0	1	2	3
Dilatation (cm)	0	1 to 2	3 to 4	5 or more
Effacement (percent)	0 to 30 percent	40 to 50 percent	60 to 70 percent	80 percent or more
Station (cm)	−3 or less	−2 cms	−1/0	+1 or more
Consistency	Firm	Medium	Soft	
Position	Posterior	Mid	Anterior	

The Bishop Score is an attempt to numerically assess the "ripeness" of the cervix as well as the station and position of the fetal caput, all of which should be helpful in assessing risks and the wisdom or need for the induction of labor. Induction of labor by any means, including the rupture of membranes, would be ill advised unless the Bishop Score were six or more.

OBSTETRICAL ANALGESIA AND ANESTHESIA

Epidural Block

In modern obstetrics the need for analgesics in labor has nearly disappeared, and in large medical centers, it is now rare to order analgesics for a patient in labor. Under ideal conditions, a continuous epidural block anesthesia is best; however, this is only obtainable in certain centers. (A description of this technique is beyond the scope of this book.)

Paracervical Block

Prior to use of epidural blocks, a paracervical block was sometimes used. Cervical block is disfavored because of fetal complications and because the epidural is safer and more effective for a longer period of time. Paracervical block was done by injecting 10 ml of local anesthetic into both uterosacral ligaments. Unfortunately, the mother and fetus could get a quick systemic absorption of local anesthetic, and fetal bradycardia could be quite pronounced and frightening. *Fetal deaths were reported with this method of anesthesia, and thus it is no longer favored.*

Pudendal Block

Pudendal block was obtained by using a 20-ml syringe with a 20-gauge needle. The needle was inserted through an Iowa trumpet to a point overlying the tips of the ischial spines. Ten ml of local anesthetic were injected on each side (Fig. 10–1).

Trained obstetricians have occasionally used this form of regional block and were always disappointed by its failure to produce satisfactory anesthesia of the region; therefore, an average physician would have more trouble and even less success with this method. *Pudendal block is not recommended.*

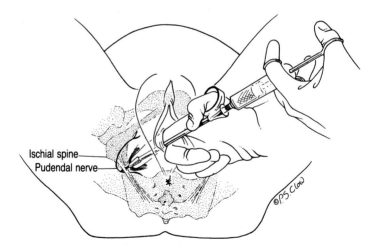

Fig. 10–1.   Pudendal block.

Local Infiltration

The third form of regional anesthesia is local infiltration into the episiotomy site. This method is used when the patient is having natural childbirth and an episiotomy is required.

Equipment

Sterile tray
10-ml syringe with 1½ inch 25-gauge needle
Local anesthetic, such as 1% lidocaine

Method

Since this type of infiltration anesthesia is used prior to an episiotomy, the operator must decide whether a midline or mediolateral episiotomy is planned. A wheal is then raised in the midline perineal skin, just posterior to the vaginal outlet. The skin and vaginal mucosa are then infiltrated with local anesthetic along the lines of the intended episiotomy. Some of the anesthetic should also be placed in the deeper tissues.

EPISIOTOMY

When the head crowns, the episiotomy is performed along the line of local anesthetic injection. It may take 10 minutes for the local anesthetic to take effect. This is not a significant delay since the episiotomy is usually repaired following completion of the third stage.

Clinical Uses

Useful to enlarge the birth canal to facilitate delivery and mandatory in a breech presentation.

Equipment

   Local anesthetic (infiltration) unless patient has epidural
      block
   Sterile gauze
   Needle driver
   Chromic catgut suture, size 00 or 000 with needle
   Scissors (some operators use bandage type of scissors to
      avoid any possible injury to the fetal presenting part)

Classification

Episiotomies may be medial (midline) or mediolateral.
The midline is preferred because it is easier to sew and
reconstruct and because of less postoperative discomfort.
Mediolateral episiotomies may be done in the presence of
a breech delivery or a short perineum because of the possibility of tear into the rectum if the midline episiotomy
were used in this situation.

Method of Repair

Repair is done using a 00 suture, beginning in the vagina
at the apex of the episiotomy and sewing the vaginal mucosa with interlocking sutures to just beyond the hymenal
ring (Fig. 10–2A). The bulbocavernosus muscles are then
approximated with 1 or 2 sutures that should be snug but
not tight (Fig. 10–2B). The skin is closed with interrupted
mattress sutures. These must approximate the skin edges
but not be too close or too tight since postoperative swelling
often occurs.

Be sure the rectal sphincter has not been torn. If so, it
must be carefully repaired before repair of the episiotomy
or perineal tear. The retracted sphincter ends are sought
with toothed thumb forceps, and the opposing edges sutured with 2 figure-of-eight sutures (Fig. 10–2C). Be careful
not to put any sutures through the rectum. If this occurs,

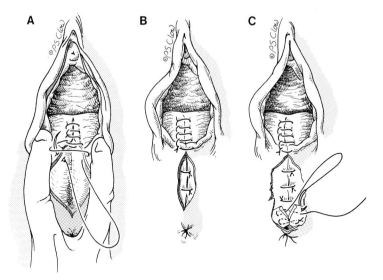

Fig. 10–2. Repair of episiotomy. **A.** Vaginal mucosa repair using continuous interlocking sutures. **B.** Bulbocavernosus muscle repair. **C.** Repair of torn rectal sphincter using figure-of-8 sutures.

an extra glove should be put on and the sutures palpated through the rectum. If the rectum has been oversewn, the sutures must be removed and the sphincter repaired again.

The mediolateral episiotomy is repaired in identical fashion, but remember that because of asymmetry, more tissue must be taken from the outer side than from the inner side when approximating both the deeper tissues and the skin in order to properly line up the structures involved.

Follow-up Care

One or 2 days after delivery, the patient may begin warm sitz baths. Sometimes an ordinary 60-watt bulb in a lamp placed some 50 cm (18 inches) from the perineum between the separated thighs will reduce pain and swelling. Be careful that no burn results from the bulb touching the skin. If extensive bruising has occurred, an ice pack to the perineum may be helpful.

Management of a Rectal Tear

Occasionally the midline episiotomy may extend into the rectum, or the rectum may be traumatized with forceps delivery. If the rectum has been entered, the same equipment and procedure for an episiotomy are used, but the rectum is oversewn with a 000 suture in a continuous fashion.

Care must be taken that the extent of the rectal laceration is known. Repair begins at the apex and works down toward the anus. The sphincter is then approximated, and the remainder of the episiotomy closure is carried out, as described in that procedure.

Precautions

After a rectal repair, the patient should not receive a rectal digital examination or enemas. Antibiotics are unnecessary. The patient may be given a bulk, mucilloid type of laxative (e.g., Metamucil). When normal bowel movement have returned and the episiotomy is healing the patient may leave hospital.

APGAR SCORING

This procedure was developed by Dr. Virginia Apgar as a measure of the general condition of newborn infants. The assessment on which the score is rated is done at 1 minute and 5 minutes after birth. To be valid, the scoring must be timed accurately and by someone trained to make the necessary observations.

APGAR SCORE TABLE			
	0	*1*	*2*
Heart rate	Absent	Less than 100	More than 100
Respiratory effort	Absent	Irregular, weak cry	Strong
Reflex reaction to flicking foot	Absent	Facial grimace	Cry with stimulation
Color	Cyanotic	Body pink, limbs blue	Completely pink
Muscle tone	Flaccid, limp	Some flexion of limbs	Active limb movements

The first scoring must be done exactly 1 minute after delivery since the most severe depression would occur at that time. A score of 10 indicates a baby in optimum condition; a score of 3 would indicate a severely depressed newborn; a score of 4 or less indicates the need for respiratory assistance. Virginia Apgar noted when talking about the score, "it is no substitute for a careful physical examination or serial observations over the first few hours of life."

POSTPARTUM HEMORRHAGE

Postpartum hemorrhage may be defined as the loss of more than 500 ml of blood in the 24-hour period following delivery. The causes of postpartum hemorrhage may be considered in 5 classifications: 1. Abnormal placental implantation and development such as placenta previa, placental abruption, and a hydatid mole. 2. Trauma during delivery that may be due to laceration of the vagina, the cervix, and the lower uterine segment. 3. Uterine atony that may be due to an overdistended uterus in a multiple pregnancy, hydramnios, prolonged labor, general anesthetic, and previous postpartum hemorrhage. 4. Small women with a small blood volume. 5. Coagulation defects due to placenta abruption, retention of dead fetus, amniotic fluid embolism, sepsis, intravascular hemolysis (toxemia), and massive hemorrhage.

If postpartum hemorrhage has occurred or if the patient is considered to be at risk, an I.V. infusion of normal saline should be started using a large bore needle (e.g., size 16 to 18). Blood should be crossmatched, grouped, and ready for transfusion. Once hemorrhage has occurred, plasma expanders (e.g., albumin) should be started at once, while awaiting blood. A coagulation screen should be done, and a blood specimen should be observed for clotting and clot stability.

If the placenta has not been expelled, it must be removed. The operator should be gowned and gloved in sterile fashion (long gloves are no longer used). For placenta removal, the patient must be anesthetized by epidural or general anesthetic. Oxytocin (20 units per liter of infusion) must be running in the I.V. If the cervix is closed, it should be dilated by inserting 1 finger, 2, 3, and then 4 fingers. The whole hand is then passed through the dilated cervix and the placenta located. The plane of cleavage should then be determined, and the hand inserted between the endometrium and the placenta, thus freeing the placenta (Fig. 10–3). It should be grasped with the fingers and removed. The vagina should then be inspected and the uterine cavity re-explored to make sure that there is no rent or tear in the uterus and that no placental fragments remain.

If it has been a difficult forceps delivery, look for lacerations under the pubic rami and over the ischial spines. Inspection of these areas should be done first to determine the full extent of possible lacerations. A weighted vaginal retractor will often help visualize vaginal or cervical lacerations or tears. If there is severe hemorrhage, adequate exposure and assistance are essential. If the laceration is extensive, assess whether or not the rectal sphincter has been torn or the rectum entered. (In such cases, refer to

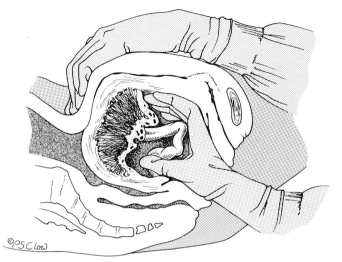

Fig. 10–3. Manual removal of placenta.

the section on rectal repair.) If the laceration is limited to the vaginal mucosa, it should be closed with a continuous interlocking suture, using 00 chromic catgut.

A hematoma may develop in the vagina. This can be determined by palpation. If a hematoma is found, it should be incised with a scalpel and the blood evacuated. Several figure-of-eight sutures (00 chromic) are then placed in the base of the hematoma. Watch the area carefully for the next 10 to 15 minutes to make sure that the hematoma does not recur.

Next, inspect the cervix by grasping it with a sponge forceps at the anterior and posterior lips, as well as at 3 and 9 o'clock positions. Lacerations tend to occur at 3 and 9 o'clock, and careful inspection of these areas is necessary, especially after forceps rotation. Repair is carried out with a continuous, interlocking suture of 00 chromic for each individual laceration (Fig. 10–4). The uterine cavity is care-

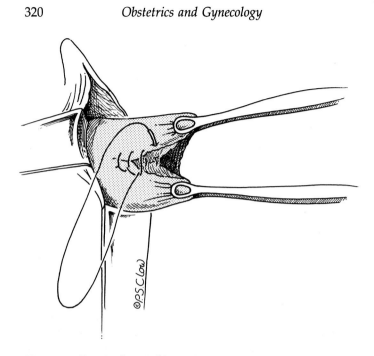

Fig. 10–4. Repair of cervical laceration.

fully palpated through the cervix. If laceration or rupture of the uterus has occurred, hysterectomy is necessary.

Precaution

Care must be used in administering I.V. ergonovine (Ergometrine) as it may cause a precipitous rise in blood pressure.

If prostaglandin $F_{2\alpha}$ is injected through the abdominal wall into the myometrium in doses of 0.5 to 1 mg, tetanic uterine contractions will result.

GYNECOLOGY

Taking of a Pap (Papanicolaou) Smear

Indications

This test is performed to screen for cervical cancer. This should be done annually once the patient becomes sexually active.

Equipment

Vaginal speculum
Wooden spatula for taking specimens
Glass slide
Spray fixation solution

Method

The vaginal speculum is lubricated with warm water; a jelly lubricant must not be used. It is gently inserted into the vagina and adjusted in order to expose the cervix. The rounded end of the spatula is used to obtain a specimen of secretion from the posterior fornix. The specimen is then spread on one-half of the glass slide. The other irregular end of the spatula is used to obtain a specimen from the cervical os. The longer portion is inserted in the cervical canal and a scraping of the endocervix is obtained by rotating the end of the spatula through a full circle. The specimen is then spread on the remaining half of the glass slide and sprayed with fixative.

For high risk patients, a cotton-tipped applicator is dipped in saline and then used as the means of obtaining a specimen from the endocervical canal. This specimen should be spread on a second glass slide and fixed. The slide is then sent to the laboratory for examination and interpretation.

Hanging Drop Test for Trichomonas

Indications

This test is performed if trichomonas vaginitis is suspected. The diagnostic accuracy is between 60 to 70%.

Equipment

Vaginal speculum
Cotton-tipped applicators
Normal saline solution
Glass slide

Method

With the vaginal speculum in place, a specimen of vaginal discharge is obtained on an applicator and mixed with a little normal saline in a small container. A drop of mixture is then placed on a glass slide under a microscope and examined under both low and high power. Trichomonads (about the size of a white blood cell) can be seen as motile organisms and the flagella noted. Trichomonads may be present but not motile; differentiation from white blood cells can be difficult. If numerous white cells appear in this test or on a Pap smear, be suspicious of trichomonas.

Insertion of an Intrauterine Contraceptive Device (IUD)

Clinical Uses

This mechanical device is used to prevent pregnancy. The ideal candidate should be parous and have only one sexual partner. Some authorities believe that an IUD should not be used in nulliparous women who have multiple sexual partners. Some advise against the use of an IUD in women who desire future fertility.

Equipment

An IUD in sterile package
Vaginal speculum
Sterile uterine sound
Gauze sponges
Povidone-iodine solution (Betadine)
Sterile gloves

Method

Note: The IUD should be inserted at the time of menstruation.

With the patient in a suitable position, a careful bimanual vaginal examination is done to ascertain uterine size and position, and the absence of signs of infection.

The vulva and vagina are carefully cleansed and prepared with the povidone-iodine solution. The position of the uterus is then ascertained, and with the cervix exposed by a sterile speculum, a uterine sound is carefully inserted through the cervical canal to determine the depth or length of the uterine cavity.

While some operators recommend the use of a cervical tenaculum, this is not necessary and may be painful. If insertion is done at the time of menstruation and no force is used, the use of a tenaculum is not considered necessary or advisable.

With the cervix exposed by the speculum, the loaded and prepared IUD is gently inserted into the endocervical canal in the direction of the uterine position and to the depth of the uterus as previously determined by the uterine sound.

There are several types of IUD's available, and with each package the manufacturer describes in detail how to insert that particular type. These package instructions must be followed, and then the general procedure outlined here may be carried out.

Following insertion of the IUD, the attached string should be cut so as to leave 2 to 4 cm protruding from the cervical os. This enables the patient to check its presence by feeling for the string with her finger inserted into the vagina.

Precaution

No force should be used to insert the IUD. If force is needed, stop the procedure. An IUD should never be used in the presence of pelvic inflammation.

Occasionally a severe vasovagal reaction occurs at the time of IUD insertion. The usual supportive measures and treatment should be instituted immediately should collapse occur.

Contraindications

Pregnancy
Abnormalities of the uterine cavity or uterine enlargement
Pelvic infection
History of ectopic pregnancy
Abnormal uterine bleeding
Patients taking anticoagulants
Patients allergic to any components of the IUD (e.g., copper)

Removal of an IUD

Following visualization of the cervix, gentle yet persistent traction is accomplished by grasping the protruding string of the IUD with suitable, long forceps clamps (e.g., Kelly or Kocher clamp). Following removal, no special after care is necessary.

An IUD should be removed if abnormal bleeding occurs,

if pelvic infection occurs or is suspected, or if undue pain is noted by the patient.

Fitting of a Vaginal Diaphragm

Clinical Uses

To prevent conception.

Equipment

Vaginal speculum
Lubricant jelly
Set of diaphragm fitting rings. These can be obtained
upon request from the manufacturer (e.g., Ortho Pharmaceuticals Ltd.).

Method

Following a careful bimanual examination to determine the uterine position and vaginal length, and to determine the absence of any significant pelvic pathology, a lubricated ring is inserted beyond or behind the cervix and fit snugly in the posterior fornix. A 75-mm size is often a good size to begin with. Different sizes may then be inserted one at a time until the correct size is determined.

The ring should reach the posterior fornix and be able to be pushed up behind the symphysis. The size that does this is the correct size for the patient. The ring must not be so large as to protrude beyond the symphysis, nor should it be so small that it does not remain in place.

When the correct size has been chosen, the examiner removes the examining fingers and asks the patient if she feels the ring.

If the correct size has been chosen, all the above criteria will be met, and the patient will be unaware of the presence of the ring in the vagina. The fitting ring is then removed and its size (diameter in millimeters) noted.

Note: The diaphragm should always be used with contraceptive jelly in order to maximize contraception. The diaphragm should be left in place 6 to 8 hours following intercourse, at which time it may be removed. No douche is necessary or advisable. Prior to each act of intercourse, the diaphragm must be inserted with contraceptive jelly and according to the manufacturer's instructions.

When the diaphragm is compressed for insertion (or when placed on a plastic inserter), two furrows are formed when the dome-up position is used. Strips of contraceptive jelly are placed in these two furrows (Fig. 10–5A), the ring is lubricated with contraceptive jelly and the diaphragm inserted dome-up. In the dome-up position, the jelly is held closer to the cervix and the diaphragm also tends to rest higher in the vaginal canal; thus it is less likely to interfere with coital sensation.

In addition, it is usually advised that contraceptive jelly be placed deep in the vagina after the diaphragm is in place (Fig. 10–5B). Details about application are found on a package insert with both diaphragm and contraceptive jelly packages. Following use and removal of the diaphragm, wash it with soap and water and dry it carefully. The diaphragm should never be boiled nor should antiseptic solutions be used; these could damage the thin rubber of the diaphragm.

When used correctly and consistently, the diaphragm jelly technique is 95 percent reliable for contraception.

A new diaphragm should be purchased once a year. The size should be checked after each pregnancy and delivery for those who wish a return to this method of birth control.

Management of Bartholin's Abscess

Usually a Bartholin's abscess is relatively asymptomatic and is 3 cm or greater in size. Initially, local hot compresses or hot sitz baths 4 times a day may be all that is required.

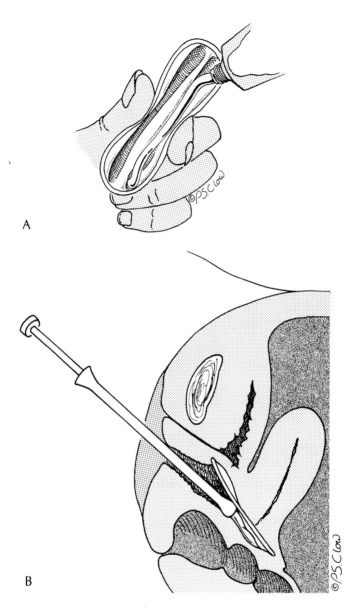

Fig. 10–5. Application of contraceptive jelly to diaphragm. **A.** Jelly is placed in furrows, and then additional jelly is used to lubricate ring for ease of insertion. **B.** Diaphragm in place with additional jelly being added.

Appropriate antibiotics are indicated. Often the infection will then settle down and drain spontaneously. If symptoms persist and the abscess is increasing in size, it should be opened. This should be done under general anesthesia, but if this is not possible, incision and drainage can be done under local infiltration anesthesia. The surgical technique is the same in both methods.

Incision and Drainage of a Bartholin's Gland Abscess

Equipment

Set for local infiltration anesthetic
Local anesthetic (e.g., 1% lidocaine)
Sharp pointed scalpel
000 non-catgut suture
¼ inch impregnated (e.g., iodoform) packing gauze strip

Method

Local infiltration is carried out gently, using the smallest bore needle possible. The vaginal mucosa is then incised, placing the incision vertically inside the introitus (Fig. 10–6A). The incision must then be made deeper in order to incise the capsule of the gland/abscess. Pus will appear and exude (Fig. 10–6B). Cultures must be taken.

The operator then gently introduces the little finger into the abscess cavity to make sure no adhesions, or a septum, are present. The gland should then drain freely.

If desired, packing may be used, but it is not necessary. If general anesthetic is used, packing is desirable, and no patient discomfort will be noted. Following insertion of the packing into the abscess cavity, the gland is sewn in four quadrants, attaching the gland to the vaginal submucosa so that drainage can occur easily (Fig. 10–6C).

If packing has been used, it should be removed within 24 hours. Sitz baths are used 4 times a day for 2 to 3 days,

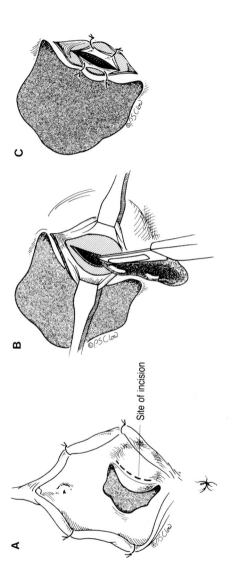

Site of incision

Fig. 10–6. Incision and drainage of a Bartholin's gland abcess. **A.** Site of incision. **B.** Drainage of incised Bartholin's gland abscess. **C.** Marsupialization of abscess sac.

or until there is no further discomfort. Intercourse should be avoided for at least 1 week after symptoms have disappeared. With recurrent Bartholinitis, the gland must be excised, but this is a major operation requiring general anesthetic.

Precautions

Sometimes brisk bleeding occurs. This can usually be controlled by local pressure and may be minimized by using a local anesthetic with epinephrine.

Management of Condyloma Acuminatum

If a patient has condyloma acuminatum, there is usually an underlying vaginitis due to trichomonas, gonorrhea, or yeast. Condylomata may be treated by local application of 20 percent podophyllin in mineral oil, by surgical excision or by cauterization.

Equipment

20 percent podophyllin in mineral oil
Cotton-tipped applicators

Method

If there are small or very few condylomata, they can be treated as an office procedure. The podophyllin is applied with the applicator only to the condyloma. The patient is advised to take a bath at home when the vulva starts to become sore. Failing that, a bath should be taken that evening to wash off the medication, even if the patient does not complain of undue pain. Follow-up should be in 2 weeks and treatment may be repeated if necessary.

Note: large or multiple condylomata should be treated surgically, by excision or cautery, under general anesthesia.

11
Ophthalmology

John Speakman

VISUAL ACUITY

An accurate record of visual acuity is an important measurement of visual function. It is useful in assessing the severity of acute problems such as an eye injury or in following the progression of a chronic disorder such as a cataract. Standard letter or number charts are available for testing acuity both for distance and close reading, and illiterate E charts or symbols can be used for children beginning about age 3.

If a standard chart is used, the vision is recorded as a fraction. The numerator records the distance from the patient to the chart in feet or meters, and the denominator records the distance at which a normal eye can see the lines seen by the patient. For example, an acuity of 20/200 means an individual can see at 20 feet what a normal eye can see at 200 feet (Fig. 11–1).

If the patient cannot see the symbols on the chart, test the ability to count fingers (Fig. 11–2). The vision may be

331

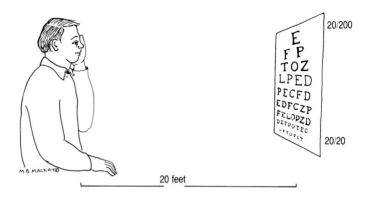

20/200

20/20

20 feet

Fig. 11–1. Visual acuity: Snellen chart.

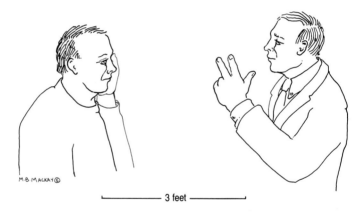

3 feet

Fig. 11–2. Visual acuity: counting fingers.

recorded, for example, as "counts fingers at 3 feet." If the vision is poor, test the ability to see hand movements. If the patient cannot see a hand moving, test for light perception, using a small pen light in a dark room, making sure the second eye is completely occluded (Fig. 11–3). Shine the light in the eye from different directions and ask

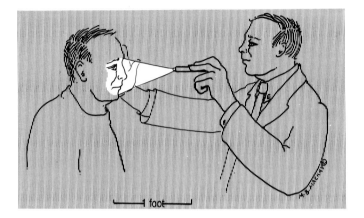

Fig. 11–3. Visual acuity: light perception

the patient to point to the light. If the patient can point to the light source, the vision is recorded as "light perception with good projection," but if the patient cannot point to the light, the vision is recorded as "light perception with no projection."

It is useful to determine if a person with reduced acuity improves when looking through a pinhole (Fig. 11–4); such a person often has a refractive error and the vision can usually be corrected with glasses. In this way, the physician can rule out serious causes of vision loss. A pinhole disk can easily be constructed by drilling a 0.5 mm hole in an opague piece of cardboard or plastic.

The pinhole disk is also a useful method of measuring visual acuity following an injury to the eye in cases where the patient's spectacles were broken or lost. This observation is helpful in possible later medicolegal action in order to record the patient's vision immediately after eye trauma.

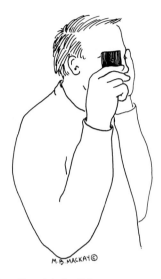

Fig. 11–4.   Visual acuity: pinhole disk.

PATCHING

Patching is used after corneal trauma to promote healing and to make an eye more comfortable. Patching is also used if an eye is severely injured, in order to avoid contamination and additional damage prior to definitive treatment.

Method

Prepare three strips of adhesive tape 1 inch × 6 inches, and place a patch over the eye, making sure the lids are closed. (Occasionally, the extra thickness of two eye patches may be necessary to keep the eye closed.) A strip of tape is first attached to the forehead above the brow, and then the cheek is pulled up as the tape is secured below the patch (Fig. 11–5A). This applies pressure to the patch and prevents the eye from opening. Additional tapes on each side are used to secure the patch (Fig. 11–5B).

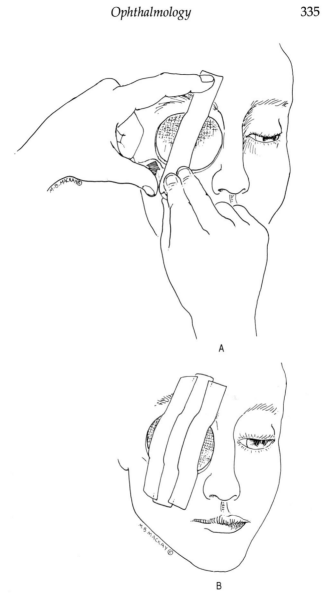

A

B

Fig. 11–5. Eye patching. **A.** Application of tape. **B.** Securing of patch.

Note: The patch must keep the lids closed, especially if corneal sensation is reduced (e.g., if topical anesthetic has been instilled into the eye) in order to avoid a corneal abrasion caused by the patch.

TONOMETRY

Tonometry is helpful in making a correct diagnosis when a patient presents with a painful red eye and blurred vision. It is also used as a screening procedure for chronic glaucoma.

Equipment

Topical ophthalmic anesthetic solution
Schiotz tonometer

Method

The tonometer is checked on the test block to make sure that the plunger and lever are moving freely. The scale reading should be zero when the tonometer is applied to the steel block. The patient is examined in the supine position and after instilling an anesthetic, is asked to fix the gaze on an object directly above the head. The lids are separated with one hand and the tonometer is applied to the center of the cornea with the other (Fig. 11–6). A conversion table in the tonometer box will give the scale readings in millimeters of mercury. A low scale reading means a high pressure. Additional weights may be slipped on the tonometer plunger if very low readings are obtained. False high pressure readings are often recorded if force is required to separate the lids. Normal pressures vary from 15 to 20 millimeters of mercury. The tonometer foot plate should be cleaned after use by rinsing it under a tap and may be sterilized by immersion in alcohol. All alcohol must be removed or have dried prior to use of the instrument.

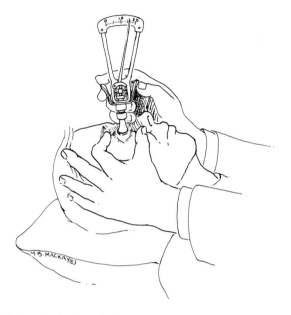

Fig. 11–6. Examination with tonometer.

CHALAZION

A chalazion is an inflammation in a meibomian gland in the tarsal plate. In the acute phase, a painful localized swelling occurs in the lid that often resolves spontaneously or develops into a chronic thick-walled cyst. A persistent cyst is treated by incisional drainage through the tarsal plate.

Equipment

Small syringe with 25- or 27-gauge short needle
1% lidocaine (without epinephrine)
Topical ophthalmic anesthetic solution
Chalazion clamp (continued)

Scalpel, fine point
Eye patch

Method

Instill a drop of topical anesthetic on the conjunctiva and infiltrate the lid around the cyst with local anesthetic (Fig. 11–7A). Apply a chalazion clamp to the lid so that the ring of the clamp is adjacent to the tarsal conjunctiva and completely surrounds the cyst (Fig. 11–7B). Evert the lid and make a vertical incision into the cyst 2 to 3 mm in length so that the contents can be expressed with a cotton-tipped applicator (Fig. 11–7C). The vertical incision should not extend to the lid margin, in order to avoid notching. Remove the clamp and apply pressure to the lid with a patch to achieve hemostasis. An occasional warm compress is the only aftercare required.

OCULAR FOREIGN BODY

A foreign body sensation may be caused by a corneal abrasion, a foreign body adherent to the cornea, or a for-

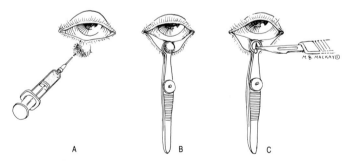

Fig. 11–7. Drainage of chalazion. **A.** Anesthetize. **B.** Apply a chalazion clamp to the lid. **C.** Make a vertical incision into the cyst. See text for more information.

eign body trapped under the upper lid or to the conjunctival fornix.

Diagnosis

Inspect the eye carefully with a flash light and magnification (e.g., a binocular loupe). A small abrasion is difficult to see but if fluorescein is instilled using 1 to 2 drops of a 1% solution or an impregnated strip (e.g., Fluor-i-strip), a defect in the epithelium will stain green. This green may be accentuated with an ultraviolet light.

Pull down the lower lid to inspect the lower fornix. Inspect underneath the upper lid by asking the patient to look down, grasp the lashes and roll the lid over a paper clip or a swab stick (Fig. 11–8A). A loose foreign body is often trapped just inside the lid margin (Fig. 11–8B). If there are multiple abrasions and numerous foreign bodies,

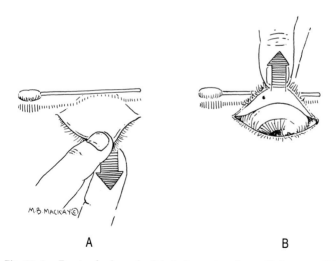

A   B

Fig. 11–8. Foreign body under lid. **A.** Inspect underneath the upper lid. **B.** A loose foreign body is often trapped inside the lid margin.

examination can be facilitated by instilling a topical ophthalmic anesthetic.

Treatment

A corneal abrasion is treated by instilling an antibiotic and patching the eye. A small abrasion will heal in 24 hours, but if half the epithelium is removed, healing may take 2 to 3 days.

A loose foreign body can usually be gently removed from the conjunctiva or from the cornea using a cotton-tipped applicator. This can sometimes be done by rolling the cotton tip rather than rubbing the tip at the site of the foreign body. Flushing the conjunctival sac with normal saline (or even tap water) may remove gross contamination.

If a foreign body is adherent to the cornea, it is usually necessary to instill an anesthetic, and if it is embedded in the superficial layers of the cornea, a sharp instrument such as a sterile spud, No. 19 needle, or dental burr must be used to remove the foreign material. A topical anesthetic is instilled and the patient is placed supine on a table or in a chair with a head support. The patient is told to fix his gaze on an object with the uninvolved eye, in order to reduce unexpected eye movements. The physician holds the instrument used to remove the foreign body like a pencil, supporting the wrist on the cheek; gentle scraping will remove the embedded material (Fig. 11–9). A residual rust deposit is often easier to remove 24 hours later. After removing the foreign body, an antibiotic is instilled and the eye is patched. Healing is usually complete in 48 hours. Increasing discomfort or a gray infiltrate around the foreign body site suggests the presence of an infected ulcer and indicates more intensive antibiotic treatment. If the patient with a foreign body symptom gives a history of hammering metal, a skull radiograph should be taken to check for a radio-opaque intraocular fragment.

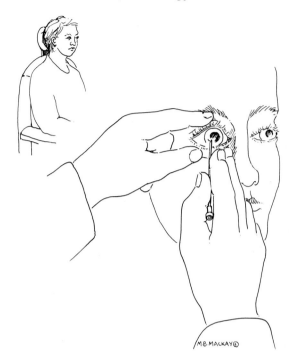

Fig. 11–9. Removal of embedded foreign body.

Note: A large corneal abrasion or the removal of an embedded foreign body may be extremely painful and require general sedation. A topical anesthetic will relieve the discomfort temporarily but should not be used frequently for pain relief as it will inhibit the healing of an epithelial defect. The cornea is approximately 1 mm thick and is not easily penetrated during removal of a superficial foreign body if due care is taken.

CORNEAL EXPOSURE

Persistent exposure of the cornea leads to corneal ulceration, infection, and scarring. It occurs in patients with a seventh nerve paresis (e.g., Bell's palsy), thyroid exophthalmos, and commonly in unconscious patients, for example, during general anesthesia, or for unconscious patients in intensive care units who suffer from severe head trauma.

Method

Minor degrees of exposure can be controlled by instilling ointments that prevent drying, e.g., Lacrilube or tear substitutes.

Adhesive tape is commonly used to close the lids during general anesthesia. If more prolonged closure is required, a 4-0 suture inserted through the skin near the lid margin of the upper lid can be pulled down and taped to the cheek (Fig. 11–10). Medication can be instilled in the eye by lifting the suture.

Tarsorrhaphy

Persistent exposure with evidence of ulceration is corrected by performing a tarsorrhaphy, which permanently closes the lids.

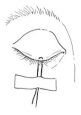

Fig. 11–10. Temporary lid closure.

Equipment

Topical anesthetic, lidocaine 1%
Syringe 10-ml and needle No. 27
Scalpel
4-0 silk
Needle driver
Rubber pegs made by splitting the tip of a fine catheter

Method

A topical anesthetic is instilled in the eye and the lid margins are infiltrated with local anesthetic. The epithelium of the outer (lateral) third of the edges of the lids is roughened with a sharp knife (Fig. 11–11A). One or two sutures (e.g., 4-0 silk), passed through rubber pegs, are used to bring the lid margins together (Fig. 11–11B and C). In 2 weeks when the sutures are removed, a permanent adhesion results between the lid margins, which reduces exposure of the cornea. If lid function returns, the adhesion can be divided with scissors. In severe cases of exposure, it may be necessary to close the medial ⅓ of the lid margins as well.

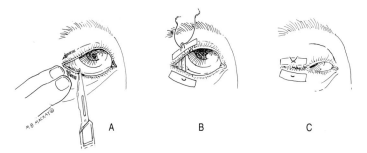

Fig. 11–11. Tarsorrhaphy. **A.** The outer (lateral) third of the lid edges is roughened with a sharp knife. **B.** One or two sutures passed through rubber pegs. **C.** The lid margins are brought together.

ENUCLEATION

A badly injured eye, a blind painful eye, an eye containing a tumor, or a donor eye for corneal grafting may require enucleation. This procedure is usually done under general anesthetic, but adequate local anesthesia can be obtained by a retrobulbar injection of 10 ml of 1% procaine or lidocaine, without epinephrine. A donor eye is normally removed from a cadaver within 12 hours of death.

Equipment

Lid speculum
1% lidocaine
10 ml syringe and No. 27 needle
Dissecting scissors
Toothed forceps
Muscle hook
Enucleation scissors
Needle driver
Absorbable 4–0 suture

Method

If local anesthesia is employed, inject 5 ml of anesthetic behind the globe entering the lower temporal quadrant of the orbit through the lower lid (Fig. 11–12A). Wait five minutes, insert the lid speculum and obtain additional anesthesia by injecting 2 ml behind the globe through the conjunctival fornices in each of the remaining quadrants (Fig. 11–12B).

The conjunctiva is incised for 360° just outside the cornea and blunt dissection is used with scissors to free the globe from adhesions to periorbital tissue (Fig. 11–12C). A muscle hook is passed circumferentially around the globe in order to pick up the attachments of the rectus muscles that are located about 5 mm from the cornea in the 12, 3, 6 and

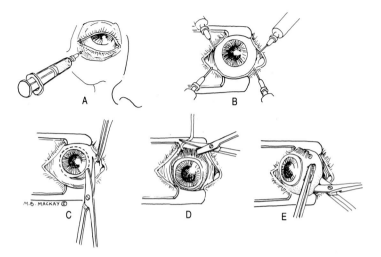

Fig. 11–12. Enucleation of the eye. **A.** Anesthetize. **B.** Insert the lid speculum and obtain additional anesthesia. **C.** Conjunctiva is incised for 360°. **D.** A muscle hook is passed around the circumference of the globe. **E.** Enucleation scissors are used to free any remaining loose posterior adhesions. See text for more information.

9 o'clock positions (Fig. 11–12D). The stump of the medial rectus muscle is left long so that the globe can be manipulated with a heavy forcep or hemostat. Passing the muscle hook more deeply in the upper nasal quadrant will pick up the superior oblique muscle and in the lower temporal quadrant will pick up the inferior oblique muscle. Enucleation scissors are then used to free any remaining loose posterior adhesions, and if the eye is rotated laterally, it is possible to feel the optic nerve attached to the back of the eye (Fig. 11–12E). The scissors are used to sever the optic nerve; this permits the eye to be withdrawn from the socket. Bleeding is controlled by pressure with gauze pads. If available, a ball implant is inserted into the socket, and

the conjunctiva is closed using a continuous suture of 4-0 chromic catgut.

If a donor eye is used for a corneal transplant, it should be placed in a sterile jar on a layer of gauze soaked in saline. The eye should be kept cold and transported in an ice filled cooler available from an eye bank.

BASIC EYE EQUIPMENT

General

Eye pads
1 inch adhesive tape
Fluor-i-strips
1% lidocaine
Pinhole disk
No. 26 needles, 1½ inch
10-ml syringe

Instruments

Tonometer
Spud
Chalazion clamp
Scalpel (small curved blade)
Small dissecting scissors
Needle driver
Silk sutures 4-0 and 6-0
Muscle hook
Fine and heavy toothed forceps
Binocular magnifier
Lid speculum
Absorbable suture 4-0

BASIC EYE MEDICATIONS

Antibiotic

10% sulphacetamide
Chloramphenicol
Polymyxin B-Neomycin-compound (Neosporin)
Gentamicin
Two of the above as drops or ointment

Steroid

Dexamethasone

Cycloplegic

1% atropine

Pressure Reducing Agents

Pilocarpine 2%
Timolol Maleate Ophthalmic 0.5% (Timoptic)
Acetazolamide
Mannitol 20% intravenous

Topical Anesthetic

Proparacaine HC1 0.5% (Ophthetic)

Tear Substitute

Methylcellulose 0.5%
Ocular lubricant (e.g., Lacrilube)

12
Orthopedics

Adult Orthopedics
James F. Kellam

Any physician who treats patients with extremity injuries must understand these basic principles: splintage and closed reduction and external immobilization.

SPLINTAGE

A patient with a suspected extremity injury should not be transported without a splint applied. The term "to splint" means to immobilize an injured extremity, spine, or pelvis, in an anatomical alignment by using prefabricated splints, slings, or plaster of paris. The reasons for splintage are obvious: the procedure relieves pain and prevents further injury to the surrounding soft tissue structures.

Techniques of Splinting

1. Prior to splinting, the injured extremity requires assessment by a thorough physical examination. Neu-

rovascular injury or compartment syndromes should be suspected.

2. Inspection of the extremity on all aspects for open wounds is required.
3. Radiographic evaluation is not necessary at this stage.
4. Alignment of the limb is carried out. This will provide axial alignment but is not an attempt at a closed reduction.
5. Realignment may be performed by gentle traction with or without appropriate analgesia, depending upon the clinical situation.
6. Appropriate padding (a soft towel or material such as abdominal padding or absorbent cotton) should be applied to the extremity.
7. Where possible, the splint should extend one joint above and one joint below the suspected injury.
8. The splint should fit firmly against the padding and be bandaged to the limb with flannel. Tensors or elasticized bandages should be avoided because they tend to constrict if swelling occurs.
9. Any open wound should be irrigated, major debris removed, and a sterile dressing applied.

The following represent specific methods of splinting common injuries:

Cervical Spine Injuries

The initial method used to stabilize the cervical spine is the application of inline immobilization. The physician places one hand on either side of the patient's chin with one or two fingers below it, maintaining the head in a neutral position (Fig. 12–1). Traction should *not* be applied. If necessary, hold a handful of the patient's hair, and with gentle traction, stabilize the cervical spine. This technique can be used in the acute resuscitation phase of trauma patients. Inline immobilization must be used until a lateral

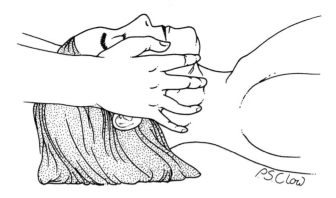

Fig. 12–1. Inline immobilization of the cervical spine.

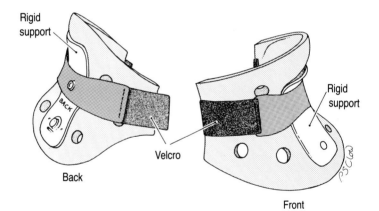

Fig. 12–2. Philadelphia collar.

cervical spine radiograph, which includes the C7-T1 junction, indicates the absence of fracture or dislocation of the cervical spine.

More rigid immobilization may be obtained by using a Philadelphia collar, a commercially available splint. It comes in two halves that are secured by Velcro straps

(Fig. 12–2). The posterior shell may be flattened and slid under the patient's neck, while an assistant applies inline stabilization. When this is completed, the anterior shell is placed over the front of the patient's neck and chin and secured with the Velcro straps (Fig. 12–3).

An alternate technique for immobilization of the cervical spine is to place 5 kg sandbags on either side of the head to maintain it in a neutral position. The head is then taped across the forehead directly to the bed or spinal board

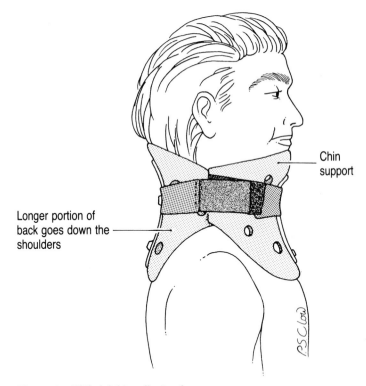

Chin support

Longer portion of back goes down the shoulders

Fig. 12–3. Philadelphia collar in place.

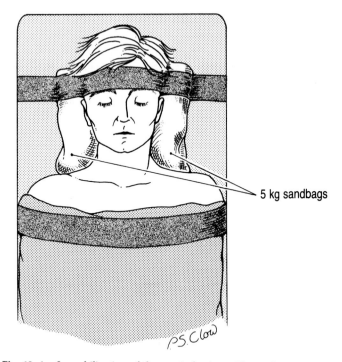

Fig. 12–4. Immobilization of the cervical spine with sandbags.

(Fig. 12–4). These techniques are the most suitable for cervical spine immobilization if transport of the patient is required.

Thoracolumbar Spinal Injuries

The splintage of the thoracic and lumbar spine is best accomplished by placing the patient on a long, rigid spinal board. Logrolling is the only acceptable way to turn a patient suspected of a spinal injury. This maneuver requires a minimum of three people: one at the head to maintain longitudinal stabilization, one at the side of the body to turn the trunk, and one at the feet to turn the legs. The aim of logrolling is to move the body as a whole so that one segment does not precede or drag behind another. This procedure should be done in unison under the control of the one person at the head, who directs the operation. This technique will allow the safe placement of x-ray film or spinal board, or for examination of the patient's back (Fig. 12–5).

The Upper Extremity

The Shoulder

Injuries to the shoulder, including the humerus, are best splinted with the arm at the side. The use of either a sling, collar and cuff, or Velpeau bandage is appropriate. Further splintage may be obtained by adding a bandage that straps

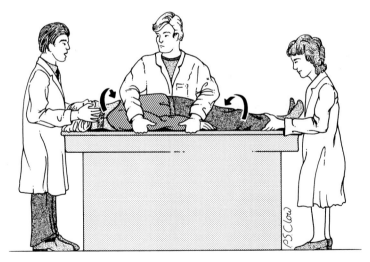

Fig. 12–5. Logrolling in suspected spinal injury.

the arm to the trunk; this creates a thoracobrachial bandage. In isolated injuries, it is useful to maintain the patient in the sitting position (see Fig. 12–20).

The Elbow

The elbow should be immobilized in the position in which it is found, using pillow splints or a well-padded posterior plaster slab. Elbow dislocations and supracondylar fractures of the elbow are usually found in a semi-flexed position. To attempt to straighten or flex the arm causes the patient extreme pain and carries the risk of subsequent neurovascular compromise.

The Forearm

The forearm may be immobilized in commercially available splints that extend from the wrist to above the elbow. Another method is to apply a posterior plaster slab, ten layers thick, over a well-padded arm, which extends from the metacarpophalangeal joints to the axilla. This plaster slab is held in place with a flannel bandage (Fig. 12–6).

The Wrist and Hand

Commercially available splints may be used for the wrist and hand. A simple forearm splint will provide enough support for the wrist. Finger fractures probably require nothing more than elevation and protection during initial assessment.

The Lower Extremity

The Pelvis

Splintage of the pelvis is almost impossible, but in massive disruption of the pelvis where the patient's general condition is unstable due to blood loss, it may be useful to apply pneumatic antishock garments in order to stabilize

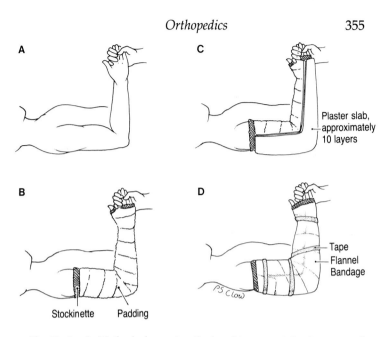

Fig. 12–6. **A.** Method of grasping the hand to support the forearm and maintain the elbow flexed at 90° for application of splint. **B., C., D.** Application of a posterior plaster slab.

the pelvis and hopefully, reduce bony displacement. This type of stabilization will tend to decrease retroperitoneal hemorrhage.

Hip Fractures

Fractures of the hip are best splinted by the application of Buck's extension traction. This is applied to the lower leg through a foam boot, or combined with commercially available skin tapes and held in place with a tensor bandage. Two or three kg of weight over the end of the stretcher or bed are suitable for immobilization (Fig. 12–7).

Dislocations of the Hip

Most hip dislocations, either anterior or posterior, require a general anesthetic for reduction. Consequently,

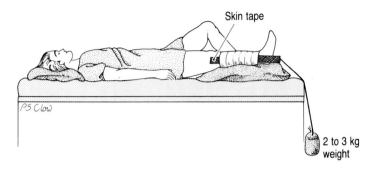

Fig. 12–7. Buck's extension traction.

they are difficult to splint in any position other than the one in which they present. Splintage should consist of allowing the limb to stay in the position in which it is found, with support from pillows, until a reduction can be carried out.

Femoral Shaft Fractures

Femoral shaft fractures are best splinted by the use of a Thomas splint and application of skin traction as described under the Buck's extension treatment. Once the skin traction apparatus has been applied, a Thomas splint is placed over the injured extremity. The rope is then tied to the end of the splint, applying the appropriate amount of fixed traction to realign the limb. Realignment, not reduction, is the goal of this method along with maintenance of realignment.

The Thomas splint comes either with a half or full ring at the proximal end of the apparatus. These rings should be checked to make sure that they are wide enough to go over a swollen thigh and to accommodate further swelling. The rings are also angled, the longer portion of the splint going to the outer side of the leg. This point should be checked to make sure that it is long enough to provide at least 15 to 20 cm of length past the foot. The splint should also have firm cloth material, such as toweling, applied between the long arms. Stockinette is insufficient because it is weak and will allow the leg to sag in the splint. In order to apply more traction, tongue depressors may be placed across the ropes where they run from the ankle to the splint. Turning the tongue depressors produces a wind-lass effect and will tighten the ropes, increasing the traction. When the appropriate increase has been obtained, the tongue depressors are taped to the splint to maintain the increased traction. (Fig. 12–8).

Knee Injuries

Tibial plateau fractures and knee ligament disruptions are best splinted with soft dressing and posterior plaster slab (Jones' bandage) (Fig. 12–9). Commercially available knee immobilizers are useful.

Dislocations are best splinted in the position in which they present unless neurovascular compromise is noted, in which case immediate reduction should be undertaken, preferably with general anesthetic.

The Lower Leg

Fractures of the tibial shaft, ankle, and foot are best splinted by the application of either commercially available splints or a well-padded plaster of paris splint.

These splints should be form fitting and should extend above the knee and be wrapped onto the extremity, taking care not to compress the leg. Careful assessment for compartment syndromes and vascular compromise, before and after application of the splint, is *mandatory.* A simple way to apply a plaster of paris splint is to let the leg hang over the edge of the bed and allow gravity to provide the necessary traction (Fig. 12–10). The padding is first applied,

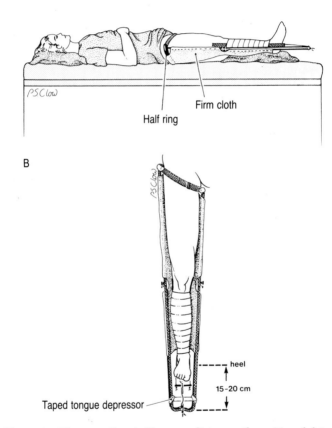

A

PSClow

Firm cloth

Half ring

B

PSClow

heel

15-20 cm

Taped tongue depressor

Fig. 12–8. Thomas splint. **A.** Thomas splint correctly positioned, lateral view. **B.** Thomas splint in position as viewed from above, right leg.

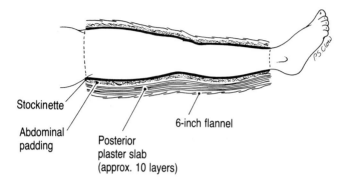

Stockinette

Abdominal padding

Posterior plaster slab (approx. 10 layers)

6-inch flannel

Fig. 12–9. Jones' bandage with knee at midpoint.

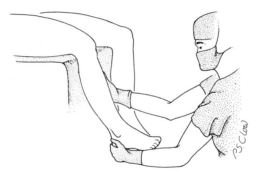

Fig. 12–10. Gravity provides traction. Realignment for lower leg fracture.

the below-knee portion of the splint applied next (Fig. 12–11), and the upper portion of the splint added with the leg elevated. Long-leg immobilization will be much more comfortable if the knee is not quite fully extended (Fig. 12–12).

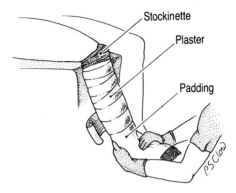

Fig. 12–11. Application of a below-knee splint assisted by gravity.

*Knee is not fully extended

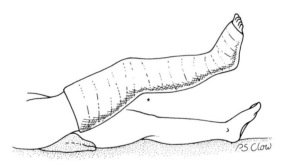

Fig. 12–12. Long-leg immobilization.

Open Fractures

Except for wound care, an open fracture is handled the same as closed fractures. Any major contamination should be removed; if a foreign object impales the extremity, it should be left in place. Debris and dirt that are on the wound surface may be removed and the wound irrigated with sterile saline. If there will be a delay in definitive debridement, irrigation should definitely be performed in the emergency department, using approximately 10 to 12 liters of saline run gently through the wound. Following this, a sterile dressing should be used and an appropriate splint applied.

PRINCIPLES AND TECHNIQUES OF CLOSED REDUCTION OF COMMON FRACTURES

The treatment of fractures requires an adequate history and physical examination followed by appropriate radiographic investigation. These techniques define the fracture. Undisplaced fractures are usually managed by immobilization alone. Displaced fractures require reduction and immobilization; this reduction may be closed or open depending upon the "personality" of the fracture. The closed method of treatment of fractures usually consists of four phases:

1. Manipulation or reduction of the fracture.
2. Application of a device to maintain reduction.
3. Immobilization of the fracture until healed.
4. Rehabilitation or restoration of function.

The closed method of fracture treatment is dependent upon the presence of a soft tissue hinge between the two fracture fragments (Fig. 12–13). Most fractures, except

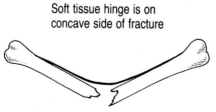

Soft tissue hinge is on
concave side of fracture

Fig. 12–13. Fracture with soft tissue hinge.

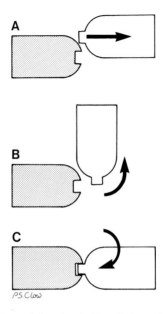

Fig. 12–14. Technique of closed reduction. **A.** Longitudinal or axial traction. **B.** and **C.** Realignment by reversing mechanism that caused fracture.

those resulting from high energy causes, will have this hinge. It is located on the concave side of a displaced fracture. The soft tissue, or periosteal hinge, functions as a guide for reduction as well as a buttress for forces applied to maintain the reduction. Without the bridge, the fracture is unstable and difficult to manage by closed techniques.

Principles of Closed Reduction (Fig. 12–14)

1. Adequate relief and control of pain is mandatory. This may be through the use of a general anesthetic, regional blocks, local infiltration, or intravenous medication.

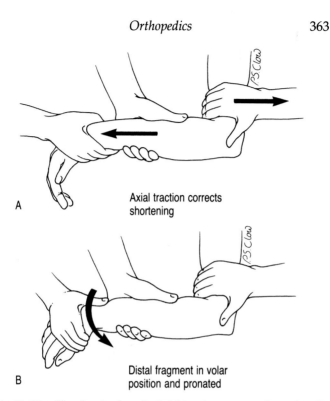

Fig. 12–15. Closed reduction. **A.** Axial traction corrects shortening. **B.** Distal fragment in volar position and pronated.

2. Reduction is accomplished by aligning the distal fracture fragment to the proximal fragment. Study the radiographs and limb to determine the displacement of the distal fragment. It is important to assess the position of the proximal fragment as well.
3. Next, longitudinal or axial traction is gently applied along the axis of the extremity. This will restore length. and is the first and most important step as most displaced fractures shorten.
4. The fracture can then be realigned by reversing the

mechanism that caused it. For example, in a distal radial metaphyseal fracture, the displacement consists of shortening, dorsal displacement with volar angulation, and a supination deformity. Axial traction corrects the shortening (Fig. 12–15A), and then the distal fragment is placed in a volar position and pronated (Fig. 12–15B).

5. Once reduction is obtained and assessed clinically, immobilization is carried out. This is usually by means of a plaster of paris cast which is well molded, taking into account the soft tissue hinge which must be placed on tension.

6. Radiographic confirmation of the reduction is then obtained.

7. Appropriate elevation of the extremity and evaluation for potential complications such as swelling or neurologic impairment are carried out. Following reduction of all fractures or dislocations, it is wise to repeat these evaluations 24 hours later.

8. Follow-up care at weekly intervals in order to evaluate the position and healing of the reduced fracture is advised.

9. Once healing is complete and confirmed by radiography the cast is removed and rehabilitation therapy instituted.

10. *Further specialized evaluation is indicated when:* reduction is not possible; intra-articular fractures are present; loss of reduction occurs following attempted reduction, and adequate function will not be obtained by closed reduction. This includes fractures of the radius and ulna, intra-articular fractures, fractures where neurologic or vascular injury have occurred, and most open fractures.

Precaution

If in doubt about any aspect of the diagnosis, reduction, immobilization or treatment of any fracture, orthopedic consultation should be obtained.

Technique of Closed Treatment of Common Fractures

The primary care physician should be able to manage these displaced fractures or dislocations:

Shoulder dislocations.
Acromioclavicular dislocations.
Clavicle fractures.
Dislocations of the elbow.
Fractures of the head of the radius.
Fractures of the distal radial metaphysis.
Fractures of the metacarpals.
Extra-articular fractures of the phalanges of the hand.
Dislocations of the joints of the hand.
Selected fracture dislocations of the ankle.
Fractures of the metatarsals and phalanges of the feet.
Dislocations of the joints of the toes.

General Considerations

1. Patient Assessment

History. Assessment of the patient should be based on the "personality" of the fracture, considering the problem with respect to the patient, the limb, and the fracture, in that order of importance. For example, it is of no use to treat the fracture if the patient is too injured to survive. In patients where this is possible, the emergency treatment of the patient comes first, the involved limb next, and finally the fracture.

Examination. Assessment of the limb is directed to open fractures, compartment syndromes, neurologic, and vascular injuries.

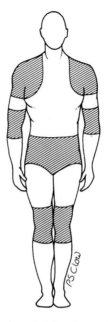

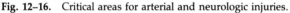

Fig. 12–16.   Critical areas for arterial and neurologic injuries.

2. Palpation of pulses prior to and after manipulation of the limb is essential. The index of suspicion for arterial injuries should be high with elbow fractures and dislocations, fractures of the distal third of the femur, and fractures and dislocations about the knee and ankle. Neurologic injuries should be suspected with dislocations of the shoulder, hip, and elbow (Fig. 12–16).

3. Radiographic assessment. Two views at 90° are mandatory for evaluation of every fracture. These must include the joint above and below the fracture. Oblique views may also be helpful. No dislocation should be reduced prior to radiograph confirmation.

The Clavicle

History and Diagnosis

Fractures of the clavicle usually occur from direct trauma or a fall on the outstretched arm. The patient presents with exquisite and acute pain in the region of the shoulder girdle and will be holding the injured arm and leaning forward to relieve the pain. Diagnosis is as simple as palpation, which will confirm the site of injury.

Method

These fractures can usually be treated adequately by sling immobilization. The use of figure-of-eight bandage may be associated with significant complications from axillary vein thrombosis, brachial plexus compression, and skin necrosis.

The use of a broad arm sling and rest in a supine position is usually best for the first 3 to 4 days. When the patient is comfortable, motion should begin in the shoulder region. In adults, the fracture will usually heal in 6 to 8 weeks.

Precautions

Some clavicular fractures will perforate through the platysmus and superficial fascia of the shoulder girdle region. Jagged bone ends at the fracture site may come to lie extremely superficially under the skin, and in this situation closed reduction or open reduction may be required to avoid skin necrosis and the complication of an open fracture.

Be wary of the massively displaced clavicular fracture as a clue to significant neurologic or vascular injury in the upper extremity. This is especially common in high energy injuries that occur with motorcycle accidents.

368   *Orthopedics*

Anterior Shoulder Dislocation

History and Diagnosis

Fall on the outstretched arm.
Forced abduction and external rotation.
Blow to posterior aspect of shoulder.

Physical Examination

Squared-off shoulder.
Palpable defect posteriorly in glenoid fossa.
Pain with passive and active motion.
Beware of neurologic symptoms and signs.

Radiographic Evaluation

Anteroposterior radiograph of the shoulder and trans-
scapular views are necessary. The trans-scapular radiograph is obtained by placing the x-ray film plate next to
the outer aspect of the patient and angling the patient at
30 to 40°. The x-ray beam is then aimed down the scapula
(Fig. 12–17A). The appearance of the scapula is a "Y" with

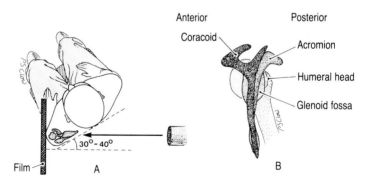

Fig. 12–17. Radiographic evaluation. **A.** Trans-scapular roentgenogram.
B. Medial view of scapula with normal placement of humerus.

the body of the scapula meeting the acromion posteriorly and the coracoid anteriorly.

The glenoid is at the junction of the three limbs of the "Y." The head of the humerus should overlie this junction (Fig. 12–17B). Anterior or posterior dislocations can easily be confirmed with this view.

Method

The safest method to obtain a reduction is by turning the patient into the prone position and allowing the dislocated arm to fall forward over the side of the stretcher. The stretcher is high enough so that a weight may be affixed to the wrist of the patient. Do not have the patient hold the weight. Starting with 1 to 3 kg, traction and gravity will allow reduction of the shoulder. Reduction is usually apparent when the patient describes reduced pain and the shoulder appears normal (Fig. 12–18).

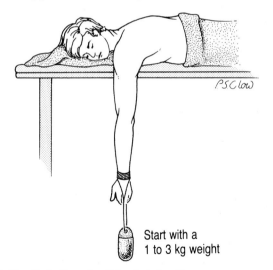

Start with a
1 to 3 kg weight

Fig. 12–18. Reduction of a dislocated shoulder.

Orthopedics

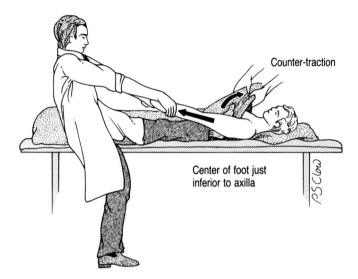

Fig. 12–19. Reduction of shoulder dislocation. Hippocratic method.

The Hippocratic method is an alternative and is performed with the patient supine. A sheet is placed across the upper lateral chest wall below the axilla and held by an assistant on the opposite side of the stretcher to allow for countertraction. The reduction is accomplished by the physician's placing his unshod foot on the lateral chest wall just inferior to the axilla. Gentle traction is then applied to the outstretched arm. With gentle traction, time, and appropriate analgesia, the shoulder muscles will relax and reduction will be obtained (Fig. 12–19).

Follow-up Care

A Velpeau bandage is used for 3 weeks, maintaining the shoulder in internal rotation and in a neutral position at the side of the body (Fig. 12–20). For the next 3 weeks, the arm is allowed to remain in a sling avoiding abduction or

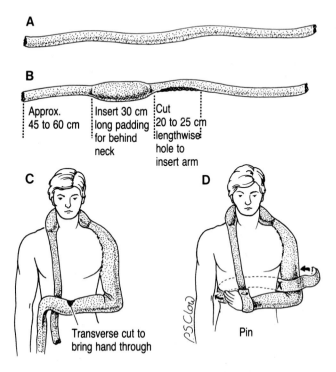

Approx.
45 to 60 cm | Insert 30 cm long padding for behind neck | Cut 20 to 25 cm lengthwise hole to insert arm

Transverse cut to bring hand through

Pin

Fig. 12–20. Velpeau bandage. **A.** 3-inch wide stockinette approximately 3 meters long. **B.** Prepare bandage. **C.** Cut small hole to bring hand through hole (C), wrap stockinette behind body. Wrap behind trunk and pin arm at X with arm tight beside body.

external rotation activities but allowing isometric strengthening exercises and pendulum motion.

Posterior Shoulder Dislocations

History and Diagnosis

Less common than anterior dislocations.

Associated with epilepsy, seizures, electroconvulsive therapy, and alcoholism.

Physical Examination

Shoulder contour appears normal.
Prominence posteriorly.
Defect in the anterior glenoid area.
Most importantly, the patient is unable to externally rotate the arm.

Radiographic Evaluation

AP and trans-scapular views.

Method

Reduction is accomplished by gentle longitudinal traction, with pressure applied posteriorly over the head.

Immobilization

Following reduction, a trial range of motion should be undertaken to determine stability. In unstable posterior dislocations, orthopedic consultation should be obtained. Stable posterior dislocations may be immobilized as mentioned under anterior dislocations.

Precautions

All these require orthopedic consultation:
1. Greater tuberosity fragment: unreduced or subacromial location.
2. Neurologic involvement.
3. Irreducible or unstable dislocation.

Proximal Humeral Fractures: Surgical Neck

History and Diagnosis

Common fracture in elderly, over 65 years of age.
Fall on oustretched arm.
Assess swelling, neurovascular status.

Assess stability by grasping the humeral head with one hand and gently rotating and abducting the arm to assess whether fragments move together.

If fragments appear to move as a unit and the patient is relatively comfortable, the fracture is impacted and stable.

Radiographic Evaluation

AP and trans-scapular views of the shoulder.

Method

The treatment of proximal humeral fractures depends upon a thorough evaluation of the physiologic and functional status of the patient. The majority of these fractures are minimally displaced, impacted and stable, and therefore may be treated in a Velpeau bandage with early motion at 10 to 14 days, as permitted by pain. Depending on the functional level of the patient, displaced surgical neck fractures should be assessed for possible further intervention.

Precaution

Be aware of the fracture dislocation because this requires operative intervention.

Humeral Shaft Fractures

History and Diagnosis

Direct blow or torsional injury such as from throwing.
Swollen tender shaft of humerus.
Angulation.
Beware of radial nerve palsy.

Radiographic Evaluation

Anteroposterior radiographs of the humerus, including the shoulder and elbow.

Method

Initial treatment involves realignment of the fracture with the patient in a sitting position. Gravity will assist the reduction. Gentle traction may be applied through the epicondyle of the humerus with the elbow at 90°.

The arm is aligned and then wrapped with soft cast padding. Plaster is placed around this in a sugar-tong or "U" fashion, starting in the axilla and bringing it down the inner

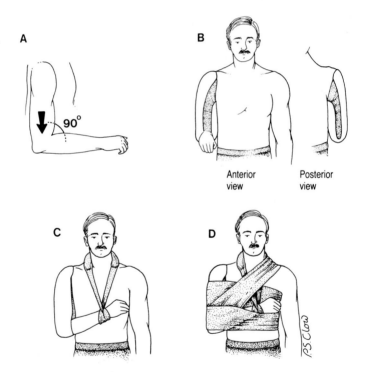

Fig. 12–21. Humeral shaft fractures: sugar-tong or "U" splint. **A.** Elbow at 90° flexion. **B.** Anterior view and posterior view. **C.** Collar and cuff. **D.** Thoracobrachial bandage.

aspect of the arm, under the elbow, and then up over the lateral aspect onto the shoulder (Fig. 12–21A & B). This is wrapped on the arm. The wrist is suspended by a collar and cuff and the arm bound to the body by a thoracobrachial bandage (Fig. 12–21C & D).

For 6 to 8 weeks, the patient should be assessed frequently for hygienic reasons, cast checks and radiograph evaluation. At 6 to 8 weeks, the use of a functional cast brace in the upper extremity may be instituted.

Precaution

Radial Nerve Injuries. Closed radial nerve injury seen initially will usually resolve. Radial nerve injuries caused by reduction require orthopedic or neurosurgical consultation.

Dislocations of the Elbow

History and Diagnosis.

Common dislocation is posterior or posterolateral. Caused by fall on outstretched arm.

Beware of neurovascular injury.

Examination shows loss of the isosceles triangle between the two epicondyles and the olecranon.

Decreased range of motion.

Elbow held in partial flexion.

Radiographic Evaluation

AP and lateral views of the elbow.

Method

Reduction is obtained by traction. An assistant applies countertraction to the humerus, while the physician applies traction to the forearm by grasping the wrist and proximal forearm. Longitudinal traction is exerted in the

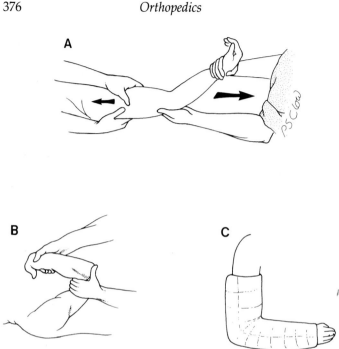

Fig. 12–22. Reduction and immobilization of elbow dislocation. **A.** Elbow is moved through a full range of motion. **B.** Stable reduction is confirmed. **C.** Posterior plaster of paris splint is applied.

position where the arm lies. Posterolateral displacement is corrected, and then the elbow is flexed with pressure over the proximal forearm and posteriorly over the olecranon to disengage the coronoid and push the olecranon back into position. Reduction occurs with palpable "clunk" (Fig. 12–22). Following reduction the elbow is moved through a full range of motion to assess stability.

With a stable reduction, a posterior plaster of paris splint is applied at 90°. Close observation for compartment syndrome or vascular compromise should be undertaken.

With stable dislocations, begin motion at 5 days; the splint is removed several times a day for this. Between 10 to 14 days, a sling or collar and cuff is substituted, allowing increased motion.

Precaution

These conditions require orthopedic consultation: Unstable elbow dislocations, and elbow dislocations with mechanical block after reduction; fracture dislocations of the elbow: arterial or neurologic injuries plus or minus compartment syndrome.

Fractures of the Radial Head

History and Diagnosis

Elbow pain following fall on outstretched arm. Difficulty with flexion, extension, supination, and pronation. Tenderness over the radial head. Rapid effusion of elbow joint.

Radiographic Evaluation

AP and lateral views of the elbow.

Method

Assessment of the range of motion is mandatory. With full flexion, extension, supination, and pronation, this injury may be managed with a sling or posterior slab for comfort, and early motion begins between 5 to 7 days.

If, in the acute injury, range of motion is difficult to test, then aspiration of the joint and subsequent infiltration with lidocaine or other appropriate local anesthetic is required. Following satisfactory anesthesia of the joint, full supination, pronation, flexion, and extension should be obtained. If this is so, the fracture may be treated non-operatively with early motion. A posterior slab and sling for 5 to 7 days is used followed by use of a sling alone, which encourages early motion.

Precaution

These conditions require orthopedic consultation: inability to regain full supination and pronation, major displacement of the radial head, and an associated dislocation.

Fractures of the Distal Radial Metaphysis (Colles' Fracture)

Fractures of the distal radial metaphysis have long been treated with a cavalier attitude. Abraham Colles' original description in the elderly osteoporotic bone represents the true Colles' fracture. Patients under 60 years of age or extremely active elderly people will require perfect reduction and stabilization in order to maintain good wrist and distal radioulnar joint function. Therefore, in assessing this fracture, one must take into account the age, functional activity, and type of fracture (intra-articular or extra-articular in nature).

History and Diagnosis

Fall on the outstretched arm: osteoporotic older group.
High velocity or energy injuries in people under 60 years.
Neurologic assessment, especially median nerve.
Dorsal swelling: dinner fork deformity.

Radiographs

Minimum of AP and lateral views plus oblique. Assess for intercarpal or carpal injuries.

Method

Anesthesia. Colles' fracture may usually be treated, if displaced, by reduction under hematoma block or regional anesthesia. The hematoma block is the injection of a local anesthetic directly into the fracture hematoma.

Anesthesia is accomplished following suitable sterile preparation of the dorsum of the arm over the fracture area, by palpation of the step or fracture site. Following infiltration of the skin with local anesthetic, 10 ml of 1 to 2% lidocaine without epinephrine is injected into the fracture hematoma. The hematoma may be found by placing the needle just proximal to the suspected fracture line and by gently walking the needle along the bone until the needle plunges into the fracture site. Equal amount of hematoma and local anesthetic is exchanged (Fig. 12–23).

The area of the ulnar styloid, if fractured, should also be anesthetized. It is essential to wait 10 to 15 minutes for the local anesthetic to take effect.

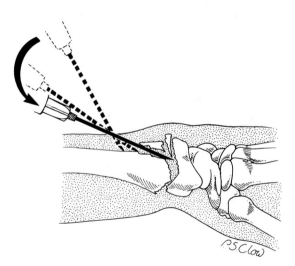

Fig. 12–23. Fracture of the distal radial metaphysis. Hematoma block with local anesthesia.

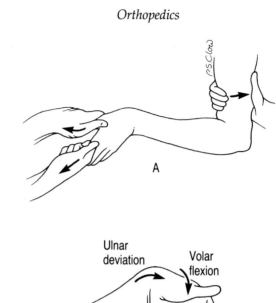

Fig. 12–24. Fracture of the distal radial metaphysis. Mechanics of reduction. **A.** Longitudinal traction to thumb and index finger. **B.** Increase angulation.

Reduction.

1. Longitudinal traction: an assistant supports the arm with the elbow of the patient flexed at 90° (Fig. 12–24 A).

    Longitudinal traction is applied to the thumb and index finger by the operator.

2. Palpation of the fracture site will reveal the dorsal displacement to be gradually disappearing. Occasionally, it will be necessary to increase the angulation

and thus reduce the fracture by volar flexion and ulnar deviation and supination. In most distal radial metaphyseal fractures, however, longitudinal traction will allow reduction of the dorsal displacement and angulation.

3. Once length has been obtained, the fracture is placed in pronation and ulnar deviation, and immobilization applied (Fig. 12–24 B).

Immobilization

In acute fractures, a dorsal radial plaster of paris slab should be applied over one layer of cast padding. This provides fixation over the dorsal radial aspect of the forearm. Positions of severe deformity should not be accepted. The wrist should be immobilized in neutral flexion and extension, and mild ulnar deviation and slight pronation. The splint should be molded with pressure applied over the distal fracture fragment, in a volar direction, combined with molding behind the radial styloid (Fig. 12–25).

Quality of Reduction

Reduction should be anatomical. The aim is that the radial styloid should be 5 to 6 mm longer than the ulnar styloid with at least a neutral volar tilt (Fig. 12–26).

Precaution

These conditions require orthopedic consultation: inadequate reduction, displaced lunate facet, dorsal comminution, failure to maintain reduction, acute carpal tunnel syndrome.

The Hand

Basic Principles

The majority of injuries to the hand occur from hyper-

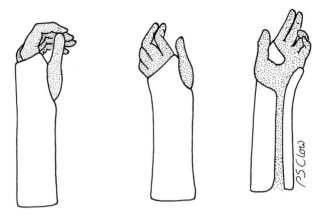

Neutral flexion and   Mild ulnar deviation
extension   slight pronation

Fig. 12–25. Fracture of the distal radial metaphysis (Colles' fracture). Dorsal radial plaster slab.

extension forces through the fingers. Consequently, most injuries are then stable in some degree of flexion and can be reduced and immobilized in this position. The major principles in the treatment of hand injuries are to obtain early motion with limited swelling and appropriate alignment of the fracture. The most important factors affecting alignment are rotation, axial deviation, and shortening.

The majority of hand injuries may be treated adequately by non-operative methods. Splinting should be in a functional position and early motion encouraged. Unless treating an acute mallet or boutonniere injury to the interphalangeal joints, splinting of any finger injury should *not* be in full extension. To avoid joint stiffness, motion is started as early as 7 to 10 days and no later than 3 weeks.

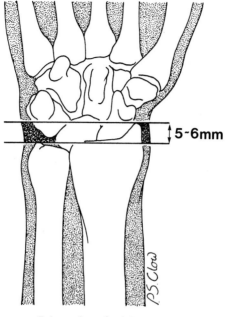

Palmar view of wrist

Fig. 12–26. Quality of reduction, Colles' fracture. Length of radial styloid vs. ulnar styloid.

Fractures of the Phalanges

Method

The involved digit should be anesthetized with appropriate interdigital blocks. Then, a reduction is affected by applying longitudinal traction and correcting axial and rotational deformities. Once reduction has been obtained, the finger is moved through an active range of motion to determine the fracture stability. If the fracture does not displace through a full range of motion, the finger needs to be dynamically splinted to the next digit by "buddy-taping." If the fracture becomes unstable during any degree of extension, then motion should be blocked by a splint. Dynamic buddy-taping is first carried out, then a dorsal plaster of paris slab is applied. The fingers are splinted in a position to maintain the reduction in flexion (Fig. 12–27). Radiographic confirmation of the reduction should be obtained. As the fracture becomes more stable during healing, motion is allowed up to full extension and full flexion.

Interphalangeal and Metacarpophalangeal Dislocations

All dislocations should be reduced by recreating the deformity and then applying axial traction to reduce the joint. Test the range of motion to determine stability and to identify crepitus in the joint. This will determine the stability and whether there are any intra-articular bone fragments. The fingers are splinted in the same fashion as fractures of the phalanges, depending upon the relative stability.

Metacarpal Fractures

These are inherently stable unless there are two or more together, or if they occur on the border digits. If stable,

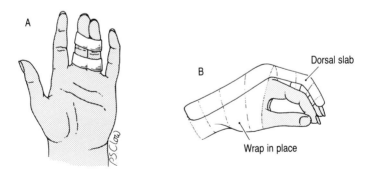

Fig. 12–27. If fracture is unstable after buddy-taping **(A)**, splint with dorsal slab to maintain reduction in flexion **(B)**.

they should be supported and protected in a bandage until healing permits initiation of gentle and increasing motion.

Soft Tissue Joint Injuries

Mallet Finger

Diagnosis

Rupture of the extensor tendon or central slip extensor tendon occurs where it inserts in the dorsal distal phalanx. There may be a small intra-articular avulsion fragment.

Method

Reduction attempted by hyperextension of the distal interphalangeal joint. Immobilization is by a dorsally placed splint over the distal interphalangeal joint which hyperextends, to a mild degree, the distal interphalangeal joint (Fig. 12–28). Splinting is maintained for a minimum of 6 weeks. At 6 weeks, the splint is removed during the day but reapplied at night. If any deformity recurs when the

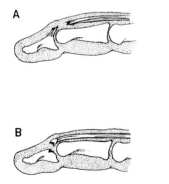

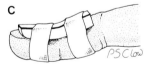

Fig. 12–28. Treatment of mallet finger. **A.** Rupture of tendon. **B.** Avulsion intra-articular fragment. **C.** Immobilization.

splint is removed, the splint should be reapplied for an additional 2 to 4 weeks.

Precaution

Large intra-articular fracture fragments (that is, greater than 25% of the joint surface) or displaced intra-articular fracture fragments require orthopedic consultation.

Acute Boutonniere Deformity

Caused by rupture of the central slip of extensor over the proximal interphalangeal joint. It is associated with volar dislocation of the interphalangeal joint (Fig. 12–29A). Precise clinical examination determines the maximal area of tenderness dorsally over the central slip. There is min-

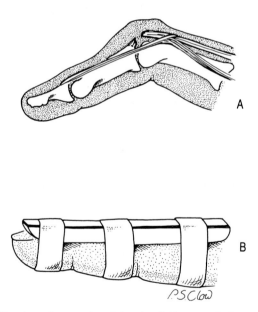

Fig. 12–29.   Acute boutonniere deformity. **A.** Rupture. **B.** Treatment with extension splinting.

imal volar tenderness, although there will be some swelling. Acute boutonniere deformity is secondary to migration of the lateral band to a flexion position.

Method

Treatment is with extension splinting (Fig. 12–29B). Close maintenance of extension splinting for 6 weeks is mandatory.

Rupture of the Ulnar Collateral Ligament of the Thumb

History and Diagnosis

Suspect with skiing injuries or falls on the outstretched hand causing abduction of thumb. Precise clinical examination demonstrates maximal tenderness over the ulnar collateral ligament of the thumb. Stress applied to the thumb will reveal instability.

Radiographs

AP, lateral, and oblique views of the thumb, particularly the carpometacarpal and metacarpophalangeal joints.

Method

Immobilization in a thumb spica or scaphoid type plaster that incorporates the thumb past the distal interphalangeal joint is necessary for 6 weeks. The thumb must be positioned so that the patient could, for example, grasp a glass (Fig. 12–30).

Fractures of the Neck of the Fifth Metacarpal (Boxer's Fracture)

History and Diagnosis

Common mechanism is striking against a solid object with a clenched fist. Be wary of the open injury about the

A   B

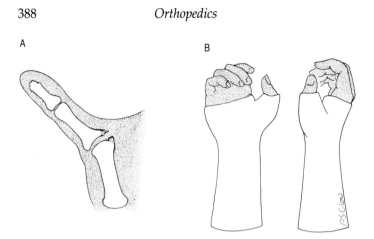

Fig. 12–30. **A.** Rupture of the ulnar collateral ligament of the thumb. **B.** Scaphoid type plaster.

metacarpophalangeal joint; this may represent a tooth laceration. Treat as a human bite with appropriate debridement and irrigation to avoid serious infection. Tenderness and swelling are noted over the neck of the fifth metacarpal, and radiographs show an impacted or stable fracture.

Method

Most boxer's fractures can be treated with observation and support. Indication for reduction is a greater than 40° angulation on a lateral radiograph. Reduction is carried out by pushing the metacarpal head and neck up using a flexed fifth metacarpal (Fig. 12–31).

Precaution

Do not immobilize the fifth finger in acute flexion at all three joints. A molded splint should immobilize the fracture with the MP joint at 60° and the interphalangeal joints slightly flexed in the position of function.

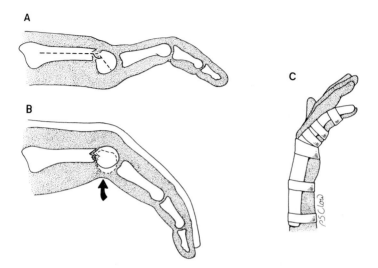

Fig. 12–31. Fracture of the fifth metacarpal neck (Boxer's fracture). If angulation is greater than 40°, reduction is necessary. **A.** Indication. **B.** Reduction. **C.** Immobilization.

Lower Extremity Injuries

The majority of lower extremity injuries require the care of an orthopedic surgeon; however, the techniques of appropriate splintage, as outlined in the first section, can be useful in preparing patients for transfer and making them comfortable until orthopedic consultation can be obtained.

Fractures and dislocations about the hip, knee, ankle, and tibia will usually require operative intervention or at least hospitalization, under the care and guidance of an orthopedic surgeon.

Dislocation of the Patella

Dislocations of the patella are uncommon and usually relocate without assistance.

History and Diagnosis

Dislocation of the patella may occur from a direct blow or a sudden flexion force across the knee, usually in 20° to 30° flexion. The patient will describe the knee as moving inward while the patella remains in position. This is a false sensation since the patella has actually moved outward and the knee has stayed in its appropriate position.

Physical examination reveals a large hemarthrosis, tenderness over the medial parapatellar retinacular region, stable ligaments of the knee, and a positive patellar apprehension sign. *Patellar Apprehension Sign:* the examiner, using the thumb, exerts lateral pressure on the medial side of the patella. In a positive sign, the patient becomes extremely apprehensive that the patella may dislocate again with this pressure. Dislocation may occur if the pressure is maintained by the examiner.

Radiography

AP, lateral, and axial views of the patella with the knee in approximately 20 to 30° of flexion. The latter view is necessary to rule out osteochondral fracture fragments.

Method

1. If dislocation is still present, gradually extending the knee to full extension and pushing the patella back into its position will usually accomplish reduction. If reduction does not occur, seek orthopedic consultation.
2. Most dislocations reduce spontaneously, but good clinical examination will confirm the history.
3. If a dislocation is suspected, then appropriate radiographs to confirm reduction and absence of osteochondral fracture should be done. Following reduction, the leg should be immobilized in a long leg cast

such as a Jones' bandage, posterior slab, or knee immobilizer. The use of crutches and weight bearing, as tolerated, is then appropriate. Static quadriceps exercises may also begin. If an osteochondral fracture fragment is found, further consultation should be sought. Immobilization is between 4 to 6 weeks; range of motion and physiotherapy exercises are encouraged following immobilization.

Fractures of the Foot

Avulsion Fractures of the Base of the Fifth Metatarsal

History and Diagnosis

An inversion injury with avulsion secondary to peroneal brevis force on the base of the fifth metatarsal. Tenderness and swelling occur over this area. Be sure to assess the ankle ligaments. The fracture is confirmed by AP and lateral radiographs (Fig. 12–32).

Method

Treatment is symptomatic, but pain may require immobilizaton in a below-knee walking cast for 4 to 6 weeks. Fractures of the shaft of the fifth metatarsal are a more serious injury and may result in non-union. Immobilization

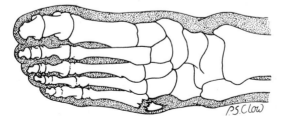

Fig. 12–32. Avulsion fracture of the fifth metatarsal base.

in a below-knee walking cast should be carried out for at least 4 to 6 weeks (Fig. 12–33).

Fractures of the Metatarsals

Isolated metatarsal fractures can be adequately managed by cast immobilization in a below-knee walking cast. Healing requires 4 to 6 weeks of immobilization. In multiple metatarsal fractures from falls, be sure that a serious dislocation or fracture dislocation through the tarsometatarsal joint has not occurred. In this unstable fracture pattern, seek orthopedic consultation.

Fractures of the Toes

These fractures can be managed using the same principles as fractures of the fingers. Splintage is difficult and dynamic buddy-taping is useful, but a simple fracture of

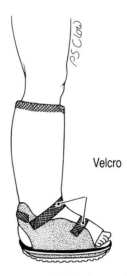

Velcro

Fig. 12–33. Immobilization with below-knee walking cast.

the fifth digit often needs no splinting. Crutches for partial weight bearing are recommended.

Ligamentous Injuries to the Lower Extremity

The two major ligamentous injuries in the lower extremity occur in the knee and ankle.

The Knee

Ligamentous injuries to the knee require prompt diagnosis and appropriate management.

History and Diagnosis

Evaluation

Mechanism of injury: How, when, and where did it occur? Swelling: How soon after injury did it occur (within 6 hours indicates hemarthrosis)?

Precaution

Beware of the bruised, indurated, boggy feeling of a knee with no contours: this indicates a major ligamentous disruption. Traumatic hemarthrosis equals 60% to 70% chance of anterior cruciate ligament injury.

History Following the Injury

Following ligamentous injury, most patients are unable to return to competitive level. Many patients (38%–65%) describe a sudden "pop" in their knees as well as a sensation of the knee "giving out."

Physical Examination

Each of the ligaments of the knee should be tested in a logical, organized fashion. The patellofemoral joint and menisci should be assessed. Inspection of the knee will

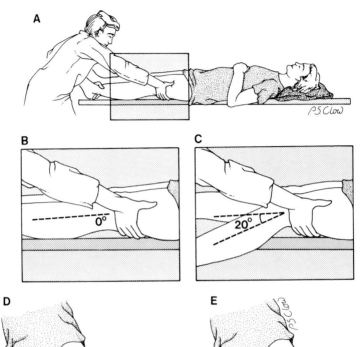

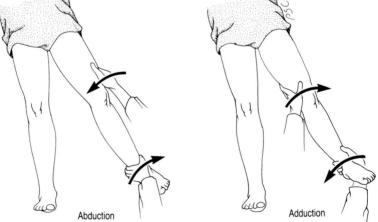

Abduction

Adduction

Fig. 12–34. **A.** Collateral ligament testing. **B.** At 0° of flexion. **C.** At 20° of flexion. **D., E.** Both tests done at 0° and 20° flexion.

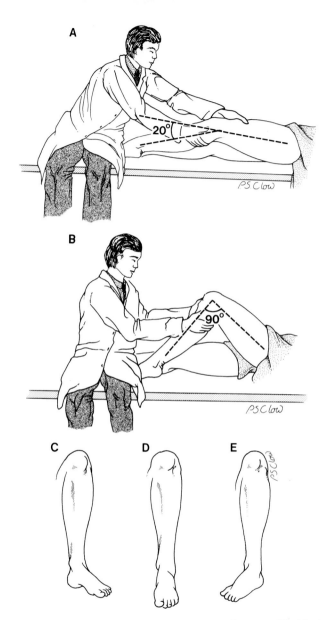

Fig. 12–35. Anterior cruciate testing. **A,** Anterior drawer at 20° of flexion. **B.** Anterior drawer at 90° of flexion. Rotatory tests. **C.** External rotation. **D.** Neutral position. **E.** Internal rotation.

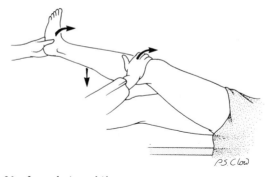

P.S. Clow

Fig. 12–36. Lateral pivot-shift test.

reveal swelling or effusion and evidence of bruising. Collateral ligament testing at 0° and 20° of flexion (Fig. 12–34). Anterior cruciate testing with anterior drawer at 20° and 90° of flexion (Fig. 12–35), rotatory tests (Fig. 12–35 C,D,E), pivot shift (Fig. 12–36), or flexion-rotation drawer sign are all advised. Meniscal tests are difficult to perform in acute knee injuries unless the knees can be flexed past 90°.

Precaution

In knee injuries, carefully check the neurovascular status. Beware of occult knee dislocation. The patellar apprehension sign usually indicates spontaneously reduced patellar dislocations.

Under no circumstances should the comment "knee too painful to get adequate examination" be written on a chart. It is mandatory that assessment of knee joint stability be carried out by a qualified physician. If determination of knee joint stability cannot be made, then referral must be made for further evaluation.

Method

If knee is stable, immobilization may be carried out through a compression dressing of absorbent cotton and flannel (Jones' bandage) or a commercially available knee immobilizer for 1 to 3 weeks. An unstable knee requires orthopedic consultation.

Lateral Ligamentous Ankle Sprains

History and Diagnosis

A common injury secondary to inversion strains. Examine for swelling, tenderness, and ecchymosis over the specific ligamentous structures involved: anterior capsule, anterior talofibular ligament, the talocalcaneal ligament, and the calcaneofibular ligament. Palpation of the entire fibular shaft must be carried out to rule out occult fractures associated with ankle injuries. Anterior drawer test of the ankle as well as varus instability testing may also be carried out.

Radiography

AP and lateral views are mandatory; however, an internal oblique or mortise view is useful to complete assessment.

Classification

This is a functional classification of ankle injuries, which in clinical examination do not have gross inversion, positive stress tests or anterior drawer sign.

Mild Sprain: minimal functional loss, little difficulty hopping symmetrically, no limp when walking, minimal or no swelling, mild point tenderness and pain on reproducing motion of injury.

Moderate Sprain: moderate functional loss, inability to toe-rise or hop-limp when walking, and localized swelling and point tenderness.

Severe Sprain: diffuse tenderness, with tenderness over the lateral and medial aspects. The patient is unable to bear weight and requires crutches.

Method

Treatment during the first 24 hours is the application of ice or a cool water bath for 10 to 15 minutes. Then wrap the ankle with a compression dressing and elevate the ankle for 12 to 24 hours. Crutches may be required to relieve pain on weight bearing. Reassess in 24 hours.

Unstable ankle or severe sprain category: plaster of paris immobilization with a below-knee walking cast for 3 weeks, and then reassess.

Mild and moderate sprains should be immobilized with adhesive strapping and weight bearing permitted as tolerated by patient's threshold of pain. Range of motion exercises should then be gently established.

Severe sprains should be re-evaluated at 3 weeks after cast removal. Range of motion exercises can be started just as in mild and moderate sprains. When all ankle injuries reach full ankle flexion and extension, and patients are without pain, can walk without a limp, and are able to toe-rise supporting the body weight, a conditioning program of calf strengthening and peroneal muscle strengthening may be started.

Precautions

Beware of the anterior tibiofibular ligament injury, the eversion injury where the foot is in a supinated position (the early phase of an unstable ankle fracture), and tenderness and swelling over the ligament on the medial side.

Unstable Ankle Injury

Stress radiographs with greater than 10° talar tilt over normal side or 20° to 25° of talar tilt signify an unstable ankle. Refer the patient to an orthopedic specialist.

Note: It is obvious that orthopedics is too vast a subject to adequately consider in one chapter; further reference is advised.

SUGGESTED READING

1. Salter, R.B.: Textbook of Disorders and Injuries of the Musculoskeletal System, 2nd Ed. Baltimore, Williams and Wilkins, 1983.
2. Adams, J.C.: Outline of Fractures, 8th Ed. Edinburgh, Churchill-Livingstone, 1983.
3. Apley, A.G., and Solomon, L.: Apley's System of Orthopedics and Fractures, 6th Ed. London, Butterworth Scientific, 1952.
4. Charnley, J.: The Closed Treatment of Common Fractures, 3rd Ed. Edinburgh, Churchill-Livingstone, 1972.

Pediatric Orthopedics
C.F. Moseley

TEST FOR CONGENITAL DISLOCATABLE HIP

Examination of a newborn's hip is necessary to discover congenital dislocation or laxity. Many clinical signs provide evidence of the dislocated hip, but diagnosis of the lax, dislocatable hip depends on the demonstration of a "clunk" that accompanies movement of the femoral head over the posterior lip of the acetabulum as it moves from the reduced to the dislocated position and back.

Method

The newborn is placed supine on a firm surface with the examiner directly caudad. The newborn should not be wearing diapers or other encumbering clothing. The hip examination should be done early so that the baby is quiet and relaxed.

The examiner grasps both legs, using one leg to stabilize the pelvis while the other side is examined. The fully flexed knee is grasped by the examiner's thumb and index finger, and the fully extended middle finger is placed on the lateral aspect of the greater trochanter. The leg can then be moved back and forth; one direction tending to dislocate the hip, and the other tending to reduce it (Fig. 12–37). The movement that tends to dislocate the hip consists of adduction of the hip and posterior pressure on the leg, which influences the femoral head to ride posteriorly over the lip of the acetabulum with a palpable "clunk." The movement

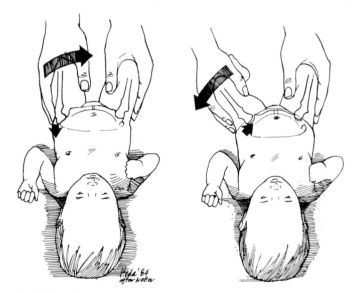

Fig. 12–37. Test for congenital dislocated hip. Baby lying on examining table as seen by an observer.

that tends to reduce the hip consists of abduction of the hip and anterior pressure on the greater trochanter, influencing the femoral head to ride forward over the posterior acetabular lip, again with a "clunk." The examiner feels a true "clunk" in the dislocatable hip, but "clicks" are usually unreliable.

REDUCTION OF DISLOCATIONS

Radial Head Subluxation

Subluxation of the radial head occurs commonly in children younger than 5 years of age. In that period, the radial head is not much larger than the shaft, and the neck is not well defined. This anatomical situation predisposes to the head slipping into the annular ligament when traction is applied to the radius, and the head may get stuck there (Fig. 12–38). The usual mechanism of injury is swinging the child by his outstretched arms. Since this tends to be a recurrent problem for a given child during the early years, and since the reduction involves a safe and easy maneuver, instruct the parents in the method of reduction.

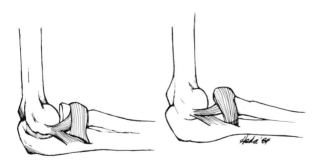

Fig. 12–38. Radial head subluxation. Normal position on left. Subluxated position on right.

Method

The physician grasps the child's hand on the affected side as if he were shaking hands. He places the other hand around the posterior aspect of the child's elbow that is flexed to 90°. With a quick motion, the child's wrist is rotated into supination while longitudinal compression force is applied to the radius between the two hands (Fig. 12–39). It is possible, if necessary, to rotate the wrist back and forth quickly between pronation and supination until the reduction occurs. The reduction may occur with a palpable "click" or it may not, but typically the child will stop crying immediately with successful reduction.

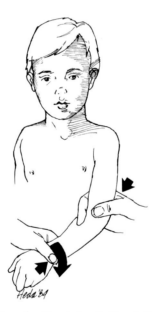

Fig. 12–39. Reduction of subluxated radial head. Procedure carried out with elbow flexed at 90°.

REDUCTION OF FRACTURES

Principles of Reduction of Epiphyseal Injuries

The Type I Fracture

Type I epiphyseal fracture passes entirely through the cartilage of the growth plate and does not actually pass through bone. The periosteum is torn on one side of the bone and intact on the other, although on the intact side, it may be stripped from the metaphysis.

Principle

If there is significant displacement of the epiphysis with respect to the metaphysis, it should not be reduced by transverse force alone since the intact periosteum forces the fracture surfaces together, and the growth mechanism of the bone could be damaged.

Method

The first step is to disimpact the fracture by restoring the angulatory deformity that occurred at the time of the fracture (Fig. 12–40A). This angulatory maneuver should result in the concave side of the angle being in the direction of the displacement of the epiphyseal fragment. Once disimpacted, the epiphyseal fragment can be easily reduced onto the metaphyseal fragment, but without the crepitus usually associated with reductions since the fracture surfaces are cartilaginous (Fig. 12–40 B, C). Finally, the angulatory deformity can be reduced (Fig. 12–40 D). This type of fracture is stable once reduced and should be immobilized in a cast that is molded to prevent recurrence of the angulatory deformity.

Type II Fracture

The type II fracture is similar to the type I except that a fragment of the metaphysis is fractured off and is part of the epiphyseal fragment.

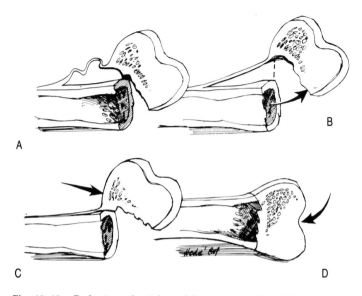

Fig. 12–40. Reduction of epiphyseal fracture, type I. **A.** Displacement of fracture fragment, periosteum intact on one side. **B.** Disimpact the fracture by traction and increase the deformity. **C.** Distal pressure to engage one cortex. **D.** Rotation to complete the reduction.

Method

The principles and method of reduction of a type II fracture are the same as for the type I (Fig. 12–41). Neither of these fractures can be over-reduced; the type I because of the intact periosteum, and the type II because of the metaphyseal fragment of bone.

The Type III and Type IV Fractures

In both types, the fracture involves the articular surface, and in the type IV, it passes through the growth plate as well. Both of these factors necessitate open reduction to the anatomical position and internal fixation, if there is any

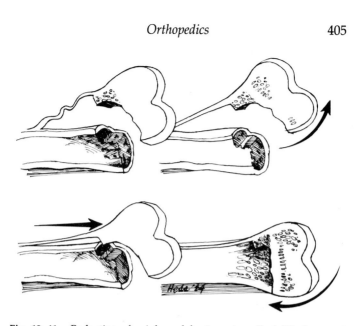

Fig. 12–41. Reduction of epiphyseal fracture, type II. **A.**Displacement of fracture fragment that includes fragment of metaphysis. **B.** Disimpact the fracture by traction and increase the deformity. **C.** Distal pressure to engage one cortex. **D.** Rotation to complete the reduction.

significant displacement. Even slight displacement following attempted closed reduction should not be accepted.

PRINCIPLE OF REDUCTION OF GREENSTICK FRACTURES

Greenstick fractures happen only in young bones because of their greater ability to undergo bending deformation without breaking. The fracture typically occurs in the shaft of one of the forearm bones with the other bone either fracturing or bending. In the greenstick type, a true fracture begins on one cortex of the bone and propagates toward the other side of the shaft. Before the fracture is complete, however, it stops propagating and instead of breaking, the opposite cortex bends and this becomes the new resting shape of the bone. If attempts are made to bend the bone back to its original shape, it will tend to spring back to the deformed shape and reduction will be lost. In the treatment of these fractures, therefore, something must be done to prevent the bent cortex from interfering with the maintenance of reduction. This portion of the bone cannot be bent straight again since the procedure would involve slight over-reduction during the manipulation; this is impossible due to the abutting together of the fractured cortices on the other side of the bone.

Method 1

The deforming effect of the plastically deformed cortex can be obliterated by completing the fracture through the unfractured cortex. This is easily done by increasing the angulation in the direction of the original fracture; bending in the opposite direction is more difficult. By completing the fracture, the injury becomes a fracture of both bones of the forearm and is treated as such.

Method 2

In certain situations, it may be possible to exert continuous force on the bone to maintain the reduction in spite of the elastic force of the unfractured cortex. This can oc-

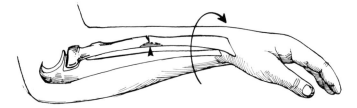

Fig. 12–42. Reduction of greenstick fracture of the radius.

casionally be done by a snug and well-molded cast, but this approach has a high failure rate. When the injury involves one of the forearm bones, it is usually the radius that suffers the greenstick fracture, and it is usually angulated with apex anteriorly. In this situation, the greenstick angulation can often be satisfactorily reduced and the reduction maintained by simply pronating the forearm maximally and immobilizing the arm in full pronation in an above-elbow cast, extending to the metacarpal heads (Fig. 12–42).

SUGGESTED READING

Rang, Mercer.: Children's Fractures. Vol. 2., Philadelphia, J.B. Lippincott, 1983.
Tachdjian, M.: Pediatric Orthopedics. Philadelphia, W.B. Saunders, 1972.

13
Pediatrics

J.B.J. McKendry

HEEL PUNCTURE TO OBTAIN CAPILLARY SAMPLE OF BLOOD

Capillary blood may be used to measure bilirubin and to screen for phenylketonuria (PKU) and hypothyroidism in the newborn. Many laboratories can estimate concentration of sugar, calcium, urea, creatinine, and other constituents in capillary blood.

Equipment

70% isopropyl alcohol (rubbing alcohol)
Disposable lancet
Capillary tubes for collection
Sterile gauze
Plasticine or similar material for sealing tubes

Method

Wash the child's heel with warm water; this will cause dilatation of capillaries. Rub the heel with an alcohol soaked pledget, then dry with gauze. Puncture the edge of heel with the lancet.

Wipe away the first drop of blood and take samples as bleeding occurs. Do not squeeze heel; this dilutes the sample with interstitial fluid. Collect blood in capillary tubes and seal them with plasticine. Stop bleeding with pressure applied using a dry sterile gauze (Fig. 13–1).

TO OBTAIN A BLOOD SAMPLE AND/OR START AN INTRAVENOUS INFUSION IN INFANTS AND TODDLERS

If a child is considered possibly septic, a blood sample should be obtained for culture before starting an antibiotic. Blood may be required for testing the concentration of blood sugar, electrolytes, calcium, phosphorus, and other constituents as determined by history and physical examination. Two people are usually required for the procedure, one to restrain and reassure the patient, the other to perform the procedure. In all intravenous punctures, the needle is pointed in the direction of the blood flow.

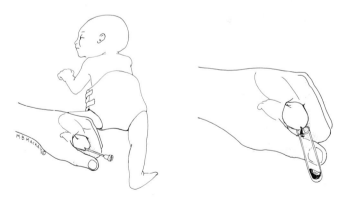

Fig. 13–1. Heel puncture to obtain capillary blood sample.

Veni-Puncture Using Straight Needle for Drawing Blood from Antecubital Fossa

When it is necessary to obtain a blood sample from a child, the first site to consider is the antecubital fossa. When this site is not possible, other sites may be tried.

Equipment

No. 21 needle
70% isopropyl alcohol to cleanse puncture site
Dry wipes
Syringe 5 ml or 10 ml, depending on sample volume required
Tourniquet

Method

Place tourniquet around patient's arm just above elbow. Feel for an appropriate sized vein on the flexor surface. Clean site with 70% alcohol wipe, and dry skin with a sterile wipe. Grasp patient's arm with elbow extended underneath the veni-puncture site and gently retract the skin. With the bevel side up at about 30° angle, insert the needle with syringe attached through the skin and into the vein. Place the thumb over the hub of the needle and gently pull the barrel of the syringe until the amount of blood required is obtained. Remove the tourniquet; withdraw the needle and syringe, and place a dry cotton wipe over the puncture site and press to stop bleeding (Fig. 13–2).

Veni-Puncture Using a Mini-Catheter with Attached Needle for Starting an Intravenous Infusion

If required, a sample of blood can be taken prior to starting the infusion. The usual sites are scalp veins in infants,

A

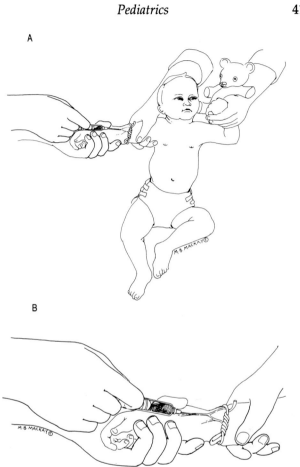

B

Fig. 13–2. A. Veni-puncture using straight needle for drawing blood from antecubital fossa. **B.** Detail.

veins on dorsal aspects of hands, veins on dorsal and ventral aspects of forearms, and veins on dorsum of feet.

Equipment

No. 21 or No. 22 mini-catheter
70% alcohol to cleanse the puncture site
10-ml bottle of normal saline
5-ml syringe
Tourniquet
Adhesive tape strips

Method (Using limbs)

Fill 5-ml syringe with normal saline and attach mini-catheter to syringe and fill it with saline to eliminate air. Choose I.V. site, select a vein, and apply tourniquet on the limb above the site. (For scalp sites see next section.) Cleanse site as described previously. Hold mini-catheter needle with bevel up at a 40° angle with the skin. Pierce skin just slightly to the side of the vein and advance needle about ½ inch subcutaneously.

Decrease the angle of the needle and advance it over the vein and enter the vein. There is a definite resistance felt as the vein is pierced. If successful, blood will flow into the tubing. Remove the tourniquet. Push 1 ml of saline into the vein to ensure the needle is within the vein lumen. Secure the mini-catheter by placing ½ inch width tape sticky side up, under the catheter, criss-cross the ends and fasten to the skin. Apply the proper size padded splint to the underside of the limb and to the limb proximal and distal to the I.V. site. Remove the syringe and attach the I.V. infusion, preferably using a system that minimizes the danger of excessive fluid intake (e.g., Buretrol by Travenol Co.). Curl the catheter tubing on itself to avoid accidentally pulling out the needle by taping the curl to the splint (Fig. 13–3).

A

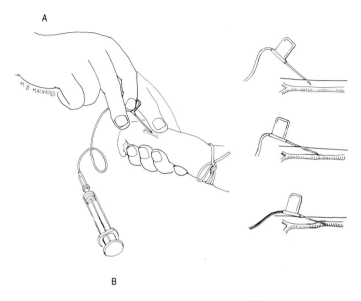

B

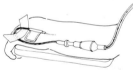

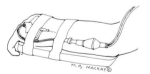

Fig. 13–3. Veni-puncture using a mini-catheter with needle attached for starting an I.V. infusion.

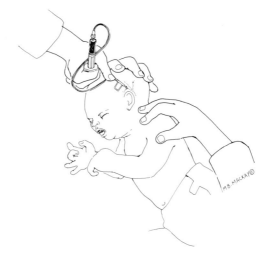

Fig. 13–4. Scalp vein puncture.

SCALP VEIN PUNCTURE

In infants, especially premature ones, the veins of the scalp are generally the best sites for puncture. If the head is held over the edge of the examining table, slightly below the level of the body, the veins usually distend, especially if the baby cries. Some physicians have found that putting an elastic around the infant's scalp until the needle is in the vein will distend a number of veins that are not evident even when the infant cries. The mini-catheter method is best for obtaining a blood sample or starting an intravenous infusion (Fig. 13–4).

VENOUS CUT-DOWN

When intravenous fluids are essential and several attempts at percutaneous puncture are unsuccessful, a venous cut-down should be done using local, infiltration anesthesia. The vein used is the internal saphenous vein.

Equipment

> A cut-down sterile tray containing a special L-shaped probe, fine scissors, sutures, No. 4 polyethylene catheter, sterile towels
> 5% povidone-iodine (Betadine)
> 70% isopropyl alcohol (rubbing alcohol)
> 10-ml normal saline
> Padded retaining splint
> Adhesive tape
> 000 silk ligature
> 5-ml syringe
> Syringe, needles and 2% procaine for local anesthesia

Method

Using adhesive tape, fasten lower limb with ankle extended to padded splint. Cleanse ankle with Betadine and rubbing alcohol. The operator, after washing hands, putting on a gown and sterile gloves, places sterile towels around operative site while an assistant holds the limb steady. Following infiltration with local anesthetic, a short (one cm) horizontal skin incision is made in front of the medial malleolus. Using the L-blunt probe, the exposed internal saphenous vein is mobilized and ligated distally. Using a ligature, the vein can be extracted to the surface, and with the fine scissors, a tiny "nick" is made in the outer surface of the vein large enough to allow threading of the catheter about 2 cm into the vein lumen. A ligature is placed around the vein and tied to hold the catheter in the vein. Three ml of normal saline in the 5-cm syringe are carefully pushed into the catheter to prove the patency of the system. The free end of the catheter is attached to a

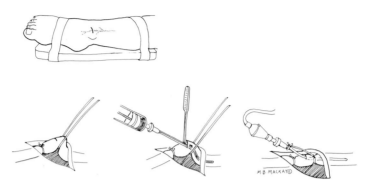

Fig. 13–5. Venous cut-down.

needle connected to the intravenous tubing and bottle of intravenous solution (Fig. 13–5).

UMBILICAL VEIN CATHETERIZATION IN THE NEWBORN

If a replacement transfusion is necessary or if unable to start a necessary intravenous infusion by percutaneous puncture, catheterization of the umbilical vein can be done.

The undressed infant is placed under a radiant heater and restrained by an assistant, while the operator cleanses the umbilical stump (after removing the cord clamp or tie) with 5% povidone-iodine followed by 70% isopropanol. Using sterile technique (gown, mask, gloves), drape the area. The operator cuts the umbilical cord just proximal to the clamped area. Usually the cut ends of the two small umbilical arteries and the slightly larger umbilical vein can be identified (Fig. 13–6C).

A 3.5-mm radiopaque umbilical vessel catheter is inserted into the vein and gently threaded along the vein for a specific distance (Fig. 13–6A and B). Dark venous blood will appear at the tip of the catheter. If the catheter is in an umbilical artery, the blood is usually brighter and pulsatile. A suture using 0000 ligature is used to secure the catheter in the vessel. The catheter is attached to an apparatus adapted for obtaining venous blood specimens or to deliver intravenous fluid (Fig. 13–6C).

LUMBAR PUNCTURE

A lumbar puncture (L.P.) is necessary to confirm a suspected case of meningitis in a child. A delay in instituting appropriate antibiotic therapy for bacterial meningitis can result in serious complications. Check the eye grounds with an ophthalmoscope for papilledema before doing the procedure. If papilledema is present, a consultation with a pediatric neurosurgeon should be obtained.

Equipment

1½ inch, No. 22 L.P. needle (infant)
2½ inch, No. 20 L.P. needle (child)
5% povidone-iodine (Betadine) for cleansing L.P. site
70% isopropyl alcohol (rubbing alcohol)
Four tubes for collecting specimens
Sterile towels, gown, gloves, cap
2% procaine injectable solution for anesthetizing the skin

Method

Feel for the correct intervertebral lumbar space. The fourth lumbar vertebra is on a line that traverses the iliac crests. The puncture may be made just above this vertebra (third interspace) or just below (fourth interspace). Held by an assistant, the child should be on his side, back flexed with knees and chin approximating on the edge of the examining table. The site should be cleansed with Betadine and followed by alcohol. After washing the hands, the

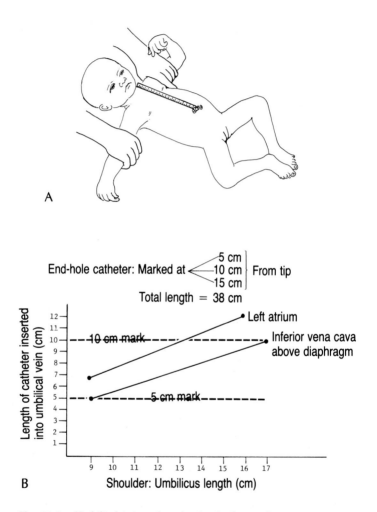

Fig. 13–6.   Umbilical vein catheterization in the newborn.

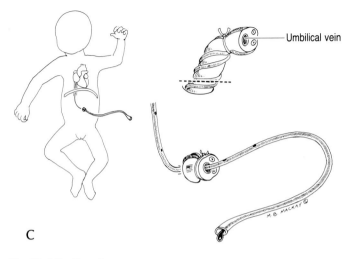

Umbilical vein

C

Fig. 13–6 *Continued.*

operator should be gowned and gloved. The patient should be draped with sterile towels to expose the puncture site.

The skin at the projected L.P. site is infiltrated with 0.25 ml of local anesthetic solution. The L.P. needle with the stylet in place in introduced into the skin over the intervertebral site in the midline and directed toward the umbilicus. A definite resistance is felt as the dura is punctured. The stylet is removed and cerebrospinal fluid appears. If no fluid appears, rotate the needle about 90° and retract slightly. If fluid is bloody, a traumatic tap can be differentiated from a true subarachnoid hemorrhage by comparing the amount of blood in the two successive specimens taken.

One specimen (0.5 ml) for each of three tubes is obtained for examinations: cell count, culture, estimation of concentrations of sugar and protein. Withdraw needle and apply

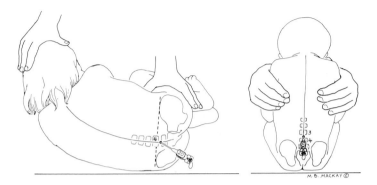

Fig. 13–7. Lumbar puncture.

a sterile gauze dressing over the puncture site. A baby may be held in a sitting position with the chin and neck flexed by an assistant. The flexed position should be maintained as briefly as possible since holding the baby in this position does interfere with normal breathing and compromises the oxygenation of the circulating blood (Fig. 13–7).

SUBDURAL TAP

If a subdural hematoma is suspected in an infant, a subdural tap should be performed if the anterior fontanelle is still open.

Equipment

Safety razor for shaving area of scalp
5% povidone-iodine (Betadine)
70% isopropyl alcohol
Sterile drapes
Short No. 20 spinal puncture needle
Two collecting tubes

Method

Shave area of scalp over puncture site. Using sterile precautions (gloves, gown, and cap) cleanse fontanelle area with Betadine and rubbing alcohol. Place sterile drapes around the site. Insert needle perpendicularly ½ cm lateral to lateral angle of the fontanelle. There is a definite resistance-release felt as it pierces the dura. Allow the fluid to drain by gravity and obtain necessary specimens. If the tap is negative, one drop or no fluid at all appears (Fig. 13–8).

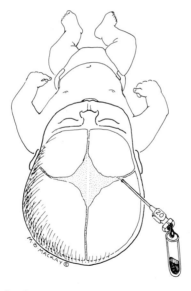

Fig. 13–8. Subdural tap.

TRACHEAL INTUBATION IN THE INFANT OR CHILD WHEN OTHER METHODS OF STIMULATION OF BREATHING ARE NOT EFFECTIVE

Equipment

Infant laryngoscope
A Portex tube (available in diameters appropriate for age of the infant or child)

Age	Size Range
Newborn	*3.0–3.5 mm*
6 months	*3.5–4.0 mm*
1 year	*4.0–4.5 mm*
2 years	*4.5–5.0 mm*
4 years	*5.0–5.5 mm*
8 years	*6.0–6.5 mm*
12 years	*7.0–7.5 mm*

Method

An assistant holds the supine infant's head slightly extended. The operator gently places the tip of the laryngoscope at the back of the tongue and then very gently, with the blade almost parallel to the line of the trachea, pushes the tip distally until the vocal cords are viewed. The tip of an appropriate sized Portex tube is then inserted between the cords, about 1 to 2 cm into the trachea.

The laryngoscope is removed and assisted respiration is instituted. The Portex tube is held in the final position by adhesive tape fastened to the face. Some operators insert the Portex tube through a nostril into the pharynx and then, using Magill forceps and a laryngoscope, into the trachea (Fig. 13–9).

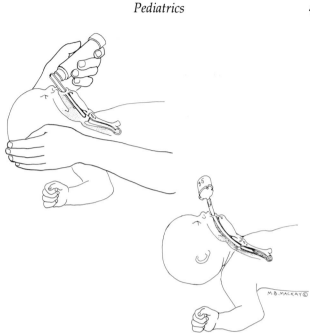

Fig. 13–9. Tracheal intubation in the infant or child when other methods of breathing stimulation are ineffective.

GAVAGE FEEDING

A small baby who does not require intravenous fluid but is sucking poorly and unable to take sufficient feeding orally can be fed by gavage until adequate sucking is established.

Equipment

No. 5 or No. 8 soft polyethylene nasogastric tube
25-ml syringe to hold milk feeding

Method

Measure total distance from infant's ear to nose to umbilicus, and mark this distance on the feeding tube. Insert tube gently through a nostril, with head slightly flexed, and continue until the mark on the tube is at the tip of the infant's nose. Check to see that the tube is in the stomach and not in the trachea, by aspirating a little stomach secretion. Alternatively, some air can be injected into the feeding tube and the operator, with a stethoscope on the abdomen, can hear a popping sound as the air enters the stomach. If baby gags or chokes, withdraw catheter since it may be in the trachea.

Allow 1 ml of the feeding into tube, and if no distress develops, continue the feeding by gravity. Where the infant requires continuous gavage feeding, the tube can be left in the stomach but should be changed every second or third day. If used only intermittently, it can be inserted for that specific feeding (Fig. 13–10).

COLLECTION OF A URINE SPECIMEN FOR CULTURE IN AN INFANT OR CHILD

In investigating a patient with a suspected sepsis or fever of uncertain origin, urine culture is usually indicated.

The external genitalia are washed with normal saline. In the female, a free flow of saline or distilled water into the interlabial fold will reduce the likelihood of a false positive result. For the infant, a sterile plastic urine collector bag with an adhesive rim (several types are available) is fitted over the genitalia, and the baby is diapered. When the infant voids, the specimen should be cultured immediately. If the baby does not void within an hour, a new bag should be used (Fig. 13–11).

For the older child, after cleansing the area, a clean catch midstream specimen can be obtained in a sterile container.

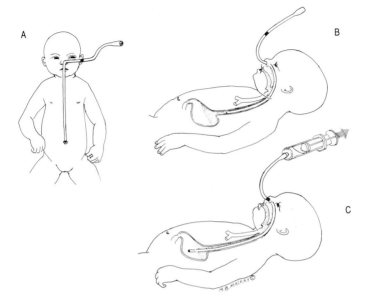

Fig. 13–10. Gavage feeding. **A.** Prior to insertion, measure total distance from infant's ear to nose to umbilicus and mark this distance on the tube. **B.** Insertion of the nasogastric tube up to the distance marked on tube, in **A. C.** With the tube in place, gentle aspiration confirms its position in the stomach.

CIRCUMCISION: Infant

Indications

Infant circumcision is usually done for religious or cultural reasons. There are few medical reasons for circumcision of a healthy, newborn male. If the foreskin is long, tight and very adherent, especially to the external urethral orifice, a circumcision may be indicated.

Equipment

Aqueous antiseptic solution
2 small mosquito forceps (sterile)

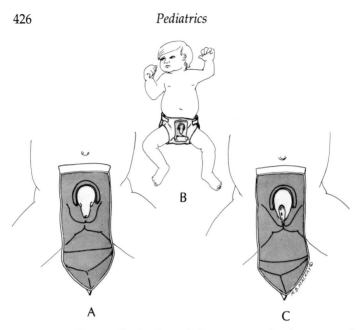

Fig. 13–11. Urine collection in an infant, an example of one type of collector bag. **A.** Position of bag in male infant. **B.** Collector bag held in place by diaper. **C.** Position of bag in female infant.

Gomco circumcision clamp (sterile) size 1.3 cm for full-term infant, 1.1. cm for premature infant
Scalpel (sterile)
Blunt probe (sterile)
Sterile 2 × 2 gauze
Petrolatum gauze, if desired
Sterile towels or small operative field drape
Padded restraint board is useful

Method

The infant is restrained by flannelette bandages around the legs and restraint board. An assistant should be available to comfort the infant and restrain the arms. Plastic form-fitting boards with Velcro restraining cuffs are available commercially.

The penis and local area are cleansed with antiseptic. With the thumb and forefinger, the foreskin is gently retracted. The blunt end of the probe is then used to free carefully the foreskin from the glans. A mosquito forceps is clamped along the line of the proposed dorsal slit. The

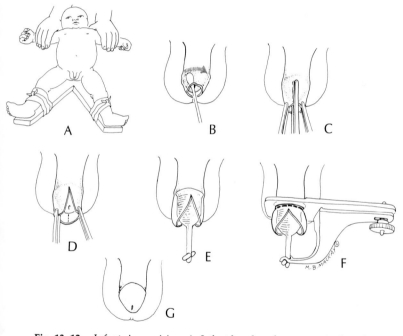

Fig. 13–12. Infant circumcision. **A.** Infant bandaged to a restraint board. **B.** Blunt end of probe used to circumferentially free the foreskin. **C.** Forceps clamped along line of proposed dorsal slit in foreskin. **D.** Grasping foreskin at site of dorsal slit. **E.** Bell portion of Gomco clamp inserted over glans, under foreskin. **F.** Clamp in position; bell portion over glans and outer portion over foreskin. After tightening clamp and waiting 5 minutes, the foreskin is cut along the area of the dotted line. The glans is protected by the bell portion of the clamp. **G.** Circumcised penis.

forceps is removed and a dorsal slit of about 0.5 cm is made in order to allow the bell portion of the Gomco clamp to be applied between the foreskin and the glans. The clamp is positioned to allow removal of about ¾ of the foreskin and tightened for 5 minutes, and then the foreskin is cut free along the clamped line with a sterile scalpel (Fig. 13–12).

A dry gauze (some physicians prefer petrolatum dressing) is then gently wound around the penis at the site of the circumcision. Twenty-four hours later, the dressing can be removed and petrolatum gauze applied daily for 2 to 3 days.

It is best to wait 2 to 3 days after birth to perform circumcision, but as long as the baby has been given Vitamin K_1 oxide, the procedure may be done anytime. Circumcision for the premature infant is delayed until the baby weighs 2.3 kg (5 lbs).

Post-operative bleeding can usually be controlled by clamping the local bleeding point or, if there is general oozing, by wrapping the penis carefully using a 1-inch gauze bandage, being careful that the bandage is not constrictive. If the bleeding continues, the infant should be given 1 mg of Vitamin K_1 oxide intramuscularly after a sample of blood has been obtained to determine a possible coagulation defect. If a significant blood loss has occurred, or if oozing is not controlled readily by local measures, a transfusion of fresh, whole, compatible blood (20 ml/kg) should be given without delay and a consultation with a pediatric hematologist obtained.

14
Physiotherapy

Charles M. Godfrey

With the prescription of any type of medical regimen, it is necessary to consider the purpose of the therapy, the possibility of success, alternate therapies, and possible side effects. These considerations apply to physical therapy as well as any other treatment programs.

The principle purpose of physical therapy is to restore normal function. This may be accomplished by initially reducing pain; subsequently the patient undergoes a number of activities such as movement, stretching or exercise programs to decrease muscle spasm, or to re-education to normal patterns of movement. To reach this goal, various methods may be used.

HEAT

Heat is frequently applied to reduce pain and promote ease of movement in preparation for either a program of stretching or exercise. Various agencies can be used to increase tissue temperature; many have the same physiolog-

429

ical effect and the choice of method is usually one of convenience to the patient or therapist.

Convection types of heating such as infrared bulbs, and conduction devices such as hot packs, hot wax, and hot water baths can be applied simply and in the home.

Infrared bulbs are inexpensive and can be purchased in the drug store. The red colored bulb has no advantage over the white.

Hot packs can be a heavy towel soaked in hot water, wrung out, and put in a plastic bag and applied to the area. Cover this with another towel to conserve heat.

Hot wax can be made using paraffin wax brought to 120°F (50°C) in the upper half of a double boiler. Add 1 ounce of mineral oil to each pound of wax. When this mixture has liquified and mixed, dip the involved area into the wax for 2 seconds and then remove; then dip again until 10 layers are built up. Alternatively the liquid can be applied with a paint brush, with serial applications, over the lumbar spine. Leave on for 20 minutes. Remove and re-use.

Hot water baths: a tub full of hot water may be drawn to tolerance temperature, immerse the body in the tub and put a sheet of plastic over the surface of the water to conserve heat. *Caution:* excessive heating may be inadvisable in older, debilitated patients, or those with peripheral vascular disease.

When instructing the patient, make sure to specify that the application is for 20 minutes followed by movement. More elaborate heating apparatus such as short wave diathermia provides little advantage in spite of the theoretical claims that it has deeper penetration. The application of ultrasound waves, particularly to hip joints, lumbosacral or cervical joints may result in deeper heating patterns; however, there is little or no evidence that suggests this can be more effective in reducing pain than the surface heating methods. Sometimes the application of infrared leads to a feeling of stiffness in the joints that may discourage the patient from movement and obtaining the desired results of therapy.

COLD

Various agents can be used to cool tissues. The easiest method is simply to grind up ice and put it in a plastic bag, applying it to the joint, as in an acute flare-up in rheumatoid arthritis. Cold is usually indicated for the first 48 hours following an acute trauma in order to reduce the amount of swelling and pain. Cold can also be used as an alternate means to control pain in chronic conditions.

MECHANOTHERAPY

Various agents are used for stretching or positioning a patient in order to regain range of movement and restore function. Most commonly traction can be used for the painful cervical spine resulting from an acute extension-flexion injury or posterior joint strain. The repositioning of the cervical spine while under traction may reduce the symptoms of a radiculopathy, most likely on the basis of reduction of pressure about the emerging cervical root. Traction is usually applied with the head in a few degrees flexion; however, the main indication of successful application is that it feels comfortable. If the patient complains of discomfort during the procedure, traction should be removed or reapplied in a different posture. Devices can be obtained for the application of traction at home; this is desirable because it can be repeated several times during the day with minimal loss of the patient's time (Fig. 14–1).

A home traction apparatus can be purchased at most pharmacies. It is mounted over the top of a door and applied

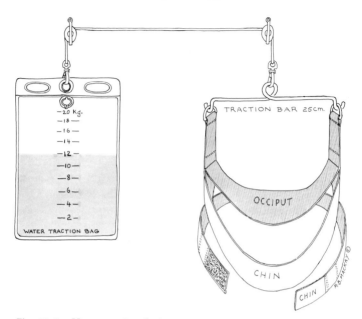

Fig. 14–1. Home-traction device.

for 20 minutes with the head in a comfortable position. Apply a hot pack at the same time to the neck (Fig. 14–2).

The use of oscillating traction apparatus, where the traction is applied for a few seconds and then relaxed in a cyclical manner, offers no specific advantage and sometimes causes the patient more discomfort. The chief reason for application is that a greater distracting weight (20 to 30 kg) can be applied to the cervical spine; however, most patients receiving cervical traction do well with a distraction weight of 6 to 16 kg. Lumbar traction may be applied in the treatment of chronic lumbosacral strain, but application through a series of pelvic and thoracic belts is difficult. A more effective means of treatment is to apply the distracting force by lifting the lower limbs into the air at 90° flexion to the

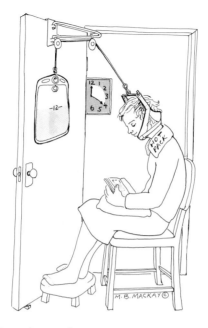

Fig. 14–2. Hot pack on neck.

lumbar spine while the body is in a slightly forward flexion posture. This applies traction specifically to the L5 to S1 and L4 to 5 posterior joints.

Lumbar traction can be applied by elevating the foot of the bed 15 cms and suspending the supine patient from the foot board by applying soft holding lines about the ankle. The gravitational weight will provide some lumbar distraction. Avoid cutting off the circulation with these holding lines (Fig. 14–3).

Pulley therapy, where the arm is abducted or forward flexed by a rope passing over a pulley and going to the normal side, can increase the range of passive movement about the shoulder girdle. Generally it should be applied

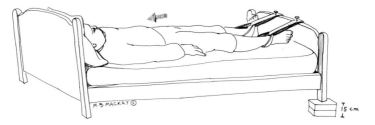

Fig. 14–3. Lumbar traction.

for 2 or 3 cycles to as complete a range of movement as possible and should not be used continuously—that is pulling up the arm 20 or more times per session. Pulley therapy is portable and can be erected and operated by the patient at home (Fig. 14–4).

MASSAGE

Massage is the movement of soft tissues to reduce fibrous tissue contractures and stretch elastic tissues. Applied properly, massage can greatly relieve pain about a chronically strained joint and can increase the range of movement. Fibrous tissue massage, where the therapist applies force to a fascial plane, can be effective in increasing the range of movement. Other types of massage such as gentle stroking may be also used.

Fibrous tissue massage can be done using the thumb to press and move tissues about a joint. A patient can do this or another member of the family can be taught to administer the massage.

EXERCISE THERAPY

Exercise prescriptions are usually unspecific and ordered indiscriminately without rationale of application. Exercise

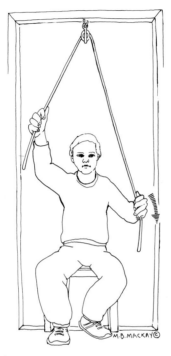

Fig. 14–4. Pulley therapy.

therapy philosophy is based on the use of isometric exercises, which are reputed to cause minimal damage to the joint and may be applied in a graduated manner to increase muscle strength. While this seems to work, many patients fail to respond to therapy and may show less strength increment.

In general, the slogan "no pain, no gain," which applies to athletes in training, also applies to patients who are in a restorative program. Certainly most of the exercise programs prescribed are inadequate and vague.

A major area where exercises are beneficial is in the low

back for chronic pain. A series of abdominal exercises in which the supine patient does a curl-up with the knees bent and the feet held tightly to the floor can be valuable (Fig. 14–5). This can follow tensing exercises that isometrically contract the rectus abdominis and lateralis; however, inasmuch as they do not overstress the muscles, the value of the last exercises is debatable. The curl-up can also be done with the patient on his side. Extension type exercise is not usually prescribed for the lumbar spine, except in post-fracture cases or osteoporosis. With osteoporosis, flexion exercises are usually interdicted.

One of the major areas requiring exercise is the quadriceps, particularly in older people who are beginning to suffer knee instability, usually concurrent to osteoarthritis. These patients should be given a program of isokinetic

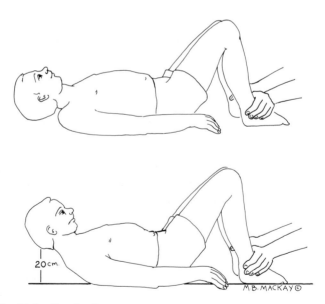

Fig. 14–5. Exercise therapy.

exercises instead of isometric. Isokinetic exercises are performed on special equipment such as Cybex, which controls the rate of movement at the knee and maintains a standard resistance throughout the exercise. Isokinetic exercises can also be used in the upper extremities and in the lumbar spine. Restoration programs using isokinetic exercises can be designed more specifically because a power profile is developed by the muscle rather than a single strength measurement.

Recently, considerable interest has been shown in eccentric exercises where the muscle contracts while lengthening, which is opposite to what happens with concentric exercises that shorten muscles. Eccentric exercises can produce a faster rate of muscle force development in a shorter time. This may be associated with temporary increased discomfort. Eccentric exercises usually have to be designed specifically for the patient, for example, for the quadriceps muscle, it may be necessary to instruct the therapist on how to apply the exercise that would have to be done manually, but devices are now available which permit eccentric exercises.

Frequently exercises are prescribed in order to increase range of movement rather than simply increase power. It is necessary that *these* exercises be done without causing significant pain. For example, in a frozen shoulder, it is necessary for the patient to mobilize the glenohumeral joint by a system of gravity-assisted exercises. In doing this, it is equally necessary not to stress the joints to such a degree that a significant amount of pain is perceived, which is associated with further tearing of the pericapsular tissues resulting in further tethering of the joint.

Range of movement exercises are particularly important in looking at the femoroacetabular joint and in the joints of the foot, hand, and cervical spine. With the cervical spine, it is important that range of movement exercises be carried out while the patient is flat on his back, rather than seated in a chair. This has the advantage of off-loading the vertebral joint by the weight of the skull.

Definitions

   Isometric exercise: the muscle is contracted but the joint does not move.
   Isotonic exercise: the muscle is contracted and the joint moves through its full range of movement without control contraction speed.
   Isokinetic exercise: the muscle is contracted against resistance through the joint's full range of movement at a constant speed.
   Eccentric exercise: the muscle contracts but gets longer instead of shorter.
   Range of movement exercise: the joint is put through as full a range of movement as possible.
   Gravity assisted exercise: the joint is put through a full range of movement with the assistance of gravity. This is a minimal muscle contraction exercise.

SPLINTING

Just as complete bed rest may be ordered for an acute condition, resting a local joint problem may be necessary. A patient with a lumbosacral strain may continue working if he is fitted with an abdominal binder-type corset. This raises the intra-abdominal pressure and provides a rigid balloon that supports the back, reducing movement between the vertebrae. This is usually the binder of choice compared with a more extensive apparatus such as a Harris brace.

Elastic bandage support about the knee or ankle is useful to maintain mobility while awaiting the effects of treatment to resolve an underlying condition. This support is frequently applied in association with carrying a cane in the contralateral hand.

Carpal tunnel stenosis with resultant nocturnal paresthesia can be helped by applying a simple splint which holds the wrist in approximately 15° of flexion and is worn at night. The acute rheumatoid joint, particularly radiocarpal and metacarpal, can be relieved of pain and morning stiffness by the application of night resting splints that support those areas.

Most of these splinting devices are temporary and designed to protect the joint during recovery. Pre-formed splints of materials such as aluminum or plastic are available from most surgical supply houses. Light splints can also be formed with 5 to 6 layers of plaster of paris bandages and should be placed on the patient and formed with the limb in the desired position, making sure that some padding with material such as flannelette bandage covers the plaster. This is done by placing the wet plaster strip on a piece of flannelette bandage that is somewhat longer and wider than the plaster strip and then folding the bandage edges over the wet plaster. This splint is then molded to the forearm and held in place with a temporary bandage. When dry, the splint can be removed, stored, and then reapplied when desired and appropriate.

CONTRAINDICATIONS TO PHYSICAL THERAPY AND SOME ASSOCIATED DAMAGES

Until recently, most physical therapy that was carried out was comparatively harmless and did not have the potential for damaging a patient. Exercises were usually kept well within the range of comfort, and it was unlikely that the patient would suffer; however, with the interest by physiotherapists in manipulation and overstressing muscles, potential dangers increased.

Physiotherapists are inclined to work in two ways. The traditional way is to carry out the treatment as prescribed by the physician. If there are some questions or concern as to the appropriateness of the therapy, then a therapist's call to the physician usually results in an agreement, and a change is made. The second way is for the physiotherapist to receive a patient on referral and then to choose and carry out a treatment that may well include manipulation or some other procedure. The physician may not have considered this as a possible treatment, and therefore has not written it as contraindicated on the prescription form.

Naturally these problems have to be faced by both the physician and the allied health worker, and arrangements must be made so that each party understands what the patient requires.

Similarly in dealing with joints where there is a gross restriction of movement, a certain amount of force may be required, but overuse of stretching techniques may further damage the joint. It is necessary that the therapist speak to the physician in order to determine the limits of treatment.

A common problem is that the therapist may switch from one treatment to another without informing the physician, and in turn the physician may think that the changes were premature and not carried out in a time frame compatible with the type of lesion. This problem requires a frank discussion between both parties.

THE PHYSICAL THERAPY PRESCRIPTION

A physician does not send a patient to a drug store for "medicine"; similarly a physician does not send a patient to a physiotherapist with a prescription saying, "Treat as you like." If the physician is uncertain of how to treat the patient, the patient should not be sent for therapy. Any therapy that deviates from the assessment of the problem may result in injury. This is unlikely, but it is still the responsibility of the physician who sent the patient. It is therefore necessary that physicians and therapists clarify the purpose of sending a patient to the physiotherapy office. Is this visit a referral, one where the treatment of the patient is turned over to the members of an allied health profession, or is it a prescription?

These problems can usually be solved by proper communication between therapist and physician that results in a clear understanding, usually put in writing, as to what should or should not be done for a specific patient. This communication is particularly valuable as physical therapy and drug therapy are frequently combined in treatment.

Patients like physiotherapy. "It does not upset the bowel movements, it is good for the liver and never lowers the white blood count as it has little or no side effects." Therefore it is necessary for the patient to be prepared to leave the therapy at the earliest opportunity. Because there is a shortage of treatment facilities, therapists should demonstrate do-it-yourself programs for the patients to do at home. Patient education for the treatment of chronic low back pain, chronic obstructive pulmonary disease, postoperative hip surgery, osteoporosis, and a variety of other conditions is mandatory.

Any patient receiving physiotherapy should return to the physician 3 to 4 weeks later to check improvement and to make sure that the home treatment program has been maintained.

Physical therapy associated with proper chemotherapy can be a potent agent in the recovery of patients with musculo-skeletal disorders, and it frequently improves morale. Physical treatment has several advantages inasmuch as hands are laid upon the patient during treatment. The morale effect, however, should not obscure the fact that specific procedures in physical therapy result in a significant improvement of the patient's condition.

15
Respirology

G.M. Davies

INHALATION THERAPY FROM A NEBULIZER

Indications

This therapy is useful in relieving bronchospasm. Inhalation of broncho-reactive drugs, especially the beta-agonist drugs such as albuterol, terbutaline, isoetharine, metaproterenol, and fenoterol may be delivered by a cartridge nebulizer or via compressed air passed through a solution in a chamber, e.g., a Wright nebulizer. Cartridge nebulizers deliver drugs adequately except in the very sick or in patients who are unable to coordinate hand and inspiration. Demonstrate the use of the nebulizer to all patients.

Method

Cartridge Nebulizer. The cap of the nebulizer is removed, and the apparatus is shaken 2 or 3 times. The mouthpiece is held either away from the open mouth or between the teeth with the lips apart. The patient exhales normally and then starts a slow deep breath. The cartridge is depressed soon after starting the inhalation and the breath completed, then held for 2 or 3 seconds (Fig. 15–1).

Wright Nebulizer with Compressed Air Pump (e.g., Maximist). For home use, a compressed air pump may be provided to bubble air through a solution of a drug held in a bubble nebulizer. Beta-agonist drugs may be administered by this route. The patient breathes normally while the face mask is in place and continues breathing normally until the nebulizer is dry (Fig. 15–2). The pump mechanism is not portable, and has no advantage over the cartridge nebulizer but ensures delivery of the drug if the patient cannot cope with the hand held inhaler.

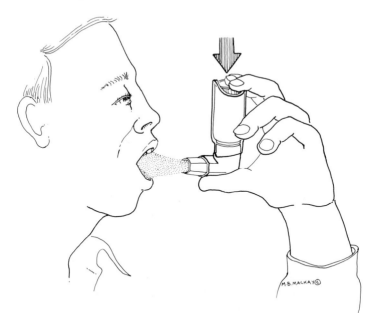

Fig. 15–1. Cartridge nebulizer.

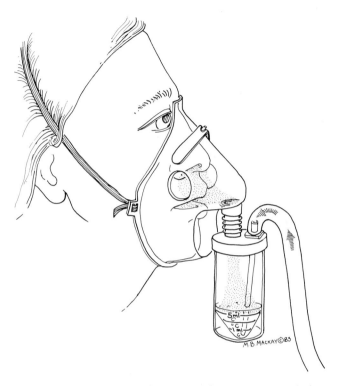

Fig. 15–2. Wright nebulizer with compressed air pump. Five ml of normal saline with addition of ½ to 1 ml of drug solution.

OFFICE PULMONARY FUNCTION TESTING

Indications

Simple pulmonary function tests of airflow carried out in the physician's office are unreliable as diagnostic tools but have some value in following the progress of pulmonary disease, especially the obstructive conditions. The variety of apparatus available is considerable; some produce a spirogram on graph paper, others yield only figures. All apparatus is subject to deterioration in accuracy over time and should be checked in a laboratory at least once a year. The most conveniently measured indices are:

Vital capacity: VC

Forced vital capacity: FVC

Timed forced expiration, usually volume at 1 second: FEV_1

Peak expiratory flow: PF

Forced expiratory ratio: $FER = \dfrac{FEV_1}{FVC}$

Maximum mid-expiratory flow rate: MMEFR (Fig. 15–3).

All these values vary with patient efforts and must be compared with predicted values corrected for age, sex, and body weight. A conclusion about the pattern of any abnormality found may not be drawn unless other values,

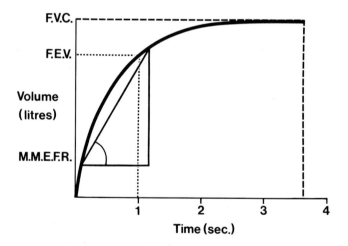

Fig. 15–3.   F.V.C. = Forced vital capacity.
F.E.V. = Forced expiratory volume in 1 second.
M.M.E.F.R. = Maximum mid-expiratory flow rate (liters per second).

such as lung volumes and gas transfer, which require a more sophisticated laboratory, are available.

Method

Spirogram. The patient stands beside the apparatus. A nose clip is fitted to obstruct nasal gas flow. The patient is instructed to inhale to the maximum. Place the mouthpiece between the lips so that no gas leaks, and then ask the patient to exhale as hard as possible and to continue the effort until no further air can be blown out. At least three separate measurements should be obtained and the best values recorded.

Peak Flow Rate (Wright). The procedure is the same but full expiration need not be achieved. The peak flow meter may be given to the patient to take home and the peak flow recorded at different times of day. This can be of value in establishing patterns in asthma.

Precautions

Over interpretation must be avoided. Especially with the peak flow meter, the patient's practice may improve the values achieved without true change in status.

TUBERCULIN TESTING (OLD TUBERCULIN TESTING, OT TEST)

Indications

Skin testing with purified protein derivative of Mycobacterium tuberculosis antigen is valuable in assessing past or recent infection with Mycobacterium tuberculosis hominis. It is not always positive in active mycobacterial disease and is weakly positive in some nontuberculous mycobacterial infections. A positive test does not necessarily indicate active tuberculosis; it is important, however, if discovered in those who are contacts of patients with active cases. A conversion of test results from negative to positive indicates invasion by the organism sometime between the tests, except if BCG (bacille Calmette Guérin) is given in the interim, or if it is the first pair of tests applied.

About 4 to 5% of noninfected subjects will have OT conversion by the test itself. In screening populations at risk (e.g., hospital workers), a first negative test should be followed by a repeat test in 2 to 3 weeks; a "conversion" at this point does not likely indicate infection.

In primary tuberculosis, the OT test takes 6 weeks to become positive; a conversion does not rule out active primary disease at the time of first injection.

Method

The OT test is traditionally carried out on the palmar aspect of the left forearm. The skin is cleaned and 0.1 ml of standard extract from a graduated thin 1-ml tuberculin syringe fitted with a 25-gauge hypodermic needle, and a dilution of 1:2000 (5 tuberculin units) is injected intradermally. An intracutaneous wheal is raised; if the injection is subcutaneous, the test is invalid. The test must be read in 48 to 72 hours. Reactions at 16 to 18 hours are frequent and irrelevant.

A positive test consists of an area of induration surrounded by a patch of erythema. The diameter of the indurated area must be measured with a transparent ruler; a positive test yields a diameter of induration of 10 mm or more. Lesser areas of induration are equivocal; large areas do not necessarily indicate active disease (Fig. 15–4).

Precautions

Old tuberculin must be kept refrigerated; it has a limited life span indicated on the label.

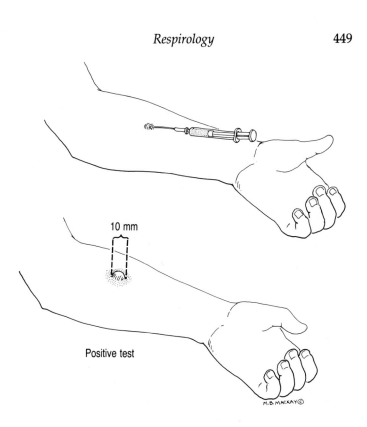

Fig. 15–4. Tuberculin testing (Old tuberculin testing, O.T. test). **A.** Intradermal injection of 0.1 ml of standard extract. **B.** After 48 to 72 hours a positive test reveals induration of at least 10 mm.

THORACOCENTESIS (ASPIRATION OF PLEURAL FLUID)

Indications

Pleural effusions have many causes, but it is almost always necessary to obtain a sample for diagnostic purposes; often fluid may be drained for therapeutic reasons. Unless the cause of the effusion is known, samples should be submitted for tests. Thoracocentesis is easily and safely carried out in the practitioner's office.

If the cause of the effusion is not known and if the specimen obtained is not obviously purulent, closed pleural biopsy also may be attempted safely. Biopsy of the parietal pleura has a low diagnostic yield, but may detect carcinoma or tuberculosis.

Preparation

The operator should scrub his hands and wear sterile surgical gloves; a mask is not necessary. The patient's back should be cleansed with glutaraldehyde, Cetrimide or Betadine solution and the lower chest covered with a sterile towel that may be tucked into the belt.

Leaning forward, the patient sits comfortably on a chair or couch and rests the folded arms on a support, such as a chair back. The extent of the effusion is determined by percussion, and a site selected for needling that is close to the upper level of dullness and between ribs. The most convenient site is usually posterior or lateral. It is safer not to introduce the needle too low as the level of the hemidiaphragm is not known with accuracy (Fig. 15–5).

Equipment

Skin marker
5 ml of 1% lidocaine without epinephrine
5-ml syringe, 20-ml syringe, 50-ml syringe for large effusions
Hypodermic 25-gauge and 18-gauge needles
Thoracocentesis needles (optional)
Spencer Wells or other scissors clamp
Three-way tap (for large effusions) with extension tube and a jug
Sterile specimen bottles (some with Heparin)
Adhesive dressing

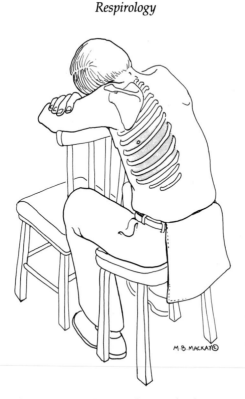

Fig. 15–5. Thoracocentesis. Seating of patient for thoracocentesis. Sterile towel is tucked into patient's belt. Thoracocentesis needle is introduced close to the upper level of dullness caused by effusion.

For Pleural Biopsy
Abrams' needle
20-ml syringe
Scalpel
For Suspected Empyema
30-ml radiopaque solution (meglumine diatrizoate, e.g., Hypaque)

Method

A site for aspiration is selected just above the edge of a rib, thus avoiding the intercostal nerve that clings to the inferior surface of the rib.

A subcutaneous bleb of anesthetic is introduced. The hypodermic needle (25-gauge) is then gradually advanced; before each advance, the syringe is drawn back to see if fluid is aspirated; if no fluid is aspirated, ½ ml of local anesthetic is introduced. The needle is then advanced a few millimeters and the aspiration and injection is repeated.

With experience, the operator may feel the needle passing through subcutaneous fascia and then muscle layers. When the full reach of the needle is attained, an 18-gauge needle is substituted and the anesthetic introduction is continued. In all but the most obese patients, the needle will reach parietal pleura, which may also be identified by feel. Once this is pierced, fluid will be drawn back into the syringe barrel and local anesthesia is complete.

The needle is then withdrawn and a fresh syringe (20 ml or larger) and a fresh needle (18 gauge) is substituted. The syringe is passed back along the same track until fluid is aspirated back into the syringe. When the needle tip is just within the pleural space, a clamp is placed across the needle, flush with the skin to prevent inadvertent movement of the needle deeper into the thorax. Prevention of unnecessary needle movement also improves patient comfort and procedure safety (Fig. 15–6). The syringe is then filled with fluid for analysis. Repeated aspiration is facilitated by the interposition of a three-way tap that allows fluid to be flushed into containers without removing the syringe or needle (Fig. 15–7). If the needle is too small, a larger one may safely be passed as long as the clamp is applied to prevent too deep insertion.

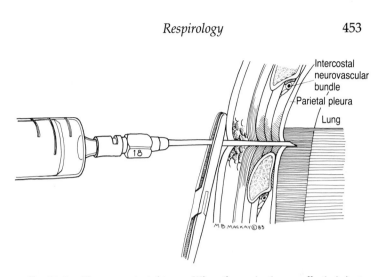

Fig. 15–6. Thoracocentesis biopsy. When the aspirating needle tip is just within the pleural space, a hemostat is clamped on the needle to prevent deeper penetration of the needle.

Specimens

    Fluid for cytology and cell count—Heparin bottle
    pH, glucose, amylase—Plain bottle
    Proteins—Heparin bottle
    Culture—Plain bottle
    AFB—Plain bottle (acid fast bacillus)
    Anaerobic culture—Special container

Precautions

After the thoracocentesis, the breath sounds in the upper zones should be compared. A loss of breath sounds on the side of the procedure may indicate a pneumothorax.

If pus is aspirated, an adequate sample is taken, but it is not necessary to attempt further drainage. If a radiograph facility is available, 30 ml of Hypaque should be injected into the empyema and the needle withdrawn. An upright

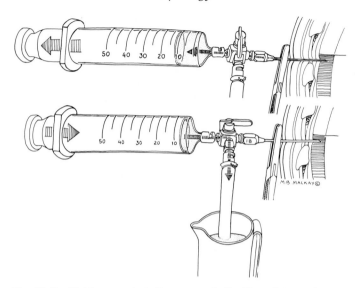

Fig. 15–7. Fluid removal via 3-way tap. **A.** Position of stopcock to aspirate fluid. **B.** Position of stopcock to flush fluid from syringe into container.

chest radiograph will then show the lower limit of the pus and guide the surgical placement of tube or rib resection.

Large quantities of fluid may be removed at one session for therapeutic reasons. To be safe, no more than 1 liter should be removed at one session, and if the patient starts to cough, the aspiration should be stopped, as further withdrawal of fluid may lead to unilateral pulmonary edema. If the needle is advanced too far, there is a risk of damage to the visceral pleural surface of the lung and pneumothorax. This risk is minimized by clamping the needle so that the tip is just within the pleural cavity.

If the patient feels faint, the procedure should be stopped. Premedicate a very nervous patient with 0.6 mg atropine subcutaneously. If the needle meets bone, it

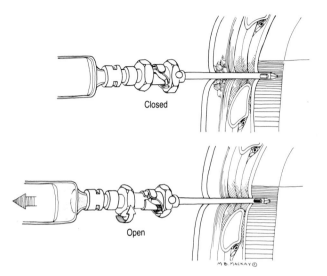

Fig. 15–8. Closed pleural biopsy. When the Abrams' needle is in the pleural cavity, the hub is twisted to open the port and aspiration of pleural fluid confirms that the needle and its port are within the cavity, beyond the pleura.

should be pulled back and reintroduced a little higher so that it passes *above* (not just below) the rib. The intercostal bundle is fairly well protected by a flange, and damage to it is unusual.

CLOSED PLEURAL BIOPSY

A sample of parietal pleura may be obtained at the time of thoracocentesis by Abrams' needle biopsy.

The anesthetized site is incised for ½ cm with a pointed scalpel. The subcutaneous fascia must also be pierced. A 20 ml syringe is attached to the Abrams' needle, which is held in the closed position. The needle is then pushed with

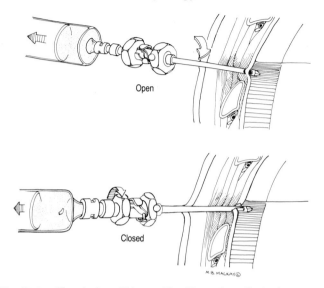

Open

Closed

M.B. MACKAY©

Fig. 15–9. Closed pleural biopsy. The Abrams' needle in the open position is withdrawn until it catches the pleura and fluid flow stops. The hub of the needle is then rotated to close the port, thus snaring a biopsy sample of pleura.

a screwing motion into the chest above the anesthetized track. Force is required, and the needle will suddenly slip into the thorax.

The needle is then opened and the syringe drawn back. Fluid in the syringe will confirm that the biopsy port is within the pleural cavity. With the syringe needle open, it is turned so that the biopsy port points along the intercostal space (never upwards) (Fig. 15–8). Pass the needle along the space with a hooking motion and pull it back until it catches. The syringe is pulled back until the fluid flow stops. Keep the pressure up and then close and withdraw the needle (Fig. 15–9). On opening the needle, a piece of tissue may be found within the port; this is removed with a needle or washed out with the fluid in the syringe, and submitted in formalin for histologic examination.

After the procedure is finished, all needles are withdrawn and a dressing (such as an adhesive bandage) is applied to the site. Suture of the small incision needed for pleural biopsy is not necessary.

Specimen:

Biopsy—Formalin or glutaraldehyde
Biopsy culture—Saline

16
Rheumatology

Hugh Little

ASPIRATION/INJECTION OF JOINTS AND BURSAE

Clinical Uses

Aspiration. When joints or bursae are swollen they should be aspirated to determine if there is intracapsular fluid, to determine the nature of the fluid, and to relieve symptoms. An acute monoarthritis/bursitis must be aspirated. The swollen joints of a chronic polyarthritis should be aspirated if there is any suspicion of infection or if the symptoms warrant.

Injection. Joints are injected with radiographic materials (dye or gas) as part of an arthrogram. This is carried out in a radiology department. Joints are commonly injected with corticosteroids and occasionally injected with radio-active colloids to control sterile inflammation. The use of an intra-articular/bursal corticosteroid is indicated when the joint or bursa is inflamed, the inflammation is sterile, and the symptoms are severe and unlikely to respond to less invasive treatment.

Indications

Joints requiring aspiration and injection should show the following clinical signs. Redness and heat may be undetectable. The swelling distends the capsule and the whole capsular surface is tender. Depending on the amount of fluid, the capsule may be tight as a drum, soft as a ripe plum or the effusion may be small enough to move around the joint (bulge sign). The inflamed joint has restricted movement in all of its normal planes. As the joint is actively moved toward the limit of range, the capsule gets palpably firmer, and the patient exhibits some guarding due to pain. A gentle push beyond the range achieved actively elicits stress pain. Inflammation causes stress pain in all directions.

The most specific evidence of intra-articular/bursal inflammation is the presence of inflammatory synovial fluid, i.e., turbid, yellow, watery. This is in contrast to normal synovial fluid which is clear, colorless, or light yellow and has the viscid consistency of sugar syrup.

Contraindications

Aspiration. There is no contraindication to joint or bursal aspiration. Infection of the surrounding skin or soft tissues is a relative contraindication since this procedure could introduce infection into the joint. If there is any suspicion that the joint is infected, it should be aspirated.

Injection. Traumatic effusions may require aspiration but should not be injected with corticosteroid since this drug may delay healing. Infected joints and bursae should be treated with systemic antibiotics and drainage; however, intra-articular injections of antibiotics are not required. The drainage must be sufficient in order to keep the joint free of inflammatory exudate. Repeated aspiration is satisfactory in most cases and lessens the likelihood of secondary infection. If the joint is too deep to be adequately assessed (i.e., hip) or the exudate cannot be adequately evacuated, a surgical drainage should be carried out.

Corticosteroid Dosage. There are many preparations of corticosteroid suitable for intra-articular injection. Some preparations are combined with other substances to prolong their action. All compounds are effective and the dosage schedules are described in the prescription information. I use methylprednisolone 40 to 80 mg for a large joint/bursa, i.e., hip, shoulder, knee and ankle, and 20 to 40 mg for a medium sized joint/bursa, i.e., wrist, elbow, and 10 to 20 mg for the small joints of the hands and feet.

Precautions

If a joint or bursa is thought to be infected, aspiration should be carried out with mask, gloves, and drapes to minimize the possibility of a confusing contaminant. If infection is clearly not an issue, the physician should use the same care and precautions that apply for a venipuncture or an intramuscular injection.

Disposable needles ensure sterility and sharpness but the steel is soft and the slightest touch in a vial or bottle can result in a bent point. Always use a new needle to puncture the skin.

Careful analysis of inflammatory fluid (turbid, yellow, watery) will give important diagnostic information. Inflammatory fluid should be sent for culture by aerobic and anaerobic techniques, and an aliquot should be put into special gonococcal medium. The fluid should be smeared and stained for immediate bacterial identification, and the cells should be differentiated and counted. A smear should be searched for crystals under polarizing microscopy. Assays of sugar, protein, and complement components are helpful occasionally.

The patient should rest the joint for 24 to 48 hours after corticosteroid is injected. This minimizes the loss of steroid to the systemic circulation via lymphatics and thus improves the local anti-inflammatory effect. Some physicians advocate absolute bed rest for several days after a steroid injection into a weight-bearing joint. There is little evidence to support this practice but it may lessen the patient's demands for repeated injections.

Occasionally a patient will have an adverse reaction to the corticosteroid preparation 11 to 24 hours after the injection. This is a transient phenomenon and should be treated expectantly with analgesics. The local anti-inflammatory effect of the corticosteroid usually requires 24 hours for noticeable improvement.

Equipment

Skin cleansing solution (soap and water)
Skin sterilizing solution (absolute alcohol, iodine)
Drapes, gloves, mask
Local anesthetic (1%, 2% lidocaine)
Needles
No. 25 (to inject small joints and tendon sheaths)
No. 22 1½ inch (to inject large, deeper joints, tendon sheaths, and bursae; to aspirate inflamed joints)
No. 18, 1½ inch (to aspirate large joints with osteoarthritic effusions)
LP needles (needed occasionally for hip or trochanteric bursae in the obese)
Large bore needle No. 14 or No. 16 (needed occasionally for viscous fluid or fluid with many fibrin bodies)
Biopsy needle (occasionally needed)
Syringes (small for injections, large for aspirations)

Containers for aspirate (sterile for culture, heparinized for cell count, plain for biochemistry)

Glass slides and polarizing microscope (smear for gram stain; search for crystals)

Note: Not all of the above equipment is required for every aspiration and injection, but these resources should be available.

Method

The skin is cleansed and prepared with antiseptic solution. The solution to be injected is drawn up into the syringe. A new disposable needle is used to enter the joint.

Local anesthesia is seldom required unless the patient is very apprehensive or a needle larger than No. 18 is used.

The landmarks and procedure for the common joints, tendon sheaths, and bursa are described subsequently. Careful aseptic technique should be used. The aspirate from an undiagnosed inflamed joint should be handled carefully to avoid contamination prior to culture.

TEMPOROMANDIBULAR JOINT

Landmarks

The mandibular condyle is identified immediately anterior to the tragus of the ear and below the posterior part of the zygomatic arch. As the mouth is opened and closed, the condyle can be felt to move forward and down (Fig. 16–1).

Method

The patient bites on the knuckles or fingers of the opposite hand. This opens the joint so that a space can be

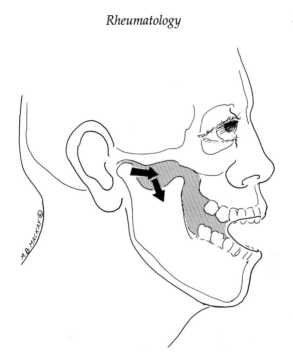

Fig. 16–1. Temporomandibular joint landmarks.

palpated between the temporal bone and the mandibular condyle. The needle is inserted into that space, pointing slightly anteriorly and downward (Fig. 16–2).

CLAVICULAR JOINTS

Sternoclavicular

Landmarks

The examiner places the tip of one finger in the suprasternal notch and the tip of the adjacent finger on the proximal clavicle. While the patient slowly protrudes and retracts the shoulder girdle, the fingers approximate until the

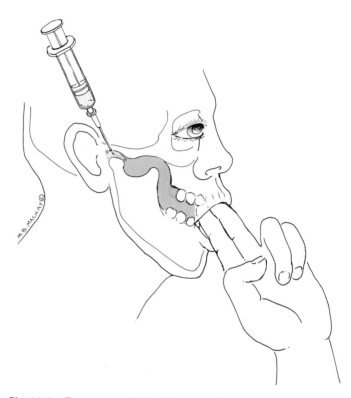

Fig. 16–2.　Temporomandibular joint procedure.

narrow joint space is identified. The medial surface of the clavicle is covered by an articular disc, so that the movement of the clavicle is better felt anteriorly (Fig. 16–3).

Method

The patient is positioned recumbent on a firm surface. A narrow pillow or rolled sheet is placed under the upper thoracic spine so that the shoulder girdle is allowed to fall back. The needle is inserted from the front, angled slightly

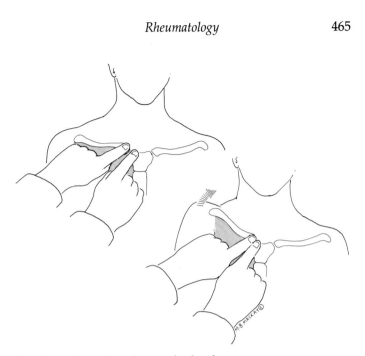

Fig. 16–3.   Sternoclavicular joint landmarks.

laterally. The needle should enter the joint just lateral to the upper corner of the sternum (Fig. 16–4).

Acromioclavicular Joint

Landmarks

The examiner places one finger on the lateral clavicle and the adjacent finger on the acromion. While the patient slowly moves the shoulder up and down, the fingers approximate until the joint space is identified. There may be a palpable step up from the surface of the acromion to the lateral clavicle (Fig. 16–5).

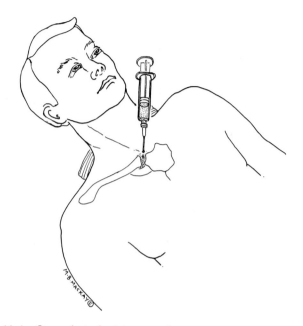

Fig. 16–4.   Sternoclavicular joint procedure.

Method

The patient is seated with the affected arm hanging. The needle is inserted into the joint space from the superior surface, angled slightly medially (Fig. 16–6).

SHOULDER

Landmarks

The tip of the coracoid is palpated just below the lateral clavicle. The physician can identify laterally the lesser tuberosity, the bicipital groove and the greater tuberosity forming the rounded lateral surface. Above this the anterior

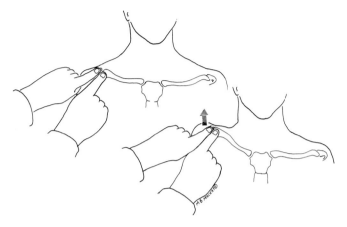

Fig. 16–5. Acromioclavicular joint landmarks.

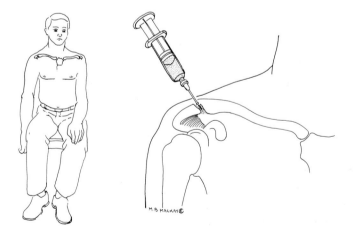

Fig. 16–6. Acromioclavicular joint procedure.

and posterior corners of the acromion are felt. Passively, internally, and externally rotating the humerus will assist in identifying the bicipital groove.

Method

The patient sits with the affected arm hanging. The joint can be entered from the back or the front.

Posterior Approach. The needle is inserted 1 cm below and medial to the posterior corner of the acromion. The needle is pointed toward the tip of the coracoid and advanced with repeated attempts to aspirate or inject until the joint space is entered (Fig. 16–7).

Anterior Approach. The needle may be directed at the bicipital tendon in its groove. The patient is seated, with the affected arm hanging. In external rotation of 30 to 45°, the groove faces forward. The groove is identified and the

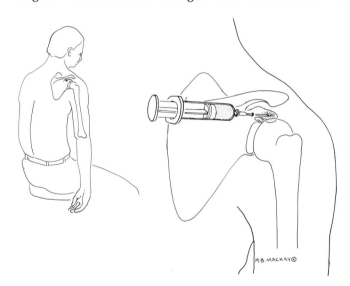

Fig. 16–7. Posterior approach to shoulder joint.

needle inserted directly from the front, lateral to the coracoid and just below the coracoacromial ligament. The joint can be entered medial to the bicipital groove by entering the skin at the same place but angling 20° medially (Fig. 16–8).

Note: The neurovascular bundle passes under the coracoid into the arm. By inserting the needle lateral to the tip of the coracoid, the neurovascular bundle will not be damaged inadvertently.

Subacromial Bursa

In middle-aged and elderly patients, the subacromial bursa usually communicates with the shoulder joint, thus the posterior approach to the shoulder, described in the previous section, is satisfactory. The normal bursa is a potential space, and a physician can be certain of puncturing it only with the aid of an arthrogram. In general, the posterolateral approach is used and the needle is angled toward the under surface of the acromion, repeatedly testing

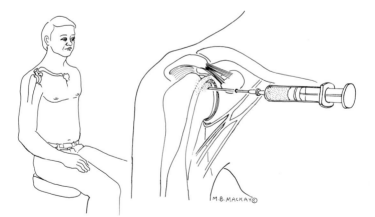

Fig. 16–8. Oblique view of anterior approach to shoulder joint.

for a loss of resistance that signals that the tip of the needle is in a potential space.

Bicipital Tendon Sheath

The bicipital tendon sheath is an out pouching of the shoulder joint, thus injecting into the shoulder is usually satisfactory. Alternatively, the anterior approach can be used, as described in the previous section; then the needle is directed slightly upward into the bicipital groove before injection.

ELBOW

Landmarks

The lateral humeral epicondyle is identified and with the arm flexed at 90°, the proximal edge of the radial head is palpable about 1 cm distal to the humeral epicondyle. When the forearm is pronated and supinated, the radial head rotates, protruding slightly with full pronation. The articular margins are slightly blunted by the radial collateral ligament, but posterior to the ligament, the joint space is easily palpable.

Elbow-Joint Method

The patient is recumbent with the arm flexed at 90° resting on the abdomen. The needle is inserted into the space between the humeral epicondyle and the radial head, just behind the radial collateral ligament (Fig. 16–9).

Humeral Epicondyles

Landmarks

The humeral epicondyles are easily identified. The point of maximal tenderness in an epicondylitis (tennis elbow)

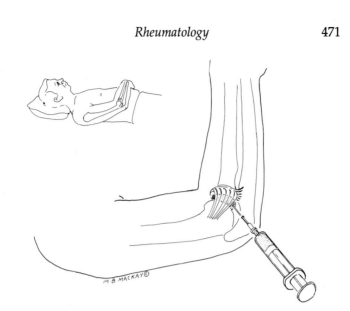

Fig. 16–9. Elbow joint procedure.

is usually found on the point of the epicondyle or just distal to the bony point over the tendinous origin of the forearm muscles.

Lateral Epicondyle

Method

The patient is recumbent with the arm flexed at 90° and resting on the abdomen. The needle is inserted through the skin just proximal to the point of maximum tenderness and advanced through the subcutaneous tissue until it approaches the bone or tendon. The soft tissues are infiltrated with the intention of placing the anesthetic and steroid on the periosteum or peritendon without actually penetrating it.

Medial Epicondyle

Method

The patient is in the lateral recumbent position with the painful elbow resting on the couch in the flexed position. The needle is inserted proximal to the epicondyle, staying anterior to avoid the ulnar nerve. The infiltration is then carried out similarly to the lateral epicondyle.

OLECRANON BURSA

Landmarks

The bursa is subcutaneous, covering the angle of the olecranon. When distended, it is easily palpable and aspiration/injection is also easy.

Method

The patient is recumbent with the elbow bent at 90° and the forearm resting on the abdomen. The needle is inserted through the skin at the back of the elbow and directed into the bursa parallel to the posterior surface of the ulna (Fig. 16–10).

WRIST

Landmarks

The tendon of the extensor pollicis longus is identified on the dorsoradial aspect of the wrist. On the radial side of that tendon is the "anatomical snuff box," the space between the distal end of the radius and the proximal surface of the scaphoid. It is easier to define if the wrist is radially deviated.

When the wrist is slightly extended another depression is apparent on the ulnar side of that tendon at the wrist. This depression has the extensor pollicis longus and the

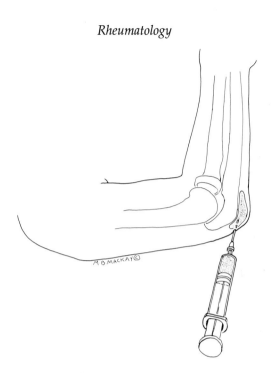

Fig. 16–10. Olecranon bursa procedure.

extensor carpi radialis longus on its radial side and the extensor indicis on the ulnar side. As the wrist is flexed, the examining finger is pushed out of the depression by the dorsal surface of the lunate.

Method

The forearm is resting on a firm surface. A small cushion is placed under the wrist so that it will rest in the neutral position. The needle is inserted into the joint just distal to the edge of the radius in either the anatomical snuff box (Fig. 16–11) or the dorsal depression (Fig. 16–12). Note that the radial artery often crosses the snuff box making this site less desirable.

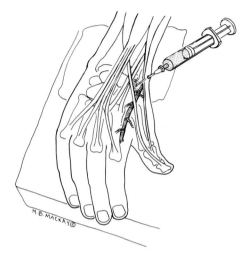

Fig. 16–11. Wrist joint procedure. Injecting the wrist joint via the anatomical snuff box. Note the proximity of the radial artery, making this approach less desirable.

METACARPOPHALANGEAL (MCP) JOINTS AND INTERPHALANGEAL (IP) JOINTS

Landmarks

These joint margins can be seen and felt on the dorso-lateral aspect with the fingers in slight flexion. In the MCP joints a slight groove is visible and a palpable step-up is noted between the metacarpal head and the proximal phalanx. The interphalangeal joints do not have a step or a groove but the articular level can be appreciated by palpation with movement.

Method

The MCP joints are entered directly through the articular groove on the radial side of the extensor tendon (Fig.

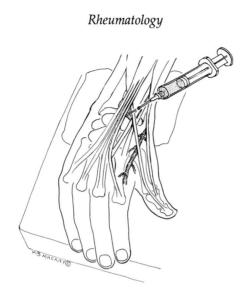

Fig. 16–12. Wrist joint procedure. Injecting the wrist joint through the dorsal depression, which is bounded on the radial side by the tendons of the extensor pollicis longus and the extensor carpi radialis longus, on the ulnar side by the tendon of the extensor indicis, and which is noted as a depression only when the wrist is slightly extended. This is the preferred approach.

16–13). The dorsal synovial pouch of the IP joints is entered from the side. The wrinkles in the skin over the dorsum of the joint form an oval. The needle is inserted through the skin at the lateral edge of that oval. The needle is directed under the extensor expansion and just above the superior surface of the bone. It is difficult to get into these joints unless they are distended (Fig. 16–14).

FLEXOR TENDON SHEATHS OF THE HAND AND WRIST

Landmarks

The flexor tendon sheaths of the index, middle, and ring fingers end in the midpalm just proximal to the main trans-

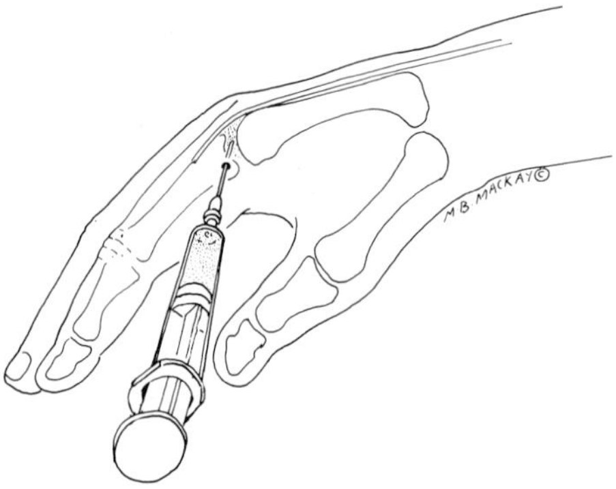

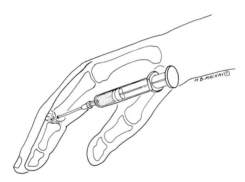

Fig. 16–13. Metacarpophalangeal joint procedure.

Fig. 16–14. Interphalangeal joint procedure.

verse skin crease. The flexor tendon sheaths of the thumb and little finger extend to the wrist. The tendons are palpable over the metacarpal eminences and are easily identifiable during active movement.

The flexor tendon sheaths at the wrist extend proximally to the carpal tunnel. The proximal border of the carpal tunnel is a line drawn from the pisiform to the tubercle of the scaphoid. This line corresponds closely to the skin crease at the proximal part of the palm.

Digital Tendon Sheaths

Method

The supinated hand should rest on a firm surface. The needle is inserted above the appropriate flexor tendon at the level of the midpalm crease, just proximal to the meta-carpal head. The needle is advanced through subcutaneous tissue and fascia until you can feel the resistance of the tendon. Slight passive extension of the finger will tug on the needle tip when the appropriate depth is achieved. The needle is then retracted slightly to clear the tip from the tendon but not from the sheath (Fig. 16–15).

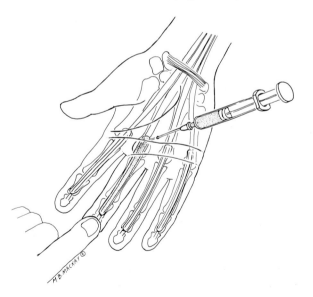

Fig. 16–15. Digital flexor tendon sheath procedure.

Wrist Tendon Sheaths

Method

The supinated hand and forearm are resting on a firm surface. A small pillow under the wrist allows it to rest in slight dorsiflexion. The needle is inserted 1 cm proximal to the palm on the ulnar side of the palmaris longus tendon. When the needle encounters the firm resistance of the flexor tendon, it is retracted slightly to clear the tip before injection (Fig. 16–16).

HIP

Landmarks

The hip is located 1 cm distal to the midpoint of a line drawn from the anterior superior iliac spine to the sym-

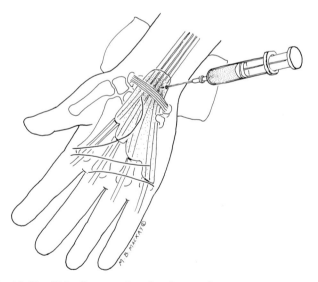

Fig. 16–16.   Wrist flexor tendon sheath procedure.

physis pubis. It is deep to the neurovascular bundle and the tendon of the iliopsoas. The femoral head is 2 cm lateral to the femoral artery.

Method

Most physicians prefer to aspirate or inject a hip with a fluoroscope (image intensifier) so that an arthrogram can be performed if there is any doubt as to whether the joint has been entered. If these facilities are not available, the following procedure should be used.

The patient is recumbent on a firm flat surface. A line is drawn from the top of the greater trochanter to the top of

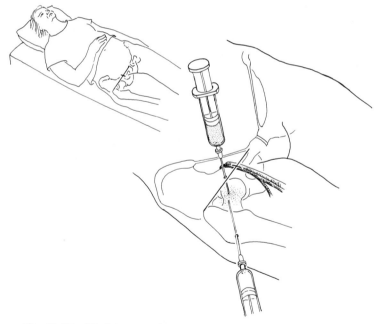

Fig. 16–17. Hip joint procedure.

the symphysis pubis. The point where the femoral artery intersects this line is marked.

The injection site is 3 to 4 cm lateral to the intersection in the average adult to avoid the femoral nerve. The needle is inserted perpendicularly. Since the capsule of the hip encloses the anterior surface of the femoral neck, the hip joint can be entered from a more lateral approach if the needle is angled slightly medially and caudally. This method avoids articular cartilage but could possibly penetrate the nutrient vessels that course along the femoral neck. This method is less direct and therefore less certain, and a longer needle is required. The lateral approach should be done with radiographic assistance (Fig. 16–17).

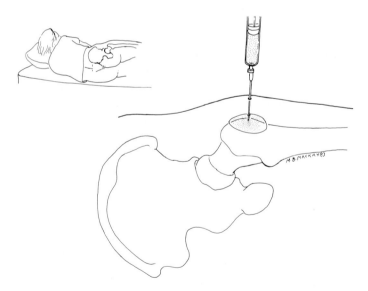

Fig. 16–18. Trochanteric bursa procedure.

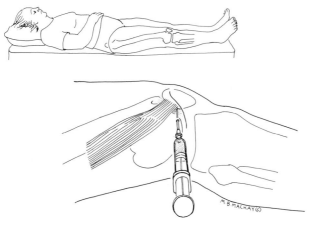

Fig. 16–19. Effused knee joint procedure.

TROCHANTERIC BURSA

Landmarks

The trochanteric bursa lies over the lateral part of the greater trochanter of the femur under the iliotibial band. With the patient in the lateral recumbent position with the painful side uppermost, the lateral aspect of the thigh is palpated. Starting at midthigh, the femur is first indistinctly palpable through the vastus lateralis. As the operator's hand moves proximally, the firm bony edge of the greater trochanter is encountered. This edge and the area immediately above it are covered by the trochanteric bursa.

Method

The patient is in the lateral recumbent position and the point of maximal tenderness over the bursa is identified. A 1 ½ inch needle for the average adult is inserted perpendicularly. As the needle is advanced through the subcutaneous tissue, the resistance of the fascia lata is en-

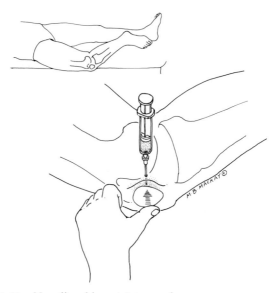

Fig. 16–20.   Noneffused knee joint procedure.

countered and penetrated. The needle is advanced slightly
to touch the greater trochanter and then slightly retracted
to clear the tip (Fig. 16–18).

KNEE

Landmarks

The suprapatellar pouch extends distally on both sides
of the patella in a horseshoe shape. The bursa communicates with the synovial space of the knee. If there is a
moderate to large effusion, the bursa should be entered at
the lateral side. In the noneffused knee, the joint should
be entered from the medial side.

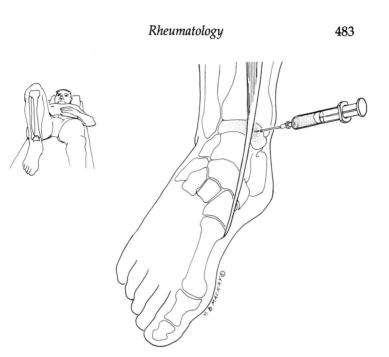

Fig. 16–21. Ankle joint procedure.

Procedure

Effused Knee. The patient is recumbent with the knee extended. The insertion of the vastus lateralis into the upper pole of the patella is identified by palpation when the patient contracts the quadriceps. The distended supra-patellar pouch forms a subcutaneous soft bulge immediately below and lateral to the insertion of the vastus lateralis tendon. The needle is directed into this bulge and under the tendon (Fig. 16–19).

Noneffused Knee. The knee is slightly bent, and the leg rests in external rotation. The groove between the patella and the medial condyle of the femur can be accentuated by gently forcing the patella medially. The needle is inserted directly into the groove (Fig. 16–20).

ANKLE

The distal edge of the tibia can be palpated medially and laterally to the extensor tendons of the foot. The dome of the talus rotates forward to become palpable just below this edge when the ankle is fully plantar flexed. In the neutral position, the talus rotates under the tibia, leaving a slight depression just below the edge of the tibia.

Method

The patient may be recumbent or sitting. The ankle is in the neutral position, and the needle is inserted 0.5 cms beyond the tibial edge and directed toward the edge of the dome of the talus (Fig. 16–21).

SMALL JOINTS OF THE FOOT

Subtalar and Midtarsal Joints. These joints should be aspirated and injected under the guidance of a fluoroscope.

Metatarsophalangeal Joints. Like the MCP joints of the hand, these joints are approached from the side, and the needle is directed into the joint under the extensor tendon.

17
Surgery

Minor Surgical Procedures
K.P. Siren

FOREIGN BODY REMOVAL

The exploration for removal of completely penetrated foreign bodies (e.g., broken needles, metal shards, and glass fragments), which will not extrude spontaneously, can be frustrating, as attempts to follow the wound path usually result in pushing the object deeper or creating false tracks. The location of the foreign body can frequently be more accurately delineated by inserting two or three syringe needles into separate sites toward the suspected locus of the body and taking two orthogonal radiographs. Incising along the path of the needle radiographically closest to the object will usually be successful.

Rings

Rings trapped by distal edema can frequently be removed without cutting by wrapping the distal phalanx with an Esmarch bandage or a 1-inch Penrose drain for about 5 minutes. This may reduce the edema sufficiently for ring removal. Alternatively, a length of string may be passed under the ring, using a small curved forceps or paper clip. The distal end of the string is then wrapped close-spaced and tightly around the digit. Lubricate the covered area with soap or petroleum jelly. The proximal end of the string is then unwound, pulling the ring distally.

Fishhooks

Barbed, embedded fishhooks can be extracted by pushing the barbed end along the arc of the hook until it exits the skin, cutting off the barbed end with wire cutters, and backing the hook out. Local anesthesia should be employed. Frequently, the barb may be removed by passing a syringe needle along the wound tract and enveloping the barb in the lumen of the needle. The hook and needle can then be backed out together.

Infected Pierced Ear Keepers

The tracts of recently pierced ear lobes, which have become infected, may be kept patent during treatment by replacing the keepers with a length of 3-0 monofilament nylon suture passed through the lobe and knotted in a loop, while the infection is treated with an antibiotic ointment.

WOUND REPAIR

Prior to the examination or treatment of non-surgical wounds, a brief history should be obtained relating to the mechanism, environment, agent, and force of the injury. Inquire into the history of previous injury to the area and note the patient's degree of keloid formation. The presence of allergies, diabetes, and the use of steroids should also be noted.

The functional state of neurologic, vascular, and motor structures distal to the wound must be assessed. While examining the wound, it is imperative to determine the extent and involvement of adjacent and underlying structures. If the wound is near a joint or tendon, it is essential to perform the examination while putting these structures through a full range of motion to assess occult injury. This may be the only way to observe an otherwise unnoticed tendon laceration.

Anesthesia can be done before wound cleansing *but must always follow appropriate neurologic examination.* Most wounds can be managed with local infiltration with 1% or 2% lidocaine, injecting via the cut surface of the wound into the immediately subdermal tissues. This method will only produce painful stimuli if injection is rapid. Extensive wounds or wounds in areas with little or no distensible subdermal tissue may require proximal nerve blocks. Lidocaine with epinephrine should only be used when active bleeding would obscure the operative field and should never be used in wounds of the fingers, toes, or penis.

Hemostasis in extremities can be achieved with a proximal circumferential Penrose drain held taut with a clamp. Vascular "bleeders" can be managed by seizing the cut vessel end with a clamp and hand tying a ligature, or by placing a circumferential figure-of-eight stitch in the area of the vessel (Fig. 17–1). Hot wire cautery, if available, is valuable in areas where cosmesis is paramount.

Wound cleansing should be by saline irrigation and debridement of avascular tissue. Use of cytotoxic agents such as soaps and detergents will only extend tissue damage and increase scar formation. Irrigation of joint spaces or tendon sheaths should not be done with a metal needle because this will cause cartilage damage. A plastic vascular

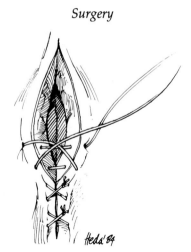

Fig. 17–1. Circumferential figure-of-eight stitch.

catheter should be used instead. Avascular tissue and foreign material may become a nidus of infection and must be removed. Minimization of scar formation is achieved by:

—careful attention to elimination of avascular tissue (including hematoma) with appropriate debridement;

—prevention of hematoma accumulation by closure in layers or proper cutaneous suture placement;

—distribution of transverse wound stress by inserting stress-bearing sutures in the deeper fibrous tissues (dermis and fascia) (Fig. 17–2);

—meticulous matching of anatomic landmarks (wrinkles, tissue-type transition zones);

—side-to-side alignment of tissue planes, especially the epidermis. Simple, interrupted sutures are adequate for most wound closures, but in areas of high transverse stress, a figure-of-eight, horizontal mattress (Fig. 17–3A), or modified horizontal mattress stitch (Fig. 17–3B) will be more resistant to tissue tearing and reduce reactive fibrosis.

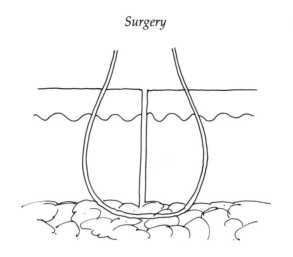

Fig. 17–2. Suture through dermis and fascia.

A Gilles corner stitch (Fig. 17–4) should be used in the tips of dermal flaps to minimize compression of the vascular supply to the epidermis of the tip.

Synthetic suture materials, such as nylon, polyglactin (Vicryl), and polyglycolic acid (Dexon), provide greater strength and homogeneity than natural material (e.g., cotton, silk, or gut) and use of the latter should be avoided if possible.

Following closure, the wound should be covered with petrolatum or tulle gras (with or without antibiotic) until the sutures are removed. A pressure dressing should be applied for 12 hours if the possibility of hematoma collection is anticipated. Although patients may bathe the repaired area, they should be advised to avoid swimming or soaking the wound while the sutures are in place and reminded of the need to use a sunscreen in exposed wounds during the first 6 months to prevent hyperpigmentation while the wound is maturing. Tetanus immunization status should always be reviewed at the time of repair.

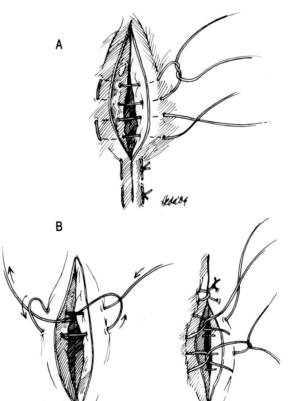

Fig. 17–3. **A.** Horizontal mattress stitch. **B.** Modified horizontal mattress stitch.

start. Back-flow of water may occur if the level of the water container is too high or the water is run in too quickly.

Note: The end of a plastic tube is replaced by a rubber catheter or cone since most plastic tends to be too hard and rigid.

MANAGEMENT OF COLOSTOMY PROLAPSE

Clinical Uses

Prevention of edema and/or necrosis. Maintenance of function.

Indications

Opening in abdominal wall is too large. Sudden increased intra-abdominal pressure (sneezing, coughing, heavy lifting).

Equipment

Rectal gloves
Water soluble lubricant
1 roll of 15-cm wide elastic bandage
Skin barrier and pouch (flexible), e.g., karaya or Stomahesive washer, wafer, or paste

Method

Remove appliance. With patient in supine position, manually replace prolapsed bowel. Apply skin barrier and pouch, which are completely flexible. Wrap the elastic bandage around patient's abdomen at level of stoma. It should be possible to insert fingers under bandage so that stomal function is not inhibited. Teach patient to reduce prolapse and apply bandage. Refer for surgical opinion.

Note: Bed rest and treatment with warm saline compresses may be necessary if edema is present before prolapse can be reduced.

18
Urology

Grant A. Farrow

URETHRAL CATHETERIZATION

Clinical Uses

Urethral catheterization provides direct bladder drainage for bladder outlet obstruction at either the bladder neck, prostate, or urethra. It is also used for neurogenic bladder, urinary incontinence, monitoring urine output, and obtaining a sterile bladder urine specimen. Strict sterile technique must be used for catheterization.

Equipment

Catheter (several types are available, depending on the
   purpose)
Aqueous skin antiseptic
Sterile towels and gloves
Kidney basin
Kelly forceps
4 × 4 gauze
Urine culture container

Lidocaine gel topical anesthesia with applicator tip
Lubricant
Closed drainage system

Various sized catheters are available to suit different situations. In general, a smaller catheter (No. 14 French) should be employed. Smaller catheters are less traumatic to the urethra and result in fewer complications such as stricture, and are more comfortable on insertion for the patient.

Catheters (Figure 18–1)

1. *Straight red rubber catheter,* No. 12 or No. 14 for simple temporary bladder emptying.

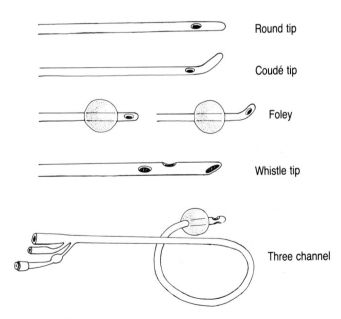

Round tip

Coudé tip

Foley

Whistle tip

Three channel

Fig. 18–1. Catheters.

2. *Coudé-tip (or Tieman) catheter.* The slightly flexed tip allows entry over an elevated bladder neck.
3. *Foley catheter.* The balloon maintains the catheter in place for continuous bladder drainage. It is available in a Tieman-tip catheter as well. The Silastic Foley catheter is less liable to encrustation and stricture formation for long-term or permanent catheter drainage.
4. *Whistle-tip catheters* or larger catheters (No. 24 French) may be employed if blood clots or significant debris are present in the bladder.
5. *A three channel (3-way) catheter* allows for continuous irrigation of the bladder.

Voiding around the catheter is usually due to catheter obstruction and/or bladder spasms. This is treated *not* by employing a larger catheter, but by irrigating the catheter to ensure patency, or by anticholinergic medication to decrease bladder spasm.

Method

Male. The patient is positioned on his back with legs slightly apart to accommodate a sterile basin. The catheter tray is prepared at the outset to allow one-handed use. The patient is draped with a folded towel (Fig. 18–2). The prepuce is retracted to allow sterile preparation of the glans penis, and the penis is grasped through the towel by the left hand (Fig. 18–3). Excessive scrubbing of the glans may precipitate a balanitis. Lubricate the distal end of the catheter and insert it with the right hand. A slight rotary motion will often facilitate insertion, and slight stretching of the penis will eliminate mucosal folds. When using a Tieman catheter, the tip must be directed anteriorly at the bladder neck. If a Foley catheter is being used, insert it completely into the bladder, inflate the balloon, and withdraw until the balloon is at the bladder neck. Obtain urine for culture and immediately attach to the closed-drainage system.

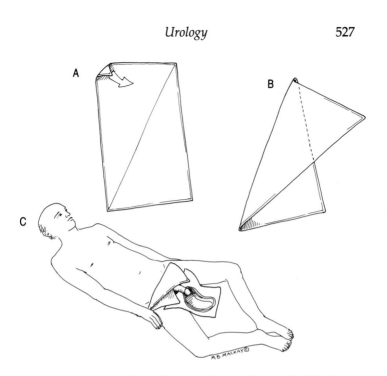

Fig. 18–2. Catheterization of the male. **A.** A sterile towel is folded over to form the shape noted in **B,** which in turn is placed on the lower abdomen to provide a proximal sterile field **C.**

Although not ordinarily necessary, local anesthesia may be used for larger catheters or for particularly sensitive and anxious patients. Prior to catheterizations, a sterile applicator tip supplied with lidocaine gel is inserted into the meatus and the entire length of the urethra is distended with the gel (Fig. 18–4). Instructing the patient to attempt to void at this stage will open the posterior urethra and facilitate complete entry of the gel to the level of the bladder.

Female. The female patient is placed in the lithotomy position; adequate lighting is directed to the perineum, and

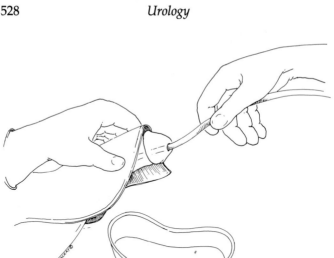

Fig. 18–3. Catheterization of the male.

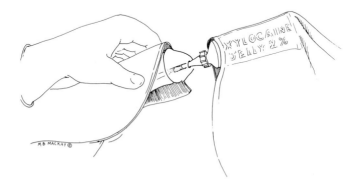

Fig. 18–4. Instilling local anesthetic.

separation of the labia with the thumb and forefinger of the left hand allows visualization of the urethral meatus (Fig. 18–5). Following sterile cleansing of the adjacent perineum, the appropriate catheter is inserted.

Catheter Guide

In situations where the catheter cannot be passed, a rigid guide is *not* recommended. This is employed in specific situations to direct the tip of the catheter, usually after prostatectomy. It is liable to perforate the urethra if obstruction is present. If a catheter cannot be inserted, the filiform and follower catheters are more effective and much safer.

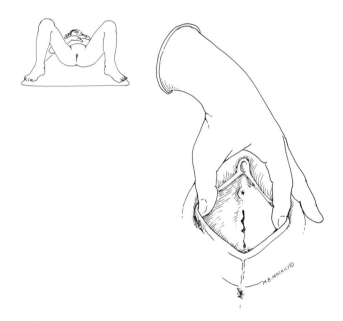

Fig. 18–5. Catheterization of the female.

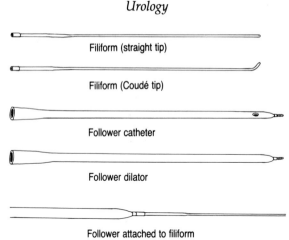

Filiform (straight tip)

Filiform (Coudé tip)

Follower catheter

Follower dilator

Follower attached to filiform

Fig. 18–6.   Filiform and follower.

Filiform and Follower (Fig. 18–6)

The penis is prepared as for simple catheterization and lidocaine gel is instilled into the urethra. A fine, flexible Coudé-tip or "pigtail-tip" filiform is inserted into the urethra using a gentle in and out and rotary motion, never forcing the filiform. Undue pressure will only create a mucosal flap. Be patient until the lumen is entered and the filiform is inserted fully into the bladder with free in and out movement. A springing back of the filiform or "catching" indicates that the filiform is curled in the urethra and must be reinserted.

Once the filiform is properly inserted, the follower is screwed snugly on to the filiform and inserted into the bladder. Progressively larger solid followers are used to dilate a stricture, while hollow followers may be taped in place to the penis to provide continuous drainage.

While an in-and-out rotary-insertion technique is employed for the filiform, the follower is inserted using steady pressure to prevent curling or kinking the filiform ahead of the follower.

After dilating the urethra with filiforms and followers, a small Foley catheter may then be inserted. If the urethra has been difficult to enter, it is often wise to leave the follower taped in place for 24 hours to allow mucosal flaps to adhere before attempting to insert a Foley catheter (Fig. 18–7).

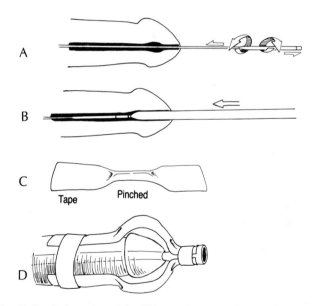

Fig. 18–7. **A.** Insertion of the filiform using a gentle in and out as well as a rotary motion. **B.** The follower is screwed snugly on to the filiform and inserted into the bladder. **C.** An adhesive bridge may be used to tape both the follower and the penile shaft. The adhesive is turned over at the midportion so it will not stick to the glans. **D.** Method of taping follower in place, using adhesive bridges (**C**) over the glans.

Intermittent Catheterization

In cases of neurogenic bladder or atonic bladder requiring prolonged bladder drainage, intermittent catheterization will allow satisfactory drainage and greatly decrease the incidence of infection. A No. 12 French catheter is passed every 8 to 12 hours, completely emptying the bladder. This allows filling and emptying of the bladder, decreasing infection and contraction of the bladder as well as allowing development of a normal voiding routine.

Self-catheterization

Teaching the patient the technique of intermittent self-catheterization allows the patient greater freedom, and decreased dependence on medical or institutional care, as well as saving time and expense (Fig. 18–8).

A clean, as opposed to sterile, technique is satisfactory, and as long as the bladder is completely emptied on each occasion, the incidence of infection is not increased. The catheter is simply washed with tap water following use, and stored in a jar of antiseptic solution, e.g., chlorhexadine.

For self-catheterization in the female, a short, rigid, slightly curved stainless steel or plastic catheter is employed (Fig. 18–9).

SUPRAPUBIC PERCUTANEOUS CYSTOTOMY

Bladder drainage may be performed suprapubically by percutaneous-needle aspiration or cannula insertion.

Indications

Acute urinary retention where perurethral catheterization has not been possible. Associated with gynecologic or urologic surgery, this technique allows the patient to de-

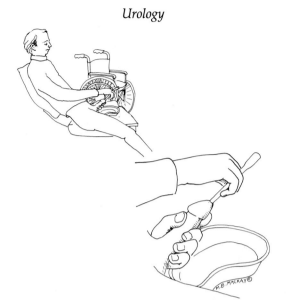

Fig. 18–8. Self-catheterization (male). The patient is able to insert the clean catheter into the neurogenic bladder with one hand supporting the shaft of the penis while the other hand inserts the catheter.

velop a voiding routine and measure residual urine to assess bladder emptying. For urethral trauma, urethral catheterization may be impossible and may cause further damage. In rare conditions, it is used to obtain bladder urine for culture.

Equipment (usually commercially available kits)

   Skin preparation antiseptic (shaving is not necessary)
   Injectable local anesthesia with syringe and needle
   Scalpel
   Needle trochar and cannula with drainage system
   Sterile drape or towel
   Silk suture

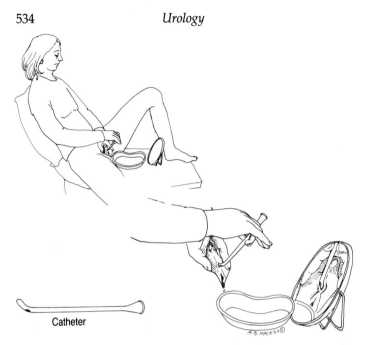

Catheter

Fig. 18–9. Self-catheterization (female). The female patient inserts the short, rigid catheter with the help of a mirror.

Method

The bladder must be distended and palpable in the suprapubic area to elevate the peritoneum and bowel away from the proposed tract into the bladder (Fig. 18–10).

Local anesthesia is injected immediately above the symphysis. Raise a skin wheal and then infiltrate down to the bladder. A point-stab incision is made in the skin, and the needle with trochar is directed into the distended bladder. Free flow of urine on removal of the stylet confirms entry into the bladder. The cannula is then passed into the bladder, and the needle removed. The cannula is attached to the skin with a silk suture, or taped to a flange, depending upon the system employed. (Be sure to familiarize yourself

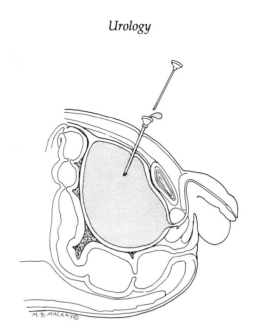

Fig. 18–10. Suprapubic percutaneous cystotomy (bladder distended).

with the manufacturer's instructions of your particular system.)

Contraindications

1. This technique is unsuitable if the bladder is not distended and not palpable above the symphysis because of the danger of entering peritoneum and damaging the bowel (Fig. 18–11).
2. Previous suprapubic surgery may cause anterior adhesion of bowel to the bladder.
3. Bladder tumors may be seeded along the cannula tract.
4. With hematuria, percutaneous cannulae are often too fine to allow irrigation of blood clot and will become occluded. Operative insertion of a large tube is indicated under these circumstances.

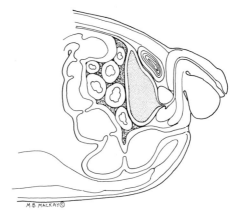

Fig. 18–11. Contraindication to suprapubic percutaneous cystotomy. A cannula inserted above the symphysis, when a bladder has insufficient urine to make it distended and palpable, would enter the peritoneal cavity and damage the bowel.

ADULT CIRCUMCISION

Indications

Phimosis, recurrent balanitis, laceration associated with intercourse, and recurrent laceration of frenulum.

Equipment

Aqueous antiseptic for skin preparation
Sterile draping
Minor surgical set including: curved mosquito hemostat forceps (4), scalpel, scissors (dissection and suture), and needle holder
4 × 4 gauze pads
Petroleum gauze strip
2 inch kling (stretch) gauze bandage
½ inch adhesive tape

2% lidocaine without epinephrine
10-ml syringe and needle for infiltration

Method

Anesthesia. General anesthesia is preferred and requires no muscle relaxation. Local anesthesia may be employed using bilateral nerve block at the base of the penis. Lidocaine 2% *without epinephrine* is injected as the block. Lidocaine 1% without epinephrine may be supplemented at the frenulum or the skin area. *Never use epinephrine solution for infiltration of the penis.*

Care must be taken not to excise excessive skin from the shaft of the penis; allow adequate skin for erection. The first step is to make an elliptical incision with slight retraction of the prepuce, ensuring redundant skin on the shaft and at the frenulum (Fig. 18–12A). A scalpel makes a smooth line.

The second step uses dissecting scissors to make a dorsal slit, extending to the skin incision anteriorly and to within 3 to 4 mm of the corona (Fig. 18–12B, C). This allows full retraction of the prepuce. Once the prepuce is fully retracted, a circumferential incision is made, using a scalpel, 3 to 4 mm around the corona (Fig. 18–12D). A tight frenular flap may be incised and closed transversely (Fig. 18–12E).

The dorsal vein is ligated, while meticulous hemostasis is secured using fine-point cautery forceps. Avoid cautery at the skin edge, which may cause areas of local necrosis. The closure is completed with 0000 chromic sutures and meticulous approximation (Fig. 18–12F).

Dressing. A firm dressing obviates hematoma under the skin flap as well as decreases post-operative discomfort.

Petrolatum strip gauze is plicated about the incision. (Plication avoids a constricting ring.) A folded 4 × 4 gauze is then held in place with a snug 2-inch kling (stretch gauze) bandage, extending from behind the corona to adjacent to

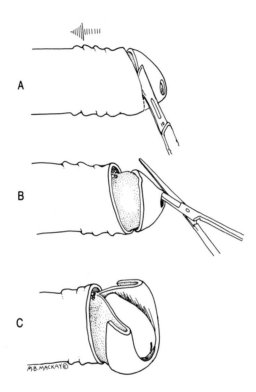

Fig. 18–12. Adult circumcision. **A.** With slight retraction of the prepuce, a scalpel is used to make an elliptical incision in the skin of the prepuce. **B.** Dissecting scissors are then used to make a dorsal slit anteriorly to the skin incision, and to within 3 to 4 mm of the corona. **C.** The result.

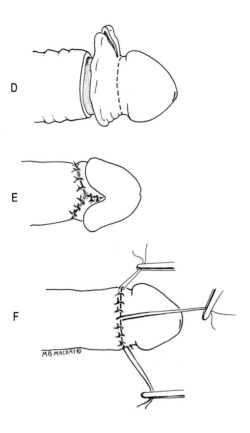

Fig. 18–12 *Continued.* **D.** The prepuce is fully retracted and a circumferential incision is made 3 to 4 mm from the corona. The prepuce is thus removed. **E.** A tight frenular flap may be incised and closed transversely. **F.** Closure of the incision, carefully approximating the edges with 0000 chromic sutures. This must be done meticulously.

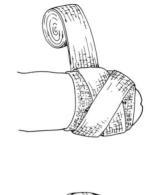

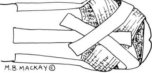

M.B.MACKAY©

Fig. 18–13. Adult circumcision. Dressing applied.

the meatus (Fig. 18–13). This is held in place with strip adhesive. All circular bandages are placed obliquely to prevent constriction. The bandage is left in place for 3 to 4 days and then may be removed in a warm bath if adherent.

VASECTOMY (BILATERAL VAS DEFERENS LIGATION)

Indications

Voluntary sterilization. Vasectomy is the simplest and most effective form of surgical contraception. It is important, however, to have an informed patient. The following facts and fables must be discussed with the patient:

1. There is no clinical evidence of increased incidence of

arteriosclerosis following bilateral vas ligation in humans.

2. There is no evidence of arthritis or other autoimmune disease associated with sperm extravasation or sperm granuloma formation.
3. There is a small incidence of impotence following vasectomy. This is purely a psychological effect.
4. Vasectomy reversal, vasovasostomy, is technically successful in 40 to 80% of cases. The reversal procedure is less likely to be successful in a patient over 30 years of age, if the time lapse since the original vasectomy is over 7 years, and if the site of the original ligation was in the convoluted segment of the vas.
5. Spontaneous reconstitution of the vas may occur in one of several thousand cases even if the procedure is performed properly. This incidence is much higher if simple ligation only is employed.

Equipment

Aqueous skin antiseptic solution
Minor surgical set including: scalpel, curved mosquito hemostats (4), Allis forceps (2), and needle holder.
Sterile drapes or towel
00 chromic catgut ligature
0000 chromic catgut suture
1% lidocaine local anesthesia without epinephrine
10-ml syringe and No. 23 needle for local anesthesia

Method

A scrub nurse assistant is valuable for this procedure.

The scrotal content is grasped with the left hand and the vas deferens (recognized as a firm round cord) is displayed under the skin between the thumb and the forefinger. This is not released until the vas is isolated and, as described later, firmly held with an Allis forcep.

Local anesthesia is injected as a wheal into the skin and infiltrated around the vas and adjacent structures (Fig. 18–14A). A 3 to 4 mm skin incision is made over the vas. Separation of the subcutaneous tissue is accomplished with a curved mosquito forceps and the vas is firmly grasped with an Allis forcep (Fig. 18–14B).

The tunica over the vas is incised with the scalpel, and the vas is isolated from adjacent structures with a curved mosquito forceps (Fig. 18–14C). The vas is then divided between forceps, removing a 1-cm segment for pathology and medicolegal purposes. Each end is doubly ligated with 00 chromic catgut ligature (Fig. 18–14D). Hemostasis is meticulously secured with 0000 ligature and the ligated ends are returned into the scrotum, holding the suture for final inspection for hemostasis, after completing the contralateral side to this stage (Fig. 18–14E).

Prior to closure, the ligated ends of the vas are widely separated by gentle traction on the testicle, and the incision is closed with 0000 chromic catgut in the muscle and skin. Pathological confirmation and negative semen analysis 1 and 2 months after ligation is documented prior to considering the procedure effective.

REDUCTION OF PARAPHIMOSIS

Paraphimosis occurs when a tight phimosis is retracted behind the corona, and the edematous prepuce cannot be reduced by the patient.

Equipment

Lubricating gel

Method

The penis is circumferntially grasped with the left hand and progressively squeezed to dissipate the edema. This

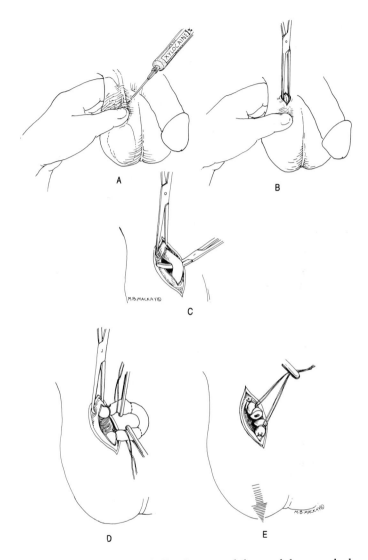

Fig. 18–14. Vasectomy. **A.** Infiltration around the vas deferens and adjacent structures. **B.** The vas is firmly grasped with an Allis forcep. **C.** The vas is isolated from adjacent structures with a curved mosquito forcep. **D.** A 1 cm segment of the vas is isolated and doubly clamped to remove this 1 cm segment. **E.** Following meticulous hemostasis, the ligated ends are returned into the scrotum.

543

maneuver takes several minutes, which allows the patient to gradually tolerate as tight a grasp as the hand can create (Fig. 18–15A). The glans is lubricated. The phimotic ring is then drawn over the corona by the fingers of each hand as the thumbs reduce the glans by counter pressure (Fig. 18–15B).

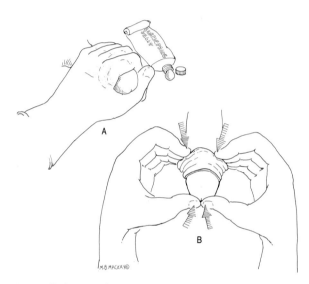

Fig. 18–15. Reduction of paraphimosis. **A.** The penis is circumferentially grasped and squeezed to reduce edema of the retracted prepuce. **B.** The lubricated glans is forced back into the prepuce when diminution of the edema makes it possible.

Urine Collection From Urinary Stoma
Enid H. Wilson

URINE SPECIMEN FROM URINARY STOMA

Purpose

To obtain uncontaminated urine for culture and sensitivity.

Indications

Suspected urinary tract infection.

Equipment

Povidone-iodine or other cleansing agent
Warm water and gauze
Sterile equipment: No. 8 or 10 catheter, gauze, water,

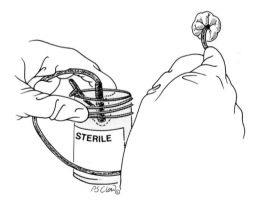

Fig. 18–16. Collection of urine from urinary stoma.

container, gloves, water soluble lubricant, and syringe with catheter tip.

Procedure

Remove the urinary collection appliance from patient, and wash the patient's skin with warm water. Put on gloves and clean stoma with povidone-iodine, working from lumen outward, using circular movements. Repeat this twice and then rinse the stoma with sterile water. Lubricate catheter tip, and insert catheter 5 to 6 cm into lumen. *Do not force catheter,* but rotate gently until it slides in. Place catheter end into sterile container (Fig. 18–16). If urine does not flow, ask the patient to change position. If urine still does not flow, attach syringe and pull back gently on plunger. After obtaining a satisfactory urine specimen, wash and dry skin and put on or replace urinary appliance.

Note: Urine taken from the pouch of the appliance is contaminated.

19
Vascular Access

Intravenous Techniques
Mary E. Archibald

The recent growth in the use of intravenous therapy brings with it a host of potential problems, e.g., microbial contamination, incompatibilities, and improper administration. These hazards are numerous but can be prevented or minimized by applying the following principles.

A calm, confident approach to the patient is helpful in minimizing apprehension. It is recommended that no more than two unsuccessful attempts at venipuncture be done by any one individual, before requesting a colleague to make further attempts.

Equipment

Containers and Administration Sets. All containers should be carefully inspected for clarity of solution, absence of cracks in bottles or punctures in plastic bags, presence of a vacuum in glass bottles, an intact seal over additive port, and the correct solution, amount, and expiration date.

547

A variety of sets is available for the administration of intravenous infusions and/or medications. The set choice depends on the type of therapy the patient is to receive. After attaching an administration set to a solution container, label the tubing or set with the start date, time, and your name.

To calculate the flow rates, the following information must be known:

—amount of solution to be infused;

—duration of administration;

—the drop factor per milliliter of the administration set used.

Example:

To obtain total hourly volume desired, divide amount of solution by time of administration, e.g.:

$$\frac{1000 \text{ ml}}{8 \text{ hours}} = 125 \text{ ml/hour}$$

The following formula should be used to calculate the flow rate:

$$\frac{\text{drop factor of set} \times \text{ml/hour}}{60 \text{ (minutes/hour)}} = \text{drops/minute}$$

e.g., $\frac{10 \times 125}{60} = 21 \text{ drops/minute} = 125 \text{ ml/hour.}$

Inaccurate flow rate is one of the most frequent problems encountered in intravenous therapy. Considerations include:

1. Device related inaccuracies, such as height of con-

tainer, pressure changes, plastic "cold flow," container overfill, flow clamps, rate of flow (increased drip rate produces a larger drop), change in needle position, and obstructed vents or airways.

2. Fluid related inaccuracies caused by the viscosity of the solution, and cold or irritating solutions that may cause vasospasm.

3. Patient related inaccuracies may relate to blood pressure, the patient's movements, clot formation in the lumen of the cannula, extravasation, kinked tubing, and vein trauma, e.g., phlebitis.

4. Administration related inaccuracies such as fluid overload, speed shock, fear and pain, extravasation, tissue necrosis, and pyrogenic reactions.

Needles and Catheters. These are commonly available and include:

Ordinary injection needles (14-gauge to 20-gauge, short-bevel)

Winged-infusion needles

Over-the-needle catheters

Inside-the-needle catheters

Guidelines for Needle/Catheter Selection. The type, gauge, and length of the device should be selected according to the therapy the patient is receiving. In general, to ensure minimal irritation to the lumen of the vein, the smallest, shortest device possible to achieve efficient delivery without complications should be used. An obvious exception would be to use large-gauge needles, often at two sites, in the case of severe shock or acute massive hemorrhage. If rapid transfusion is indicated requiring a needle of sufficiently large gauge, the administration rate can often be increased by use of a pressure infusor or by placing a blood pressure cuff around the plastic bag containing the blood to be administered, then inflating it to desired pressure. For short term therapy, 24 hours or less, and for pediatric, oncology, or geriatric patients, the winged-steel needle might be the cannula of choice. The tendency for the steel needle to infiltrate, however, is a source of concern when administering drugs that produce tissue necrosis with extravasation. For therapy of longer duration, the short, small catheter allows for greater blood flow around the tip, reducing the risk of clotting, and for more rapid dilution when cytotoxic drugs are to be infused, minimizing irritation to the vein wall. The administration of viscous solutions, such as some hyperalimentation fluids or blood, generally requires a larger gauge cannula. Blood can be administered through a 20-gauge needle/catheter, but the delivery is not as efficient as with a larger gauge device.

ADMINISTRATION

Guidelines for Vein-Site Selection

Peripheral veins should be used for routine I.V. therapy.

Hands and arms should be rotated with each restart, where possible.

For long-term therapy, as a general rule, veins of the hands should be considered first, then move up the arms for other suitable sites.

Choose a vein larger than the cannula to allow for good hemodilution. This is particularly important when administering irritating agents.

Site should be free from trauma, hematoma, phlebitis, cuts, abrasions, and infections. Sclerosed veins should be avoided.

Avoid veins located over or near areas of joint flexion. Veins in the antecubital fossa should be used for blood collection and/or cannulation of central veins only.

Consider complications such as thrombophlebitis, which can occur with the use of veins in the lower extremities.

Most hospitals allow a maximum of two venipuncture attempts per person. This policy lessens unnecessary suffering by the patient and adds to the preservation and conservation of suitable veins.

Guidelines to Assist in Finding a Suitable Vein

Apply a blood pressure cuff to the upper arm, inflated to a measurement between the patient's systolic and diastolic pressure. Alternatively, soft rubber tubing may be used as a tourniquet.

Intermittent clenching of the fist by the patient will also be helpful.

Allow the patient's arm to hang dependent over the side of the bed.

Lightly tap the skin over the venous network (do not produce pain).

If the above steps fail to help identify a suitable vein, release the tourniquet and apply heat (warm, moist towels) to entire extremity for 15 to 30 minutes. Reapply tourniquet and repeat the above steps.

Prevention of Infection or Contamination at the Intravenous Site

The person administering the intravenous must thoroughly wash the hands prior to the procedure. Meticulous preparation of the skin prior to insertion of a needle is important. After the needle/catheter has been inserted, some researchers recommend the application of a topical antimicrobial agent, such as an iodophor or polyantibiotic ointment, to the catheter-cutaneous junction. A sterile dressing should be applied over all I.V. cannula entrance sites. The I.V. dressing should be changed every 24 hours or immediately if the dressing becomes soiled, wet, or loose. When the dressing is changed, the site should be cleansed with alcohol or povidone-iodine solution and

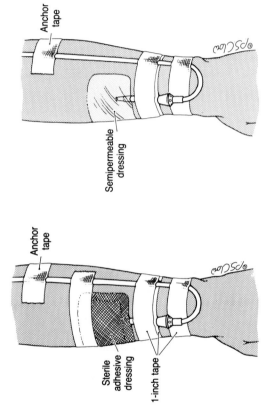

552

Fig. 19–1. **A.** Catheter in arm with regular sterile dressing. **B.** Catheter in arm with sterile transparent semipermeable membrane adhesive dressing.

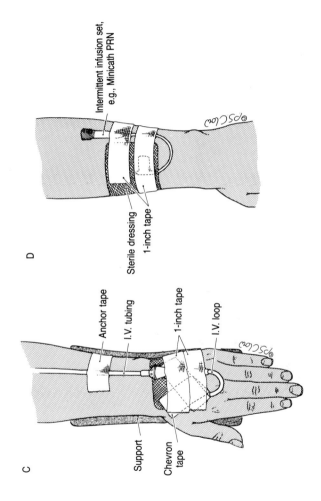

C

Anchor tape

I.V. tubing

1-inch tape

I.V. loop

Support

Chevron
tape

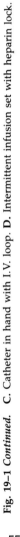

D

Intermittent infusion set,
e.g., Minicath PRN

Sterile dressing

1-inch tape

Fig. 19–1 *Continued.* C. Catheter in hand with I.V. loop. **D.** Intermittent infusion set with heparin lock.

allowed to dry, followed by reapplication of ointment and sterile dressing. Alternatively, the use of a sterile, transparent, semipermeable membrane adhesive dressing allows constant monitoring of the catheter site. This dressing can remain in place until the catheter is removed. At the first sign of pain or tenderness around the cannula site, erythema, extravasation of the I.V. fluid, infection, signs suggestive of local thrombophebitis, or any unexplained fever, the needle/catheter should immediately be removed and a new device inserted at an alternate site, if intravenous therapy is to be continued.

Skin Preparation

Preparation of the insertion site is a most important step in venipuncture technique. Chemical disinfectants available for such skin preparation include:
iodine-alcohol, iodophors, and 70% alcohol.

Shaving of the local area should be avoided as microabrasions may be caused that will make bacterial invasion more likely. When excessive hair exists, clip the hair or use surgical depilatories.

Taping Procedures

The needle or catheter should be adequately taped in order to prevent to-and-fro motion of the cannula in and out of the vein, sideways movement of the cannula, and accidental removal of the cannula by pulling on the tubing. Figure 19–1 suggests several methods that may be used to secure the catheter and protective dressing.

Employee Health and Safety

Intravenous and blood procedures can impose certain health hazards for the employee. If indicated by the patient's disease process, gloves should be worn. Care should

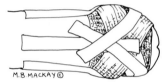

be taken at all times to avoid self-punctures with contaminated needles. Needles and syringes should be disposed of in labelled, puncture-resistant containers.

Hepatitis B antigen carriers and those suspected of having AIDS (acquired immune deficiency syndrome) should have their office and hospital records permanently "flagged" to alert staff to take special precautions when obtaining or handling their blood specimens or performing intravenous procedures.

VENIPUNCTURE

Winged-infusion Needle

Clinical Uses

Infants and children, the elderly, short-term therapy, and for small veins.

Equipment

I.V. solution, administration set and tubing label
I.V. pole or standard
Winged-infusion needle (appropriate gauge)
Tourniquet (broad)
Disinfectant solution, e.g., iodophor
Dry sterile gauze
Antimicrobial ointment (optional)
Adhesive tape, one-inch wide
Sterile adhesive bandage or dressing

Method

General Instructions for all Intravenous Procedures:
Wash hands and assemble appropriate equipment.
Identify the patient and explain the procedure.
Place the patient in a comfortable position with the patient's arm on a flat surface and lower than the heart.

Apply tourniquet and select a suitable vein by palpation. (Help the patient relax. This is most important when attempting to get good dilation of veins.)

Choose appropriate venipuncture site.

After choosing site, select appropriate needle/catheter and *release tourniquet*.

Specific Instructions for Winged-Infusion Needle:

Spike the I.V. solution container and establish drip level. Label tubing with date, time, and your name.

Connect female adapter of winged-infusion set to administration tubing. *Do not remove needle guard.* Check integrity of device.

Wash hands thoroughly.

Reapply tourniquet and cleanse site with disinfectant. *Do not touch prepped area.* If vein is palpated again, then area must be reprepped.

Prime the set. Clear all air from tubing and needle. Close clamps.

Hold needle device bevel-up. Grip wings together firmly between thumb and index finger. Remove needle guard.

Stabilize vein by anchoring it from 3 to 5 cm below the insertion site with your thumb, and stretching the skin downward against the direction of insertion.

Position needle tip directly above, or barely to one side, and parallel to the vein about 0.5 cm below proposed site of vein entry (Fig. 19–2A).

Insert needle at 30 to 40° angle through skin and underlying tissues to reach, but not penetrate, vein (Fig. 19–2B).

Decrease needle angle until almost flush with skin, approximately 10° (Fig. 19–2C). Relocate needle tip directly over vein and slowly enter vein (Fig. 19–2D). Watch for flashback of blood into clear tubing of infusion set, verifying successful vein entry.

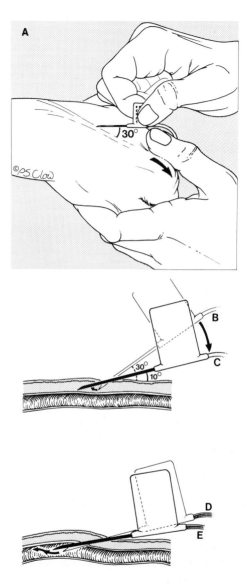

Fig. 19–2. Winged infusion needle procedure. **A.** Needle is inserted at 30° angle to reach vein. **B, C.** Needle inserted to reach but not penetrate vein. **D, E.** Needle introduced into vein and advanced.

As needle tip enters vein, slightly lift the needle tip with wings, and cautiously advance needle well into vein, with tourniquet still applied (Fig. 19–2E).

Release wings and lay them flat on skin.

Release tourniquet and open flow clamp on administration set. Observe site for patency. Adjust flow rate.

Apply antimicrobial ointment at puncture site (optional).

Apply sterile adhesive dressing over needle puncture site. Use a taping procedure that provides adequate stability and anchors needle and administration set firmly (see Fig. 19–1).

Readjust flow rate.

Label site with time, date, type and size of device, and your initials.

Document in patient's chart.

Precautions and Follow-Up Care

Same as for over-the-needle catheter.

Over-the-Needle Catheter (e.g., Angiocath)

Clinical Uses

Long term therapy, delivery of viscous liquids, e.g., blood or hyperalimentation fluids, and arterial monitoring. Allows greater mobility than needle for agitated or restless patients.

Equipment

Same as for winged-infusion needle, plus I.V. cannula (e.g., Angiocath).

Method

Follow general instructions under "Venipuncture—Winged-Infusion Needle."

Specific Instructions for over-the-needle catheter:

Spike I.V. solution container and establish drip level. *Do not remove* sterility cap on needle adapter at this time. Label tubing with date, time, and your name.

Wash hands thoroughly.

Reapply tourniquet and cleanse site with disinfectant. *Do not touch prepped area.* If vein is palpated again, then area must be reprepped.

Prime the administration set—remove the sterility cap, and remove all air from the tubing. Keep the cap from becoming contaminated. Close flow clamp and replace protective cap.

Remove cannula shield and visually inspect integrity of device.

With cannula pointed away, grasp the flashback chamber. Rotate the catheter on the needle without pushing it forward over the needle tip, thus avoiding fracture of the catheter tip.

Stabilize the vein. Anchor vein with your thumb, 5 to 10 cm below the insertion site, and stretch the skin downward against the direction of the insertion. Care must be taken to prevent contact with the cannula by the thumb holding the skin taut.

Hold the needle, bevel up, directly above and parallel to the vein. When holding the needle, do not touch the catheter hub; grasp only the plastic flashback chamber (Fig. 19–3A).

Insert needle through skin at a 40° to 45° angle about 1 cm below proposed site of vein entry (Fig. 19–3B). Do not allow catheter to touch skin surface during penetration.

After skin is penetrated, decrease needle angle until almost flush with skin, approximately 10°. *Do not touch skin.* With a slight lifting pressure, advance needle tip

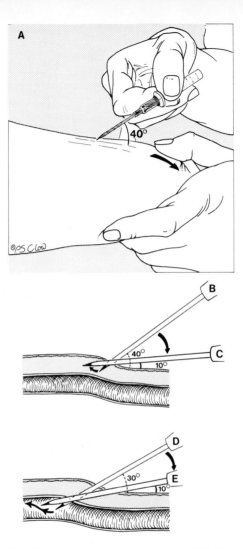

Fig. 19–3. Over-the-needle catheter procedure. **A.** With the hand grasping the flashback chamber, insert needle at a 40° angle, 1 cm below proposed site of vein entry. **B.** Skin is penetrated at a 40° angle, but angle of needle penetration is then reduced **(C)** and a slight lifting pressure is used to advance the needle toward the vein. **D.** With the needle angle again slightly increased, the vein is slowly entered, and with a lifting motion **(E)** the needle is advanced carefully.

560

about 0.5 to 1 cm to reach but not penetrate the vein (Fig. 19–3C).

With a downward motion, slowly enter vein, and watch for flashback of blood indicating successful vein entry (Fig. 19–3D).

As soon as needle tip enters the vein, again exert a lifting pressure and advance the needle another 0.5 to 1 cm to ensure catheter entry into vein (Fig. 19–3E).

Having confirmed blood return, carefully grasp catheter hub, disengage stylet about 0.5 cm (Fig. 19–4A) and while holding vein taut, and with tourniquet in place, slowly advance catheter until desired length of catheter is in the vein (Fig. 19–4B).

Release tourniquet, apply antimicrobial ointment at the

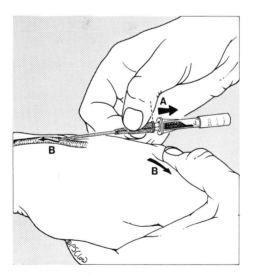

Fig. 19–4. A. When needle is sufficiently in the vein, the stylet is disengaged 0.5 cm, and while holding the vein taut, the catheter is advanced prior to release of tourniquet.

catheter-cutaneous junction and place sterile adhesive
dressing over puncture site.

Place sterile gauze or alcohol prep pad under hub of
catheter. This provides a sterile field for the connection
point and protects from contamination by touch. It will
also catch any blood that spills.

Remove protective cap from the infusion set. Grip catheter hub, remove stylet, and attach the primed infusion
set.

Open clamp and observe the I.V. site for signs of infiltration or irritation.

Regulate flow rate, discard gauze pad, and tape catheter
securely to stabilize it.

Anchor the infusion set so that there is no direct pressure
on the catheter and an accidental pull will not dislodge
it (see Fig. 19–1).

Indicate date, time, type and size of device, and place
your signature on tape at I.V. site.

Document in patient's chart.

Precautions

Strict aseptic technique during insertion, manipulation,
and management is essential in the prevention of I.V. associated infections. To facilitate good entry and prevent the
vein from rolling, the skin and vein must be held very taut
from below during needle insertion and advancement.
Only two attempts at insertion should be made by one
person. A new sterile needle is used for each attempt. If
needle placement is over or near a point of flexion, a support should be used to immobilize the area. Take care that
circulation is not inhibited. Remove and reapply support
every 8 hours.

Follow-Up Care

To maintain the I.V. site, infusion sets and extension
tubings should not be left in place longer than 48 to 72

hours. Administration sets accommodating blood, blood products, or lipid emulsions should be changed immediately after their administration.

The cannula site and complete system should be inspected hourly for signs of malfunction or complications. The skin-cannula junction should be cleansed daily and redressed. Ideally, I.V. cannulas should be removed every 48 to 72 hours, or sooner if complications arise.

Local complications to watch for include infiltration and thrombophlebitis. Systemic complications include pyrogenic reactions, air and pulmonary emboli, circulatory overload, speed shock and errors in medications or solutions.

Intermittent Infusion Set (Heparin Lock)

Clinical Uses

Allows periodic withdrawal of blood samples and eliminates multiple venipunctures. Used for intermittent I.V. injections, infusions or transfusions, without a continuous infusion, and circulatory access in emergencies. Prevents fluid overload when continuous I.V. infusion is not indicated. Allows patient mobility.

Equipment

Same as for winged-infusion needle, plus:

Intermittent infusion set (e.g., [1] Minicath PRN or [2] Angiocath PRN)

Pre-filled heparin syringe (2 ml) for flushing with 23 to 25 gauge needle, length no greater than one inch. (Heparin solution: 10 units heparin/1 ml normal saline)

Syringe filled with 0.9% NaCl (5 ml) with 23 to 25 gauge needle (optional).

Method

Prepare patient for venipuncture and insert an intermittent-infusion set as done for a winged-infusion needle or an over-the-needle catheter. Tape securely. Secure set's latex injection port away from venipuncture site. Swab latex injection port with alcohol swab before and after each injection. Check for blood backflow, then slowly instill 1 ml heparin solution to maintain patency of set until required. Remove needle and swab injection site. Recap needle and dispose in protective container.

Note: To inject medication clear lock of heparin with 1.5 ml (0.9% NaCl) solution. Administer medication. Clear lock again with 3 ml (0.9 NaCl) solution. Re-heparinize lock with 1 ml heparin solution.

Precautions

Strict aseptic technique during insertion, manipulation, and management is essential. Recent studies have shown as little as 10 units of heparin per ml of saline solution is adequate. No significant change in patient's clotting status will occur with these small intermittent doses of heparin.

To inject medications use a small needle 23 to 25 gauge and no longer than 2.5 cm. The use of larger gauge needles will cause subsequent leakage at latex port. A small amount of medication will remain in the tubing and the needle. If necessary flush out any medication with 0.9% NaCl solution.

To withdraw blood sample use no larger than 21-gauge thin-wall needle. Select different area of latex surface for each injection. Consider whether heparin could distort the results of the assay to be performed on the sample.

Follow-Up Care

To maintain patency, intermittent infusion set must be flushed with heparin solution after injection and every 8 hours if the device is not used more frequently.

This device should be removed every 48 hours or sooner if complications arise. A maximum of 12 punctures into the latex port should be allowed. Observations and care are the same as for an I.V. site.

Arterial Puncture for Blood Gas Sampling
K.P. Siren

Arteriopuncture for blood gas determination is usually performed on the femoral artery in the inguinal fold, the radial artery medial to the styloid process, or the brachial artery medial to the aponeurosis of the biceps brachii. Femoral puncture is the easiest and least complicated method, if the proper procedure is followed.

Equipment

> 10-ml syringe (glass or plastic). Plastic syringes must be low friction type; glass ones should be checked for caliber match of the plunger and barrel.
> 1 ml of 1:1000 heparin solution
> 70% isopropyl alcohol or povidone-iodine solution
> Needles: 25-gauge for radial and brachial arteries, 22-gauge for femoral artery
> Material for "capping" syringe (e.g., a cork or plastic material)
> Ice for transportation of sample (when appropriate)

Method

About 0.3 ml of heparin solution is drawn into the syringe. The plunger of glass syringes should be withdrawn to its limit, while holding the syringe needle up, allowing a few drops of heparin to trickle down the barrel of the syringe. This will provide lubrication more effectively than repeatedly sliding the plunger in and out of the barrel. The plunger is then fully reinserted to express all air and fluid. Heparin solution is quite acidic, but the amount remaining in the needle hub is sufficient to prevent blood clotting without reducing the pH of the blood sample. The needle used to draw up the heparin solution should be discarded and replaced with a fresh needle of correct size (22-gauge for femoral artery; 25-gauge for radial or brachial arteries). This ensures a fresh, sharp needle for the arterial puncture.

The skin overlying the arterial puncture site should be cleansed with antiseptic solution, and the artery axis identified by palpation. For femoral puncture, the second and third fingers should be placed co-axially with the artery to stabilize it and assist in identifying its position. With the plane of the bevel of the needle parallel to the axis of the artery to minimize muscularis trauma, penetrate the skin with a short, swift jab and then slowly advance the needle toward the artery with the needle axis at right angles to the femoral artery or 45° to the brachial or radial arterial axes, until transmitted arterial pulsations are sensed in the hand holding the syringe. Further advancement should result in visible, pulsatile entry of blood into the syringe. If blood flow is not obtainable after 5 to 10 mm of advancement, slow withdrawal may permit a collapsed artery to open. The "sewing machine" approach of multiple rapid passes to locate the arterial lumen is a poor technique.

When sufficient blood is obtained (most laboratories require a minimum of 2 ml for analysis), the syringe is withdrawn and air bubbles expressed from the syringe. The needle or Luer-Lok tip should be capped, the syringe rolled between the palms to mix the blood and heparin, and the syringe placed in ice to reduce metabolic alteration of the gases in the sample.

Digital pressure over the artery following withdrawal of the needle must be maintained at a level greater than systolic pressure for a period greater than the patient's bleeding time (usually 5 minutes) to avoid intra-adventitial hematoma, which may compromise distal arterial flow or subsequent arterial punctures. This pressure should be applied by the operator. Delegation of this task is the most important cause of morbidity and complications. Maintain pressure no less than 5 minutes.

Precautions

Advancement of the needle into structures underlying the artery (e.g., hip joint) may result in the introduction of contaminants into these structures.

Occasionally a skin plug will be cut while puncturing the skin. This will block the needle bore. Attempts to express it may leave insufficient heparin in the syringe. It is best to prepare a new syringe.

Prior to radial arterial puncture, always perform an Allen test to ensure adequate ulnar collateral circulation in case of damage to the radial artery. (Allen's Test—see page 568)

Systemic Arterial Catheterization (Percutaneous)
Ronald S. Baigrie

Intra-arterial pressure measurement and easy access for arterial blood gas sampling are the usual indications. The most common site employed is the radial artery, although the femoral, popliteal, and brachial arteries are used with varying frequency. Since the percutaneous method is similar for most superficial vessels, the radial cannulation technique is discussed in detail.

RADIAL ARTERIAL CANNULATION

Equipment

2-ml syringe with 25-gauge needle
2% lidocaine without epinephrine
18-gauge needle
Flexible cannula with central needle stylet (e.g., 5 cm Deseret Angiocath, 20-gauge; Deseret Pharmaceutical Co., Sandy, Utah).
Pressure monitoring system
Adhesive tape and sterile dressing

Method

It is advisable to ensure that adequate palmar collateral circulation exists by palpating for both the presence of an ulnar pulse as well as performing Allen's test.

Allen's Test. With occlusive finger pressure over both radial and ulnar pulses at the wrist, the raised hand is opened and closed several times by the patient in order to make it ischemic. If release of the ulnar pulse is accompanied by a rapid arterial blush of the hand within five seconds, a reasonable collateral circulation is likely. If this suffusion does not occur, it is wise to avoid cannulation of the radial artery of the tested hand.

The patient's non-dominant hand is preferred. The procedure is done using aseptic technique. Gloves and mask should be worn. The radial artery is located by palpation and the site for cannulation is located about 1 cm proximal to the distal skin crease of the wrist. The skin is punctured with a No. 25 hypodermic needle and local anesthetic (2% lidocaine) is administered. To avoid obscuration of the radial pulse, only a small amount of anesthetic is administered intradermally. Only the skin is punctured with a No. 18 hypodermic needle to ease passage of the cannula and reduce the risk of stylet occlusion by skin fragments, and cannula trauma.

With the artery stabilized by hyperextension of the wrist, a flexible cannula with central-needle stylet (e.g., a 5 cm Deseret Angiocath, 20-gauge) is introduced directly over the palpated radial artery at an angle of approximately 30° and advanced to the artery. Successful entry is evident when the stylet chamber fills with bright red blood (Fig. 19–5A). The stylet and cannula are advanced a farther 2 mm to ensure that both stylet and cannula are within the arterial lumen as evidenced by blood continuing to fill the system. The stylet is then stabilized; the cannula should advance effortlessly over the stylet into the lumen of the vessel (Fig. 19–5B). Significant resistance usually indicates that the cannula is not in the lumen and necessitates slight withdrawal of cannula and stylet or complete repositioning. The stylet is then removed and a good position confirmed by vigorous pulsation of blood from the cannula (Fig. 19–5C).

The pressure monitoring system is connected and the system flushed. The cannula is firmly secured with tape and sterile dressing and all connections are tightened to avoid leakage. The adequacy of distal blood flow to the hand is reassessed on completion of the procedure. A stopcock device should not be connected directly to the cannula for purposes of sampling since manipulation at this point can traumatize the vessel.

The cannulation site should be reassessed frequently (e.g., every 24 hours), looking for inflammation as well as the adequacy of blood supply to the hand. In the event of significant bleeding at any time, the cannula must be re-

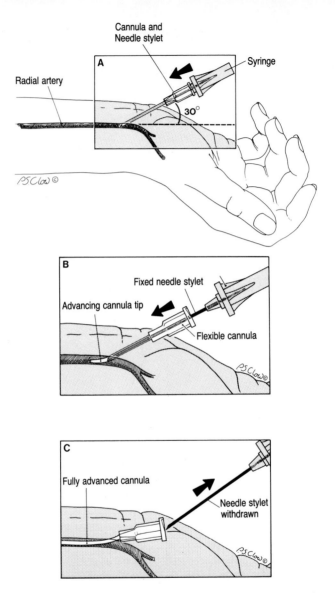

Fig. 19–5. Radial artery cannulation. **A.** Percutaneous insertion of cannula and central stylet into radial artery lumen. **B.** Advancing cannula over stylet into lumen of radial artery. **C.** Removal of stylet from cannula followed by connection to pressure tubing.

moved and local pressure applied until hemostasis is achieved.

FEMORAL ARTERIAL CATHETERIZATION

Equipment

2-ml syringe with 1½ inch, 22-gauge needle
2% lidocaine without epinephrine
Sharp-pointed scalpel
Seldinger needle and stylet (or equivalent)
Soft, flexible guidewire (may be needed)
Arterial catheter (e.g., Kifa 8 inch, No. 7 or No. 8 French)

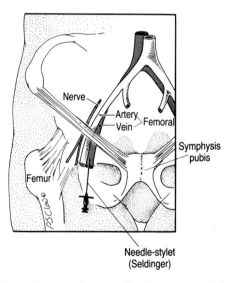

Fig. 19–6. Femoral venous (or arterial) catheterization. Pelvic diagram. Insertion of Seldinger needle into right femoral vein (or artery).

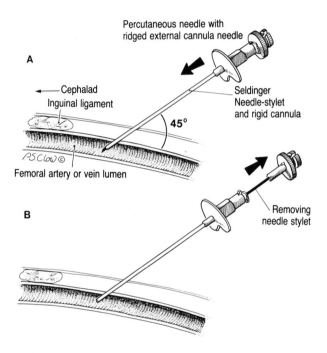

Percutaneous needle with ridged external cannula needle

A

Cephalad
Inguinal ligament

45°

Seldinger
Needle-stylet
and rigid cannula

PSClow ©

Femoral artery or vein lumen

B

Removing
needle stylet

Fig. 19–7. Femoral artery (or vein) catheterization. **A.** Needle and rigid cannula tip both located in vessel lumen. **B.** Needle stylet removed from cannula.

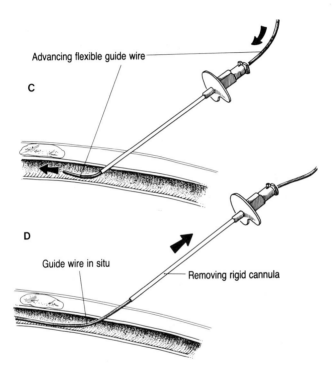

Fig. 19–7 *Continued.* C. Soft, flexible guidewire advanced well into the vessel lumen via cannula. **D.** Cannula removed from vessel and external position of guidewire.

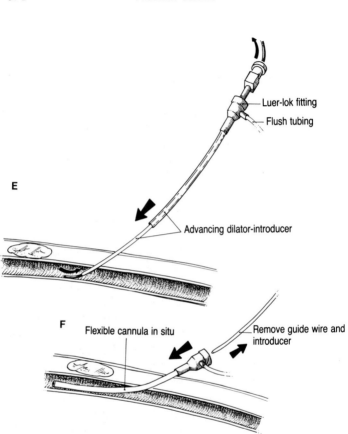

Luer-lok fitting

Flush tubing

E

Advancing dilator-introducer

F

Flexible cannula in situ

Remove guide wire and introducer

Fig. 19–7 *Continued*. E. Vessel dilator-introducer unit passed over guide-wire into vessel lumen, making sure that guidewire is visible. **F.** Final placement of cannula and removal of dilator and guidewire.

Method

The approach to this deep arterial vessel is somewhat different than the approach for a superficial artery, e.g., radial. The procedure is done using aseptic technique: mask, gloves, groin shave, iodine and alcohol preparation. The right femoral artery is preferred unless pedal pulses are not palpable, and there is evidence of significant ischemia. Local anesthetic (2% lidocaine) is used to infiltrate the skin about 3 to 4 cm below the inguinal ligament, directly over the femoral arterial pulse (similar to Fig. 19–6). Using a No. 22 hypodermic needle, the skin and subcutaneous tissue are anesthetized down to the level of the arterial adventitial tissue. A 1 to 2 mm incision is made by a scalpel in the skin only. A Seldinger needle and stylet are used to puncture the artery, entering the skin at a 45° angle from the horizontal plane in line with the anatomic lie of the vessel (Fig. 19–7A). When the vessel is punctured, the stylet is removed (Fig. 19–7B). If arterial blood is not forthcoming, the needle is slowly withdrawn until brisk arterial flow from the needle is seen. When this occurs, a soft, flexible guidewire is introduced into the needle shaft and advanced 'effortlessly' up the vessel approximately 10 cm (Fig. 19–7C). The needle is withdrawn over the guidewire and removed (Fig. 19–7D). An arterial catheter, e.g., Kifa 8 inch (No. 7 or No. 8 French) or introducer-dilator unit is threaded over the wire and advanced well into the vessel (Fig. 19–7E). The wire is removed, and the appropriate pressure tubing or stopcock is attached to the Luer-Lok end of the arterial catheter (Fig. 19–7F). Once hemostasis is ensured, the puncture site is dressed in sterile fashion. The adequacy of distal blood flow to the limb is assessed. Excessive bleeding at the puncture site or limb ischemia necessitates catheter removal and the application of local pressure until hemostasis is achieved.

FEMORAL VENOUS CATHETERIZATION

Equipment

10-ml syringe with 25-gauge needle
2% lidocaine without epinephrine
22-gauge needle, length 1½ inch
Seldinger needle (or equivalent)
Vascular catheter (e.g., Kifa 8 inch, No. 7 or No. 8 French)
Soft, flexible guidewire

Method

The femoral vein catheterization technique is identical to that of the femoral artery, except that the operator must remember that the femoral vein lies approximately 1 cm medial to the artery (nerve-artery-vein) (Fig. 19–6). The pulsating femoral artery is identified by palpation, and the preceding technique (as for femoral artery catheterization) is used to proceed to catheterize the medially adjacent femoral vein. Following puncture to an appropriate depth with the Seldinger needle, the stylet is removed and a 10-ml syringe is attached to the needle. Gentle suction on the syringe (occasionally it is necessary to slightly withdraw the needle for proper positioning in the lumen) will identify the darker, venous blood when the lumen has been entered.

The syringe is then removed, and the soft, flexible guidewire is introduced into the needle and into the vein for a distance of approximately 10 cm. The needle is gently withdrawn and the catheter inserted over the guidewire. When the intravenous catheter has been properly positioned, the guidewire is then removed, and the operator proceeds as in the arterial catheterization technique, with any necessary modifications relating to venous cannulation.

Peripheral Venous Cut-down
Peter L. Lane

Clinical Uses

Insertion of an I.V. cannula into a peripheral vein under direct vision. This may be of use when venous access is a problem by the percutaneous route or if a large line is required.

Equipment (all sterile)

Gloves
Tray with drapes
Preparation solutions
Preparation cups
4 × 4 and 2 × 2 gauze pads
10-ml syringe
Local anesthetic without vasoconstrictor
No. 18 and No. 25 needle
No. 14 scalpel blade and scalpel handle
4 small hemostats
Needle driver
1 pair of suture scissors
1 pair of vascular scissors with sharp points
Large bore venous catheter for introduction (e.g., No. 12 or No. 14-gauge catheter)
I.V. solution with blood tubing
000 ligatures (silk, catgut, or chromic)
000 silk skin sutures

Anatomy

A variety of potential sites for cut-downs are available. Choice of sites depends on patient condition and familiarity of the physician with technique in that site. The surface anatomy for each site will be described.

ANTECUBITAL FOSSA

The median basilic vein can be accessed in the antecubital fossa. The vein is usually located 2 cms lateral to the medial epicondyle in the antecubital fossa (Fig. 19–8).

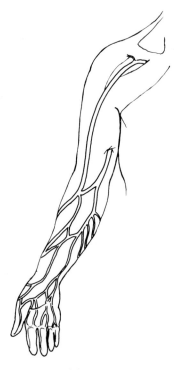

Fig. 19–8.   Venous drainage of the upper extremity.

CEPHALIC VEIN (ARM)

The cephalic vein traverses from the junction of the median basilic and median cephalic veins, just above the antecubital fossa to its junction with the subclavian vein. It can be accessed throughout most of its course over the anterior aspect of the arm over the biceps or the anterior aspect of the shoulder (Fig. 19–8).

SAPHENOUS VEIN (ANKLE)

The long saphenous vein can be accessed at the ankle. It is usually found just anterior to the medial malleolus and is superficial at this point (Fig. 19–9). The long saphenous vein can also be accessed at the saphenofemoral junction

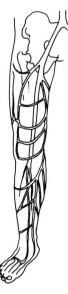

Fig. 19–9. Venous drainage of the lower extremity.

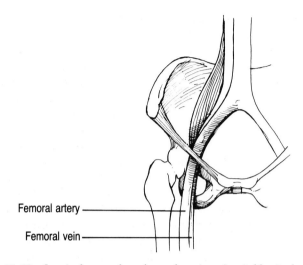

Fig. 19–10. Inguinal, or saphenofemoral, region. A suitable site for access is 3 cm below the inguinal ligament. The artery is just lateral and anterior to the vein.

Femoral artery

Femoral vein

where the vein is largest. For cut-down it is sought approximately 3 cm inferior to the inguinal ligament, just below the femoral triangle (Figs. 19–9, 19–10).

Method

The surface anatomy of the chosen site is identified. The area is prepared and draped appropriately. Local anesthetic is instilled carefully to avoid puncturing the vein and significantly distorting the anatomy. A transverse incision is made perpendicular to the long axis of the vein. The incision should be long enough to allow for adequate exploration of the area involved in case the vein is not precisely in the normal location. Depending on the site, this usually involves an incision from 3 to 10 cm in length. Once the incision is made, blunt dissection is performed using a curved hemostat, spreading the tissues parallel to the long axis of the vein.

The vein is identified and the curved hemostats carefully placed beneath the vein. Two ligatures are placed beneath the vein and pulled through, one cephalad and one caudad. The distal mobilized vein is ligated, leaving the suture in place for traction. Stabilizing the vein with the distal ligature, a small venotomy is made in the anterior surface of the vein. The venotomy is gently dilated using the blunt tip of the closed hemostats. The plastic cannula, of a size that will avoid damage to the intima of the vein, is chosen prior to insertion. The cannula is advanced (Fig. 19–11). The proximal ligature is now tied snugly about the cannula within the vein, taking care not to kink the cannula. The I.V. tubing is attached to the hub of the cannula. The hub of the cannula is then sutured in place, and the wound is closed with interrupted sutures. The cannula and I.V. tubing are taped securely in place and a sterile dressing is applied.

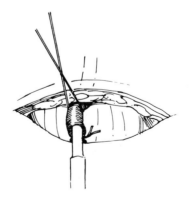

Fig. 19–11. Venous cut-down.

Precautions

In both the antecubital fossa and the inguinal region, larger arteries are close to the veins involved, although somewhat deeper. Care must be taken during dissection not to damage the arteries or small branches in the region. The veins involved are superficial, and deep dissection should not be necessary. Occasionally, particularly if the saphenofemoral site is chosen, self-retaining rake retractors can assist in visualizing structures. If, however, excessive bleeding is encountered from damage to either arteries or veins, packing the wound and applying pressure for approximately 5 minutes is usually sufficient to control hemorrhage.

Care should be taken in making the venotomy to ensure that the full thickness of the wall of the vein is incised. If not, or if the vein is insufficiently dilated, the catheter can dissect between the intima and adventitia of the vein and hence be ineffective.

Because the veins involved are relatively large, extra care must be taken with cut-down lines to ensure that they remain sutured in place and do not get inadvertently pulled out.

Meticulous sterile technique is important, as the consequences of septic thrombophlebitis in these veins can be catastrophic.

Appendix:
Positions Commonly
Used for Examina-
tion and Treatment

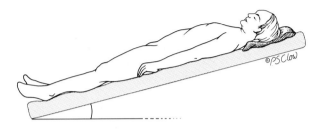

A–1. Fowler's position

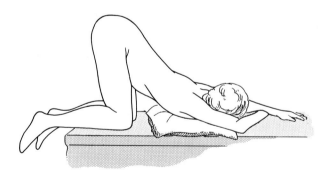

A–2. Knee-chest position

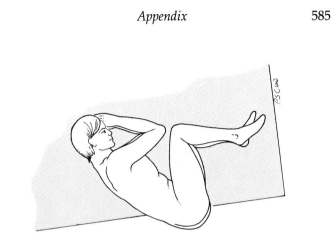

A–3. Left lateral position, at edge of examining table, seen from above

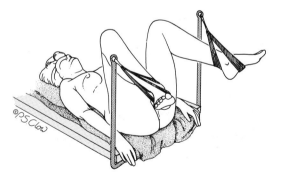

A–4. Lithotomy position, using optional stirrups

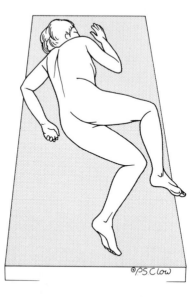

A–5.   Sim's position

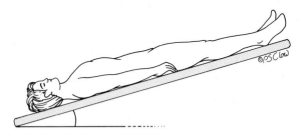

A–6.   Trendelenburg position

Index